The Medical Device R&D Handbook

Second Edition

The Medical Device R&D Handbook

Second Edition

Edited by
Theodore R. Kucklick

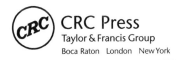

CRC Press is an imprint of the
Taylor & Francis Group, an **informa** business

Cover: Illustration of BACE heart device courtesy of Beth Croce, AMI and Jai Raman, MD.

CRC Press
Taylor & Francis Group
6000 Broken Sound Parkway NW, Suite 300
Boca Raton, FL 33487-2742

© 2013 by Taylor & Francis Group, LLC
CRC Press is an imprint of Taylor & Francis Group, an Informa business

No claim to original U.S. Government works

Printed in the United States of America on acid-free paper
Version Date: 2012926

International Standard Book Number: 978-1-4398-1189-4 (Hardback)

This book contains information obtained from authentic and highly regarded sources. Reasonable efforts have been made to publish reliable data and information, but the author and publisher cannot assume responsibility for the validity of all materials or the consequences of their use. The authors and publishers have attempted to trace the copyright holders of all material reproduced in this publication and apologize to copyright holders if permission to publish in this form has not been obtained. If any copyright material has not been acknowledged please write and let us know so we may rectify in any future reprint.

Except as permitted under U.S. Copyright Law, no part of this book may be reprinted, reproduced, transmitted, or utilized in any form by any electronic, mechanical, or other means, now known or hereafter invented, including photocopying, microfilming, and recording, or in any information storage or retrieval system, without written permission from the publishers.

For permission to photocopy or use material electronically from this work, please access www.copyright.com (http://www.copyright.com/) or contact the Copyright Clearance Center, Inc. (CCC), 222 Rosewood Drive, Danvers, MA 01923, 978-750-8400. CCC is a not-for-profit organization that provides licenses and registration for a variety of users. For organizations that have been granted a photocopy license by the CCC, a separate system of payment has been arranged.

Trademark Notice: Product or corporate names may be trademarks or registered trademarks, and are used only for identification and explanation without intent to infringe.

Library of Congress Cataloging-in-Publication Data

The medical device R & D handbook / editor, Theodore R. Kucklick. -- 2nd ed.
   p. ; cm.
  Medical device R and D handbook
  Includes bibliographical references and index.
  Summary: "Written for medical device designers, biomedical engineering students, physician entrepreneurs, and medical device entrepreneurs, this reference explains the basics on how to prototype and develop a medical device. It discusses the basics of plastics, adhesives, medical needles, and rapid prototyping as well as tips and tools to save time and money. This updated and expanded second edition includes practical advice and interviews from key opinion leaders and pioneers in the field. Extensive references at the end of each chapter enhance additional study"--Provided by publisher.
  ISBN 978-1-4398-1189-4 (hardcover : alk. paper)
  I. Kucklick, Theodore R. II. Title: Medical device R and D handbook.
  [DNLM: 1. Biomedical Technology. 2. Electronics, Medical--methods. 3. Entrepreneurship. 4. Equipment Design--methods. W 82]

610.28'4--dc23   2012023165

Visit the Taylor & Francis Web site at
http://www.taylorandfrancis.com

and the CRC Press Web site at
http://www.crcpress.com

Contents

About the Book ix
Preface to the Second Edition xiii
Editor xvii
Contributors xix

SECTION I Materials for Medical Device R&D

Chapter 1   Introduction to Medical Plastics.. 3

　　　　　　Theodore R. Kucklick

Chapter 2   Getting Stuck in a Good Way: Basics of Medical Device
　　　　　　Adhesives 29

　　　　　　Theodore R. Kucklick

Chapter 3   Introduction to Needles and Cannulae... 43

　　　　　　Theodore R. Kucklick

Chapter 4   Assessing Biocompatibility: A Guide for Medical Device
　　　　　　Manufacturers 65

　　　　　　Tom Spalding

SECTION II Processes for Medical Device R&D

Chapter 5   Catheter-Forming Equipment and Operations 93

　　　　　　Theodore R. Kucklick

Chapter 6   Basics of Catheter Assembly... 107

　　　　　　Theodore R. Kucklick

Chapter 7   Rapid Prototyping for Medical Devices.. 127

　　　　　　Theodore R. Kucklick

Chapter 8 Medical Applications of Rapid Technologies: Technology Update 167

Theodore R. Kucklick

Chapter 9 Reverse Engineering in Medical Device Design 183

Theodore R. Kucklick

Chapter 10 Prototype or Produce? How to Decide 211

Theodore R. Kucklick

Chapter 11 Elements of Injection Molding Style for Medical Device R&D 217

Theodore R. Kucklick

SECTION III Methods for Medical Device R&D

Chapter 12 Clinical Observation: How to Be Welcome (or at Least Tolerated) in the Operating Room and Laboratory 243

Theodore R. Kucklick

Chapter 13 ABCs of NDAs 251

Theodore R. Kucklick

Chapter 14 Intellectual Property Strategy for Med-Tech Start-Ups 263

Ryan H. Flax

Chapter 15 Regulatory Affairs: Medical Devices 295

Thomas Wehman

Chapter 16 510(k) Reform: The Stakes Are High 333

Sherrie Conroy

Chapter 17 Brief Introduction to Preclinical Research 347

James Swick

Contents

Chapter 18 Using Medical Illustration in Medical Device R&D 351

Theodore R. Kucklick

Chapter 19 Case Study: The BACE™ Mitral Regurgitation Treatment Device: Supplement to Chapter 18, Using Medical Illustration in Medical Device R&D 373

Theodore R. Kucklick

SECTION IV *Interviews and Insights for the R&D Entrepreneur*

Chapter 20 Interview with Thomas Fogarty, MD 379

Theodore R. Kucklick

Chapter 21 Interview with Paul Yock, MD 387

Theodore R. Kucklick

Chapter 22 Interview with Dane Miller, PhD 393

Theodore R. Kucklick

Chapter 23 Interview with Ingemar Lundquist 399

Theodore R. Kucklick

Chapter 24 Interview with J. Casey McGlynn 401

Theodore R. Kucklick

Chapter 25 Keys to Creating Value for Early Stage Medical Device Companies 413

Richard Ferrari

Chapter 26 Female Leadership in the Medical Device Industry 423

France Helfer

Chapter 27 Medical Device Sales 101 429

Devin Hughes

Chapter 28 Invention, Innovation, and Creativity: Or How Thomas Edison Never Changed the World by Creating the Light Bulb 433

Theodore R. Kucklick

Chapter 29 How to Fail as an Entrepreneur 447

Theodore R. Kucklick

Chapter 30 Raising Money for Your Medical Device Start-Up 459

Theodore R. Kucklick

Index 467

About the Book

The Medical Device R&D (Research and Development) *Handbook, Second Edition* was originally the fruition of a personal desire to see some of the practical information on how to develop medical devices compiled in one resource. I wanted to write a book that I wish had been available when I first started in medical device design.

The first edition contained three main threads, and this continues in the new edition. The first thread is practical. Many excellent books give in-depth theory on specialized medical and technology subjects in medical device engineering, but a general practical how-to manual is not available. This part of the book seeks to serve that need.

There is a great deal of practical skill, developed by intelligent and clever people, to be found in specialized areas of the medical device industry. Having worked for a succession of medical device start-up companies, each new area seemed to have its own fund of "tribal knowledge" that, for various reasons, did not seem to percolate much out of the tribe. Working for start-ups and developing products for different medical specialties were somewhat like joining a succession of guilds.

There is also little crossover between certain fields, such as engineering and medical illustration. One of the goals of this book is to collect some of the knowledge of these practical skills, such as medical device prototyping, plastics selection, and catheter construction and make them readily accessible to the hands-on designer. The skills may be well known to those who work in a specialized area, but not as well known to those outside that specialty. Some of this information is usually learned "on the job," that is, if you happen to have that kind of a job. This book brings you this type of information. Having knowledge of these practical skills can allow the designer to combine and apply these specialized techniques in new and innovative ways and can save valuable time.

Another thread is entrepreneurial. This book contains interviews with some of the top leaders in the medical device industry. These are people who know by experience how to develop innovative new medical technology and how to start and grow successful companies. All of them were unfailingly gracious and exceptionally generous with their time and insight, and they have my enduring gratitude for allowing me to interview them and pester them with my questions. Hearing these innovators share their knowledge, experience, and wisdom has been one of the most enjoyable aspects of producing this book. The insights shared represent decades of distilled top-level experience. The interviewees are people who have helped build some of the most successful companies and key technologies in the medical device industry. They share what works, and what doesn't. These interviews are valuable resources that will reward the reader with fresh insights as they are read, and re-read. Where available, there are lists of additional materials and resources about these individuals. This section will be of special interest to the designer with an idea for an innovative technology, the student, and the physician-entrepreneur.

Yet another thread in this book is historical. In my experience, I am sometimes asked to design a product that is similar to or is inspired by a device already in use. Early on, I remember an incident in which one of our scientific advisors suggested that we look at a Veress needle for ideas on how to solve a design problem. Once that suggestion was made, and the advisor left, we (the engineers) looked at each other, and asked, "What is a Veress needle?" Being new and green, I did not know, but the engineering managers in this medical device company did not know either. With apologies to Santayana, "Those who do not know history are condemned to reinvent the wheel." In the technical chapters I have made an effort to dig into the historical background of various technologies and put them in a useful context. In the chapters on needles and catheters, for example, I have compiled glossaries with detailed historical footnotes. This will help the R&D engineer understand how certain devices developed and for what purpose.

In this thread you meet fascinating personalities—often people solving a problem just like you—who, through hands-on development, have arrived at important solutions. People like Harvey, Veress, Luer, Forssmann, Sones, Tuhoy, Dotter, Gruentzig, Fogarty, Foley, and numerous others who solved important clinical problems are recognized in the 21st century for their groundbreaking contributions. It is important, as a medical device designer, to know these personalities, what they developed and why, how they sometimes collaborated, and some of the technical challenges and institutional barriers they overcame to succeed.

This new edition is organized a bit differently than the previous edition, with the topics grouped under the headings "Materials," "Processes," "Methods," and "Interviews and Insights." Taken together, this book gives the working engineer, manager, technician, designer entrepreneur, or student some of the tools to more quickly and efficiently develop innovative medical devices, and to see their role in a larger business and societal context. The first edition covered a fair bit of ground; however, it was only a start. Examples of subjects not covered were patents, the role of industrial design in medical device development, adhesives, catheter tubing extrusion, operating room procedures and protocol, new company formation, and how and where to raise start-up capital among many other important topics. Several of these topics are covered in this new edition, and more will be covered in future editions. Margins may be sufficient for some of your notes, making this your own customized handbook.

The help, support, and encouragement of the many contributors, reviewers, and collaborators involved in this project are gratefully acknowledged, along with those who have provided the opportunities and mentoring I needed to work in diverse areas of this endlessly fascinating medical device industry.

I also would like to acknowledge CRC Press/Taylor & Francis for its interest and support in publishing this title, as well as all of the work and support of the Taylor & Francis staff and editors.

About the Book

This is the beginning of what is intended to be a continuing series and is designed to be responsive to the needs and input of you, the reader. Your suggestions for future topics are welcome. Please email suggestions, feedback, and questions to editor@meddevbook.com.

Theodore R. Kucklick
Los Gatos, California

Preface to the Second Edition

First of all, thank you to everyone who purchased the first edition of *The Medical Device R&D Handbook*, and those who have included it in the reference collections at more than 100 university libraries around the world. It is because of your positive response that there is a second edition.

Since I began the first edition in 2004, there have been a number of fundamental changes to the medical device business. The medical technology (medtech) business is much more global than it was even then, and the pace is picking up. In addition to Europe, the Asian market (especially China) is growing in importance as are Brazil and the rest of Latin America. Medical applications of rapid prototyping technologies have gone from concept to mainstream products. Several companies now offer robotic surgery systems and patient-specific implants and instruments.

There are other forces at work as well. Recent health care legislation in the United States (i.e., the massive and complex Patient Protection and Affordable Care Act of 2010 [PPACA], which passed by the slimmest of margins and with great controversy) and other factors are putting increasing pressure on device manufacturers to deliver higher performance at ever-lower prices. These factors are squeezing margins, making the reimbursement landscape even more difficult, and making innovative design with the economic purchaser in mind even more important. Purchasing committees, not just surgeons, are now key decision makers in the product-adoption process. Other events have also altered the business landscape for medical device R&D: One was the unprecedented U.S. Department of Justice subpoenas and investigations of surgeon–industry relationships and conflicts of interest against all of the major companies in the orthopedic industry beginning in 2005.[*] New Comparative Effectiveness Research (CER) mandates passed in the 2008 Stimulus legislation. There are proposed changes to the Food and Drug Administration (FDA) 510(k) premarket clearance program and an ongoing National Institute of Medicine study. FDA clearances involving clinical trails are driving some innovations out of the United States.[†] Finally, the financial meltdown of 2008 has made fundraising for start-ups even more difficult, and fundamental changes to patent law are constantly passed. All of these factors are now at work, in addition to the advancements in medical device science and technology. We indeed live in interesting times.

The world of medical device R&D is bigger, more exciting, and more challenging than ever before. With every change are even more opportunities. It will take big, innovative thinking to meet the challenges going forward.

This new edition adds new material to help you meet these challenges, including material on strategic IP (intellectual property) management, OR (operating room)

---

[*] *Medical Device + Diagnostic Industry Online*, "Orthopedic Firms Settle with U.S. Justice Department," March 1, 2008, http://www.mddionline.com/article/orthopedic-firms-settle-us-justice-department-0.
[†] Robin Young, "Medical Device Innovation Leaving the U.S.," *The Life Sciences Report* (Spring 2010), previously published in *Orthopedics This Week*, http://www.wsgr.com/publications/PDFSearch/life-sciences-report/Spring10/medical-device-biotechnology-companies.htm#2.

observation protocol, how to use the new rapid-turn molding technologies available, how to use the new medical device adhesives available, and more. In addition to this new information, there are timely and practical chapters to help you start, build, and grow an entrepreneurial business, and advice on how to avoid some of the sand traps along the way.

This book would not be possible without the generous contributions of several chapters by experts in their respective fields, and I am grateful for their contributions to this new edition.

There are many other people who have helped to make my career in medtech—and this book—possible. I would like to recognize and thank them and also recognize some who are no longer with us.

First, I would like to recognize Stuart D. Edwards. Stu Edwards was the founder of several medical device companies, including Vidamed (ticker: VIDA, acquired by Medtronic), Rita Medical (ticker: RITA, acquired by Angiodynamics), Somnus (ticker: SOMN, acquired by Gyrus), Curon (ticker: CURN, now Meredi Therapeutics), Novasys, Cardiosynopsis, Advanced Closure Systems (now Neomend), Oratec (acquired by Smith & Nephew), and Silhouette Medical. I was hired by Stu to work at RITA Medical as it was being spun out of Vidamed, and I worked with Stu on a number of his start-ups. Stu was a prolific inventor, imaginative, energetic, and a hard-driving and hard-driven personality. Stu passed away April 14, 2010. (Stu's good friend and mentor, Ingemar Lundquist, who is interviewed in this book, passed in 2007.) It was working with Stu that gave me the exposure to the rapid innovation and hands-on development of medical devices across a wide range of indications, and it was during this time, I learned the spectrum of developing a medical technology, from company formation, to bench-top development, to IP strategy, to commercial product launch, and to some of the practical techniques and technologies shared in this book.

I would like to recognize Casey McGlynn, head of the Life Science practice at Wilson Sonsini Goodrich & Rosati (WSGR). In addition to these responsibilities, Casey produces the annual WSGR Medical Device Conference and recently helped establish the newer OneMedForum annual meeting. For more than 10 years, the WSGR Medical Device Conference has been one of the most important events to attend when it comes to staying abreast of trends in the industry from a business and investment point of view.

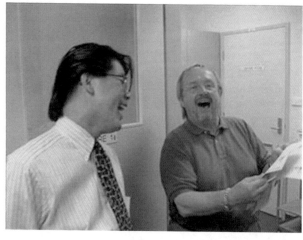

Stu Edwards (right) in Adelaide, Australia. (Photo by TRK.)

Preface to the Second Edition

This conference represents an invaluable service to the medical device community, without which I doubt I would have had the perspective to write a book like this.

I also would like to mention Paul Yock, MD, chair of the Stanford Biodesign program. Dr. Yock and Sandy Miller (former director at the Kauffman Foundation and current director of new ventures at Singularity University) helped put together a seminar called "Patents and Startups 101" a two-day "boot camp," where speakers like Dr. Tom Fogarty, Mir Imran, Rich Ferarri, and others shared information about the practical aspects of medical device entrepreneurship.* This seminar in May 2001 got me to thinking about putting a practical medical device R&D "seminar" into book form, where it could be accessible to anyone, not just the fortunate few who were able to attend these seminars in person. This was the seed of the idea for this book.

Biodesign also produced their ongoing Innovator's Workbench series, featuring medical device industry pioneers interviewed by David Cassack, managing director for Windhover Information/Elsevier. This planted the seed for the interview section in this book.

I discussed the concept of a "Medical Device R&D Cookbook" with Sandy Miller and Dr. Yock, and both encouraged me to write it as there was an unmet need and a shortage of material on the subject of practical medical device innovation and prototyping. The idea of writing such a book to me at the time was quite daunting. After pitching the book, CRC Press/Taylor & Francis took it on, which has given me the opportunity to work with Michael Slaughter, acquisitions editor, who not only has become a friend but also helps keep me on deadline.

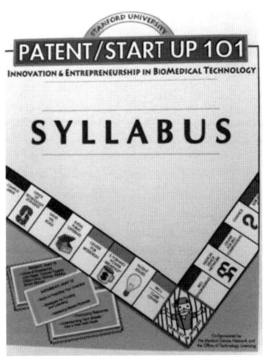

Syllabus, "Patents and Startups 101" Stanford University, May 2001.

Many years ago, Russell Conwell wrote a motivational short story titled *Acres of Diamonds*, about the endless opportunities all around us, if we are willing to

---

* Stanford Biodesign has published its own excellent book by Stefanos Zenios et al., *Biodesign: The Process of Innovating Medical Technologies* (New York: Cambridge University Press, 2010), which handles in depth many details of the needs-finding process, fundraising and company formation, and other topics complementary to *The Medical Device R&D Handbook*.

recognize them and use them. It was not hard for me to recognize that I had "acres of diamonds" all around me in the people I have described and a multitude of others. One thing that is a constant pleasant surprise to me is that those who genuinely have accomplished the most, and have the most to offer, seem the most generous in sharing their advice and insight. There are two things I would like to leave you with. First, take the time to seek out and discover the resources you already have around you, which may be far greater than you realize. Second, be a resource to others. Share what you know. Knowledge is like love, is something that increases as it is shared.

Editor

Theodore R. Kucklick has extensive experience in the hands-on design and commercial development of medical devices, including radio frequency ablation devices, microwave catheters for minimally invasive therapy, in-home diagnostics devices, surgical closure devices, battery-powered devices, disposables, gene therapy manufacturing equipment, and general surgery tools. Ted has been involved in the early stages and development and productization of devices for such companies as Vidamed, Oratec, Neomend, Somnus, Curon, Starion Instruments, Sleep Solutions, RITA Medical, AfX and Cannuflow. He is the former senior designer for RITA Medical Systems and Advanced Closure Systems (now Neomend). Ted is currently the cofounder, vice president of engineering, and chief technical officer for Cannuflow, Inc., an arthroscopic instrument start-up company, and design director for TRKD Medical Device R&D, a medical device design and development company.

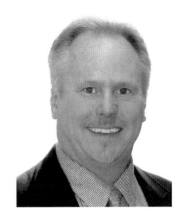

Theodore R. Kucklick

Ted has a bachelor's degree in product design and is the inventor of more than 40 US and international issued patents; he is a member of the IEEE/Engineering in Medicine and Biology Society, the Industrial Designers Society of America, and the Association of Medical Illustrators. Ted is also a founding member of the Keiritsu Forum angel investment group of Silicon Valley and a graduate of the University of California, Berkeley Haas School of Business Bio-Entrepreneurship certificate program.

Contributors

Sherrie Conroy
Penton Media
Corona, California

France Helfer
HALO Healthcare, Inc.
Irvine, California

Richard Ferrari
DeNovo Ventures
Menlo Park, California

Ryan H. Flax
A2L Consulting
Alexandria, Virginia

Devin Hughes
Devin Hughes Enterprises, LLC
San Diego, California

Tom Spalding
Pacific BioLabs
Hercules, California

James Swick
Biomedical Consulting Services
Mountain View, California

Thomas Wehman
Adel Engineering
Cupertino, California

Section I

Materials for Medical Device R&D

1 Introduction to Medical Plastics

Theodore R. Kucklick

CONTENTS

Biocompatibility 5
Biomaterials Availability..5
Materials Performance 6
Processability 6
What Is a Polymer?...7
Basics: Thermoplastic and Thermosets..7
Cross-Linked Thermoplastics 7
What Is a Medical-Grade Plastic?..8
Finding Plastics..9
Plastics for Machining 9
Plastics for Processing by Machining 11
    Acrylonitrile–Butadiene–Styrene..11
    Acrylic...11
    Polyvinylchloride 12
    Polycarbonate 12
    Polypropylene 13
    Polyethelene 13
    Acetal 14
    Nylon (Polyamide)...14
    Fluorinated Ethylene Propylene 15
High-Performance Engineering Plastics for Machining 15
    Ultem® Polyetherimide 15
    PEEK™ 15
    PTFE (Teflon®)...16
    Polysulfone and Polyphenylsulfone 16
        Polyimide Rod and Sheet (Vespel®, Kapton®) 17
    Injection-Molded and Extruded Plastics 17
        Considerations 17
Commodity Plastics 18
    ABS..18
        PC/ABS 18
        Acrylic 19
        Polycarbonate 19

        Polyethelene 19
        Polyolefin 19
        Styrene.. 19
Elastomers.. 20
    Elastomeric Plastics 20
        3Polyurethane.. 20
        Kraton® 20
        K-Resin® 20
        Monoprene® 21
        Pebax® 21
        Polyvinylchloride 21
        Ethylene Vinyl Acetate 21
Thermosets... 22
    Santoprene® 22
        Silicone.. 22
        Polyisoprene 22
        Nitrile 22
        Latex.. 22
High-Performance Engineering Plastics for Molding............................ 23
    Polyetherimide (PEI), Ultem®, PEEK®, Polysulfone....................... 23
Useful Specialty Plastic Material Forms.. 23
    Extruded PTFE (Zeus, Texloc).. 23
        Expanded PTFE 24
Sheet and Film and Foam Plastics 24
    Polyethylene Terephthalate (PET) and Polyethylene Terephthalate Glycol
    (PETG).. 24
        Tyvek® 24
        PVC and Polyethelene Film 24
        Polyester Film (Mylar®) 24
        Polyimide 25
        Styrene Butadiene Rubber Foam and Elastic Fabric (Wetsuit Material)........ 25
        Foam Sheet Material 25
Resources 25
    References: Radiation Effects on Plastics....................................... 25
Acknowledgment 26
Endnotes... 26

When working with medical plastics, there are some basic considerations: relative biocompatibility, performance, processability, bondability, cost, and availability. Using these basic characteristics as a starting point will help you sift through the myriad of available plastics to arrive at a short list of candidates that best suit your design criteria.

In addition to materials for devices, another category of medical plastics includes those that are used in packaging. These plastics need to not react with whatever is contained in them, be resistant to degradation when sterilized, and be available at the lowest possible cost.

Introduction to Medical Plastics 5

For the sake of simplicity, this chapter will organize some of the common plastics according to the more common methods of processing, as not all plastics are readily available for all processes. In the R&D environment, rapid development, cost-effective materials, and short lead times are key considerations.

BIOCOMPATIBILITY

The subject of biocompatibility could fill several books, and it does. This concept may be understood as relative biocompatibility, as the requirements for the medical devices are all different—for example, a device that does not come into much contact with a patient (such as an instrumentation case), compared with one that comes into intermittent or continuous skin contact, compared with an invasive surgical device, compared with an implantable device. Each device is biocompatible relative to the application. When choosing a material for a medical device application, biocompatibility is the first and most important consideration. If the material is not biocompatible, it may not be used, no matter what the potential performance. The most basic indicator that a material might be used is if it carries a U.S. Pharmacopeia (USP) Class VI, or medical-grade designation, or if it is marketed by the manufacturer as suitable for medical use. It is the responsibility of the designer to determine whether any particular material is suitable for its particular application.

Chapter 4, "Assessing Biocompatibility," the companion chapter in this book, provides a useful guide to understanding this topic.

Note: If a material is to be used for human use, it *must* have appropriate biocompatibility data on file *before* it is used clinically. Avoid using industrial-grade or "hardware store" materials and adhesives in *in vivo* or preclinical studies. It is good practice to use only medical-grade materials from the beginning. This way you can be more confident that you are building a device that remains usable as you move from bench tests to in vivo to clinical trials.

The amount of biocompatibility testing required varies with the class of device, duration of contact with the patient, and amount of mucous membrane or blood contact. Discuss these testing requirements with your regulatory affairs person and your testing lab *before* you begin any human clinical study. Schedule and allow enough time to conduct these tests. It is good practice to use materials that are medical grade and that you are confident will pass appropriate biocompatibility tests when doing preclinical work. Biocompatibility testing is done on the material in its *finished form*, as processed, as colored, and as it will be used in the device.

BIOMATERIALS AVAILABILITY

In response to a looming biomaterials crisis[*] precipitated by ruinous judgments against medical device manufacturers, and the associated liability exposure of suppliers of bulk raw materials, Congress passed the Biomaterials Access Assurance Act of 1998.[†] This gives a degree of protection to suppliers of materials that may become included

---

[*] Nadim J. Hallab et al., "Biomaterials Crisis Looms," *AAOS Bulletin* 45, no. 1 (January 1997). http://www2.aaos.org/aaos/archives/bulletin/jan97/bio.htm.
[†] Biomaterials Access Assurance Act of 1998, 21 U.S.C. § 1601–1606 (1998).

in medical devices. A series of liability suits based on sometimes-dubious science drove some major materials suppliers to exit from knowingly supplying materials for medical use, especially implants.[1] With the passage of this Act, the situation is somewhat improved. In some cases (e.g., silicones), smaller companies have stepped into the breach to supply these essential biomaterials, although at substantially higher cost than their industrial-grade equivalents. Ultimately, it is the responsibility of the medical device manufacturer to ensure that a material used is suitable for medical use, is properly selected for use in a well-designed product, and meets applicable regulatory and biocompatibility requirements.

MATERIALS PERFORMANCE

Under this category are such considerations as the mechanical properties of the material, its stiffness or flexibility, and its heat resistance, chemical resistance, and dielectric properties.

For example, heat resistance becomes a consideration if a device is meant for autoclave sterilization. For these applications, a heat-resistant high-performance engineering plastic like Ultem™ PEI (polyetherimide) or PEEK™ (polyetheretherketone) might be considered. If high dielectric strength in a thin material is desired, a polyimide tube or sheet may be a good choice. If ease of molding and low cost are important, acrylonitrile–butadiene–styrene (ABS) plastic may be a good choice. Determining the properties, performance, and processing of a plastic material for your application are important selection criteria.

PROCESSABILITY

Once you have found a plastic that meets your performance and biocompatibility requirements, the issue of how the plastic will be processed into its final shape needs to be considered. If a device is a one-off or low-production prototype, it will most likely be machined from a stock shape. Numerous plastics that are suitable for medical use and are available in stock shapes are described in this chapter.

One thing to keep in mind is your strategy for scaling up production if a prototype design proves successful. Think design for manufacture from the beginning. Is the material from which you are machining the part available in an injection-moldable form? Or, is a plastic that you want to injection mold available in a stock shape? Can the plastic be machined to a tolerance and surface finish acceptable for the application? Are you specifying a plastic that cannot be radiation sterilized or is not available in a form for injection molding? Planning ahead on these issues will save time, expense, and headaches down the road.

Another consideration when selecting a plastic for molding is how easy or difficult is the material to mold to get the parts you want without sinks, blushes, or blemishes. Is the part intricate with hard-to-fill thin areas? High-performance engineering plastics that are stronger and tougher, and have high heat resistance, are usually more difficult to mold and are more expensive per pound. It is important to specify the appropriate plastic for the application, and not overspecify. For example, a part that may be made in a more expensive polycarbonate, which runs hotter in the mold, may

Introduction to Medical Plastics

be made in an easier-to-mold and less expensive acrylic, at lower temperatures and cycle times, and perform just as well in the application.

WHAT IS A POLYMER?

Polymers are chain molecules. *Poly* means many and *mer* means an individual unit. Polymer means many units (mers) together (e.g., polyester). In chemistry, there is also an oligimer. *Oligi* means a few (like an oligarchy). So, an oligimer is an arrangement of a few units; monomer, one unit; and polymer, many units. Examples of monomers are styrene, methyl, and carbonate.

BASICS: THERMOPLASTIC AND THERMOSETS

Another basic distinction for plastics is whether a plastic material is a thermoplastic or a thermoset. A thermoplastic is one that can be melted. Think of thermoplastic polymer molecules like strands of spaghetti. Ones with lower molecular weight, like styrene, are shorter. Ones with high molecular weight, like ultra-high-molecular-weight polyethelene (UHMWPE), are longer. When you boil a pot of spaghetti, the noodles become soft and pliable. You can pour spaghetti into a bowl, and it takes the shape of the bowl. When it cools, it still keeps the shape of the bowl. The spaghetti can then be reheated and softened, and formed into another shape.

If you think of the length of the strands and then think of squeezing boiled spaghetti through a large funnel, you will see how plastics process differently. Spaghetti chopped up into small strands will go through easily. Noodles in long strands will be harder to squeeze through. Styrene, for example, is a short molecule that flows very easily when melted. This makes it a popular material for low-cost products that need to hold high detail, such as styrene car and aircraft models. It also easily remelts.

The other basic type of plastic is a thermoset. This is a material that is cross-linked. Unlike the spaghetti in the earlier analogy, in which the strands are separate and can be made to flow again if heated, a cross-linked plastic is more like a fishnet. The strands are hooked together. It cannot be boiled and made to flow like the spaghetti. Therefore, thermoset plastics, once they are cross-linked in an irreversible chemical reaction and form this molecular network, cannot be made to flow or melt. Examples of thermosets are epoxy, cast urethanes, and silicones.

A common example of a type of thermosetting reaction occurs when making a hard-boiled egg, in which heat causes the proteins in the egg to denature and cross-link from a liquid to a solid in an irreversible reaction.

Whether a plastic is a thermoplastic or a thermoset obviously makes a great deal of difference in how the material is processed and shaped. Thermoplastics can be melted and molded, as in injection molding. Thermosets are shaped by some form of casting. Thermoplastics assume their shape when they cool. Thermosets assume their shape when a chemical reaction causes the material to cross-link.

CROSS-LINKED THERMOPLASTICS

A special case found in some modified plastics used for medical devices is that of cross-linked thermoplastics. In this situation, a thermoplastic is irradiated with ionizing radiation to release free radicals and induce the formation of three-dimensional cross-linked structures in a thermoplastic. This modification can have a dramatic effect on the properties and performance of the plastic material. Common applications of this process in medical devices include irradiated polyester tubing for angioplasty balloons and irradiated UHMWPE for joint implants.[*]

Radiation cross-linking allows a material to be processed like a thermoplastic and then be given the properties of a thermoset. Modified Polymers Corporation (Sunnyvale, CA) offers these materials modification services to the medical device industry.

Note that radiation sterilization can cause unintentional cross-linking, stiffening, or embrittlement of some polymers. See the section in this chapter on sterilization effects on plastics for more information.

WHAT IS A MEDICAL-GRADE PLASTIC?

First, there is no such thing as a Food and Drug Administration (FDA)-*approved* material. This is a misnomer, because the FDA does not approve materials. The FDA supplies regulations and guidance for material compliance for manufacturers to follow. There are USP, International Organization of Standardization (ISO), and FDA-*compliant* materials. These are materials manufactured in compliance with particular regulations and standards.[2,†]

USP is responsible for establishing legally recognized product standards for drugs and other health-related articles in the United States. In the 1960s, methodology and requirements were established for the plastic materials used for pharmaceutical containers and closures, and these were subsequently adopted by medical device manufacturers. USP tests measure biological reactivity of plastics in contact with mammalian cell cultures (*in vitro*) and via the implantation and injection of extractables into laboratory animals (*in vivo*). Plastics are classified into one of six classes, each requiring different levels of testing. USP Class VI requires the most extensive testing. Not all plastics manufacturers wish to undertake the expense of testing their materials to this level; therefore, the number of materials meeting this classification for your application may be limited.

USP does not regulate compliance or certification of plastics tested according to its published methods. The FDA has adopted some of the tests specified by USP for regulation of medical devices.

For further information on USP test methods, consult USP 23—NF 18, Chapters 87 to 88, and contact USP at U.S. Pharmacopeia, 12601 Twinbrook Parkway, Rockville, MD 20852, at 800-822-8772.[‡]

---

[*] Sophie Rouif, "Irradiated Plastics: Applications and Perspectives for the Automotive and Electrotechnic Industries," http://www.radtech-europe.com/download/rouifpaperjuly.pdf; M. C. Sobieraj, S. M. Kurtz, and C. M. Rimnac, "Notch Strengthening and Hardening Behavior of Conventional and Highly Crosslinked UHMWPE under Applied Tensile Loading," *Biomaterials* 26, no. 17 (2005): 3411–3426.

[†] Food for Human Consumption, 21 C.F.R. Food and Drugs 170–199, http://www.access.gpo.gov/nara/cfr/ waisidx_99/21cfr177_99.html.

[‡] Boedeker Plastics Regulatory Standards and Compliance Overviews, http://www.boedeker.com/regcomp.htm#FDA (includes a good overview of several other standards, for example, ASTM, Canadian, 3A Dairy, UL, etc.).

Introduction to Medical Plastics 9

Whenever a plastic is used in a medical device in human use, even if it is advertised as a USP Class VI material, it needs to be tested by the manufacturer according to the standards relevant to the amount of contact it has with the patient. Table 1.1 describes many of these patient-contact scenarios. This is because several factors, such as the addition of colorants, processing, and the use of the plastic in combination with other materials and adhesives, can affect the biocompatibility characteristics of the material.[3]

These tests need to be done even if the same material is in use in another medical device. Using a material that is already in use in another medical device that is known to have passed biocompatibility testing can help, however, because you can have some confidence that the material will pass testing in your application.

Additionally, if any part of the material changes, such as the addition of colorant or fillers to an injection-molded part, testing will need to be done on that combination of materials even if the plastic has already been tested in its natural state, and even if the additives have been tested separately.

For more information on biocompatibility testing see Chapter 4, "Assessing Biocompatibility," which gives a quick reference to the testing to be done for several categories of medical device applications. Again, it is the responsibility of the designer and manufacturer to determine whether a particular material is suitable for its particular use.

FINDING PLASTICS

There are seemingly endless varieties of plastics under hundreds of trade names. These materials can be sorted conveniently on the "Polymer Trade Name" section of Matweb.com (http://www.matweb.com/search/SearchTradeName.asp). This tool can help you locate the manufacturer of a material in which you are interested, as well as the composition of a trade name material. Plastics.com also has a listing of materials by trade name and composition (http://www.plastics.com/tradenames.php). Plastics distributors (Port Plastics, Westlake Plastics, Polymer Plastics Corporation, Boedeker Plastics) are also good sources of information when choosing and sourcing plastic materials.

PLASTICS FOR MACHINING

This category of plastics consists of materials that are readily available in shapes that are easily set up for machining. These plastics tend to have high costs relative to weight, as most of the material is lost as chip waste during machining.*

Listed in this chapter are some of the more readily available materials suitable for machining that are sold in FDA-compliant grades. These materials are listed with plastics vendors as mechanical plastics. Check with your vendor to ensure that the material you are ordering is sufficiently FDA-compliant for your intended use.

Not all of the plastics listed here are available in USP Class VI grades. This, however, is not an issue if the application does not involve patient contact or the passing of liquids intended for patient contact.

---

* Descriptions of plastics and their stock shapes are courtesy of Polymer Plastics Corporation, Mountain View, CA.

TABLE 1.1
Biocompatibility Matrix

Device Categories   **Examples**

Device Categories		Examples
Surface device	Skin	Devices that contact intact skin surfaces only; examples include electrodes, external prostheses, fixation tapes, compression bandages, and monitors of various types
	Mucous membrane	Devices communicating with intact mucosal membranes; examples include contact lenses, urinary catheters, intravaginal and intraintestinal devices (stomach tubes, sigmoidoscopes, colonoscopes, gastroscopes), endotracheal tubes, bronchoscopes, dental prostheses, orthodontic devices, and IUDs
	Breached or compromised surfaces	Devices that contact breached or otherwise compromised external body surfaces; examples include ulcer, burn and granulation tissue dressings, or healing devices and occlusive patches
External communicating device	Blood path, indirect	Devices that contact the blood path at one point and serve as a conduit for entry into the vascular system; examples include solution administration sets, extension sets, transfer sets, and blood administration sets
	Tissue/bone/dentin communicating	Devices communicating with tissue, bone, and pulp/dentin system; examples include laparoscopes, arthroscopes, draining systems, dental cements, dental filling materials, and skin staples
		Devices that contact internal tissues (rather than blood contact devices); examples include many surgical instruments and accessories
	Circulating blood	Devices that contact circulating blood; examples include intravascular catheters, temporary pacemaker electrodes, oxygenators, extracorporeal oxygenator tubing and accessories, hemoadsorbents, and immunoadsorbents
Implant device	Tissue/bone	Devices principally contacting bone; examples include orthopedic pins, plates, replacement joints, bone prostheses, cements, and intraosseous devices
		Devices principally contacting tissue and tissues fluid; examples include pacemakers, drug supply devices, neuromuscular sensors and stimulators, replacement tendons, breast implants, artificial larynxes, subperiosteal implants, and ligation clips
	Blood	Devices principally contacting blood; examples include pacemaker electrodes, artificial arteriovenous fistulae, heart valves, vascular grafts and stents, internal drug delivery catheters, and ventricular assist devices

Source: Courtesy of Pacific BioLabs (formerly Northview Laboratories), Hercules, CA.

Introduction to Medical Plastics

Also listed are a number of high-performance engineering plastics. These are intended for particular demanding applications. The cost of these plastics can be very high relative to commodity plastics.

Most plastics in stock shapes are available only in natural (often a cream color), transparent, black, or white. Colored plastics are normally not available off the shelf. The exceptions to this are polyvinylchloride (PVC) rod and acrylic sheet and some nylon shapes.

Polymer Plastics Corporation, Mountain View, CA, has an online catalog with a quotation function for each of the standard shapes it carries (see http://www.polymerplastics.com). This can be a very useful tool when choosing a cost-effective material and when planning and budgeting a prototyping or short-run manufacturing project.

Boedeker Plastics, Shiner, TX, offers a broad range of information on plastics for medical and food processing use (see http://www.boedeker.com/agency.htm).

PLASTICS FOR PROCESSING BY MACHINING

ACRYLONITRILE–BUTADIENE–STYRENE

A terpolymer is made from SAN (styrene–acrylonitrile) and butadiene synthetic rubber. The SAN gives ABS its hardness and surface finish, and the butadiene gives it its toughness.

Commonly available plastic in sheets to 4 inches thick and rods up to 6 inches in diameter, it can easily be bonded and laminated to form thicker sheets and assemblies. Because of its reasonable cost and ease of machining, it is a popular material for computer numerical control (CNC)-fabricated prototypes.

Rod: 0.250 to 6.000 inches
Sheet: 0.062 to 0.250 inches
Plate: 0.250 to 4.000 inches
Standard color: Natural (cream), black

ACRYLIC

Acrylics were actually one of the first medical device plastics[4] and are still commonly used in molding of anaplastic prosthetics.[*] Acrylic is basically polymethyl methacrylate (PMMA). It is one of the most readily available plastics, found at signage and hobby shops. It is rigid, clear, very machinable, and bondable. One popular method of bonding acrylic is solvent bonding with methyl chloride. Acrylic is available in nearly unlimited varieties of rod, sheet, and plate shapes, and a variety of colors. Acrylics are especially suitable for light pipes and optical applications.

---

[*] For more information on anaplatological modeling, see Robert L. McKinstry, *Fundamentals of Facial Prosthetics* (Clearwater, FL: ABI Professional Publications, Vandamere Press, http://www.abipropub.com/fundfapro.htm), which contains detailed how-to information on numerous medical modeling techniques.

One project I worked on required a clear tube, 12 inches in diameter, for a hyperbaric chamber that needed to be clear for observation. I was able to locate this shape, preformed in acrylic, in an appropriate wall thickness, and had parts fabricated at reasonable cost at an acrylic fabrication shop.

Acrylics for signage and display may be used for bench testing and prototypes; however, care must be taken to identify a medical-grade version before using it in any clinical trials. Commercial-grade acrylics may contain UV (ultraviolet) inhibitors for weatherability, flame retardants, impact modifiers, and other chemicals that render them unsuitable for clinical use.

Polyvinylchloride

PVC is available in both rigid and flexible forms, depending on whether plasticizers are added. PVC is commonly used for water pipes.

The major disadvantages of PVC are poor weatherability, relatively low impact strength, and fairly high weight for thermoplastic sheet (specific gravity of 1.35). It is easily scratched or marred, and it possesses a relatively low heat distortion point (160_i).

Unplasticized PVC is produced in two major formulations: type I (corrosion resistant) and type II (high impact).

Type I PVC is the most commonly used PVC, but in applications for which higher impact strength than that offered by type I is required, type II offers better impact properties, with a slight loss in corrosion resistance. In applications requiring a high temperature formulation, polyvinylidene fluoride for high-purity applications (PVDF) is usable to approximately 280°F.

Rod: 0.250 to 12.000 inches
Sheet: 0.032 to 2.000 inches
Hollow bar: From 0.562 inches inner diameter (I.D.) to 0.625 inches outer diameter (O.D.)
Hex bar: 0.432 to 2.000 inches
Standard color: Gray, white, clear

PVC rod is available from Gehr Plastics (http://www.gehrplastics.com/products/pvc/pvc.htm) in 10 different colors and up to 6 inches in diameter.

Note: PVC is one of the few mechanical plastics available in stock shapes in colors.

Polycarbonate

Polycarbonate (PC) is an extremely tough plastic, commonly sold under the trade name Lexan®. It is the toughest transparent plastic available. It is very useful for prototype medical devices, especially if UV cure bonding is to be used. It is available in rod, plate, and sheet. It bonds readily.

Although more than a dozen performance characteristics of PC are utilized singly or in combinations, seven are most commonly relied on. These are high-impact strength, water-clear transparency, good creep resistance, wide-use temperature range, dimensional stability, abrasion resistance, hardness, and rigidity despite its ductility.

PC tends to discolor with radiation sterilization. Radiation-stable grades are available.

Rod: 0.250 to 6.000 inches
Plate: 0.375 to 4.000 inches
Sheet: 0.030 to 0.500 inches
Film: 0.003 to 0.030 inches
Tubing: 0.250 inches I.D. to 4.000 inches O.D.
Standard colors: Optical clear, black, gray

POLYPROPYLENE

Polypropylene (PP) is a lightweight, inexpensive polyolefin plastic with a low melting temperature, making it popular for thermoforming and food packaging. PP is flammable; therefore, look for a flame retardant (FR) grade if fire resistance is required.

Rod: 0.250 to 14.000 inches
Sheet: 0.060 to 2.000 inches
Tubing: From 0.060 inches I.D. to 2.000 inches O.D.
Standard color: Opaque white, natural

POLYETHELENE

Polyethelene (PE) is a material commonly used in food packaging and processing. UHMWPE has a high abrasion resistance, low coefficient of friction, self-lubrication, nonadherent surface, and excellent chemical fatigue resistance. It also retains high performance at extremely low temperatures (e.g., with liquid nitrogen, at −259°C). UHMWPE starts to soften and lose its abrasion resistance characteristics around 185°F.

Because UHMWPE has a relatively high expansion and contraction rate when subjected to temperature changes, it is not recommended for close tolerance applications in these environments.

Because of its high-surface-energy nonadherent surface, PE can be difficult to bond. Assemblies may most readily be put together with fasteners, interference, or snap fits. Loctite Corporation makes a cyanoacrylate adhesive (CYA) (Loctite Prism® surface-insensitive CYA and primer) to bond these types of plastics.

UHMWPE also is used in orthopedic implants with great success. It is the most common material used in acetabular cups in total hip arthroplasty, and in tibial plateau components in total knee replacements, bearing against highly polished cobalt–chrome.[*] Note that material suitable for orthopedic implant use is a specialty

---

[*] For detailed information on UHMWPE in orthopedic applications, see Steven Kurtz, *The UHMWPE Handbook* (New York, Elsevier Academic Press, 2004). See also the related website at www.uhmwpe.org.

material, not the industrial-grade version. A medical-grade UHMWPE is marketed by Westlake Plastics (Lenni, PA) under the trade name Lennite®.

ACETAL

Delrin® by DuPont is one of the best-known acetals, and most designers refer to this plastic by this name. Acetals are synthesized from formaldehyde. Acetal was originally developed in the early 1950s as a tough, heat-resistant nonferrous metal substitute.* It is a tough plastic with a low coefficient of friction and high strength.

Delrin and similar acetals are difficult to bond and are best assembled mechanically. Delrin is commonly used in machined medical device prototypes and close tolerance fixtures. It is highly machinable, making it popular for machined device prototypes that require strength, chemical resistance, and FDA-compliant material.

One drawback of Delrin is its sensitivity to radiation sterilization. This tends to make acetals brittle. Snap fits, plastic spring mechanisms, and thin sections under load may crack and break if radiation sterilized. If acetal parts are to be sterilized, consider using EtO, Steris, or autoclave, depending on whether the device contains any sensitive components, such as electronics.

Acetals are sold by Westlake Plastics, BASF, and Celanese. DuPont markets an improved acetal, DelrinII® with improved properties. Westlake Plastics markets an FDA-compliant grade under the trade name Pomalux®.

NYLON (POLYAMIDE)

Nylon[5] is available in 6/6 and 6/12 formulations. Nylon is tough and heat resistant. The identifiers 6/6 and 6/12 refer to the number of carbon atoms in the polymer chain; 6/12 is a longer-chain nylon with higher heat resistance. Nylon is not as machinable as ABS or Delrin, as it tends to leave stringy swarf on the edges of a part that may require deburring.

Nylon 6, most commonly known as cast nylon, was first developed before World War II by DuPont. It was not until 1956, however, with the discovery of chemical compounds (cocatalysts and accelerators), that cast nylon became commercially viable. With this new technology, the speed of polymerization was greatly improved and the steps necessary to achieve polymerization were reduced.

Because there are fewer processing limitations, cast nylon 6 provides one of the largest arrays of sizes and custom shapes of any thermoplastic. Castings are available in rods, tubes, tubular bars, and sheets. They range in sizes from as small as 1 lb to as large as 400 lb per part.

Hydlar® is a high-performance version of nylon 6/6 reinforced with Kevlar fiber for use in bearings and bushings. Note: Filled and fiber-reinforced plastics of this kind are generally *not* FDA compliant.

---

* See http://www2.dupont.com/Phoenix_Heritage/en_US/index.html for the history of Delrin®, Nylon, and many other DuPont plastics and their inventors.

Introduction to Medical Plastics 15

Rod: 2.00 to 20.000 inches
Plate: 0.250 to 4.000 inches
Tubular bar: From 2.00 to 20.000 inches O.D.; unlimited I.D.

FLUORINATED ETHYLENE PROPYLENE

Fluorinated ethylene propylene (FEP) has all the desirable properties of tetrafluoroethylene (TFE) (polytetrafluoroethylene [PTFE]), but with a lower survival temperature of 200°C (392°F). Unlike PTFE, FEP can be injection molded and extruded by conventional methods into rods, tubes, and special profiles. This becomes a design and processing advantage over TFE. Available in rods up to 4.5 inches and sheets up to 2 inches, FEP fares somewhat better than PTFE under radiation sterilization.

HIGH-PERFORMANCE ENGINEERING PLASTICS FOR MACHINING

Note: These high-performance engineering plastics may be more limited in availability (special order). Some can also be quite expensive.

ULTEM® POLYETHERIMIDE

Ultem 1000 is a thermoplastic polyetherimide high-heat polymer designed by General Electric for injection-molding processing. Through the development of new extrusion technology, manufacturers such as A. L. Hyde, Gehr, and Ensinger produce Ultem 1000 in a variety of stock shapes and sizes. Ultem 1000 combines excellent machinability and provides a cost-savings benefit over PES, PEEK, and Kapton in high-heat applications (continuous use to 340°F). Ultem is resistant to autoclave sterilization.

PEEK™

Polyetheretherketone (PEEK), a trademark of Victrex plc (UK), is a crystalline high-temperature thermoplastic that offers excellent thermal and chemical resistance properties and outstanding resistance to abrasion and dynamic fatigue. It is recommended for electrical components for which a combination of high continuous service temperature (480°F) with very low emission of smoke and toxic fumes on exposure to a flame is required.

PEEK meets Underwriters Laboratories (UL) 94 V-0 requirements at 0.080 inches. This product is extremely resistant to gamma radiation, even exceeding the resistance of polystyrene. The only common solvent that will attack PEEK is concentrated sulfuric acid. Hydrolysis resistance of PEEK is exceptional and it can operate in steam up to 500°F.

PEEK is also a very hard plastic. PEEK tubing can be sharpened to a point that can pierce tissue. It is an excellent insulator. It also has stiffness that approaches that of metal tubing. PEEK is highly biocompatible, being used in demanding applications, such as orthopedic implants and heart valves.

Victrex plc supports medical device manufacturers closely through their Invibio subsidiary. It supplies medical device manufacturers with implantable-grade PEEK-OPTIMA® and medical-grade PEEK-CLASSIX™ polymers.

PTFE (Teflon®)

TFE or PTFE (polytetrafluoroethylene), more commonly known as Teflon, is one of the three fluorocarbon resins in the fluorocarbon class composed wholly of fluorine and carbon. The other resins in this group, also referred to as Teflon, are perfluoroalkoxy fluorocarbon (PFA) and FEP.

The forces binding the fluorine and carbon together provide one of the strongest known chemical linkages in a compact symmetrical arrangement of atoms. The result of this bond strength plus the chain configuration is a relatively dense, chemically inert, thermally stable polymer.

TFE resists attack by heat and virtually all chemicals. It is insoluble in all organics with the exception of a few exotics. Its electrical properties are excellent. Although it has high impact strength, its resistance to wear, tensile strength, and creep resistance are low in comparison with other engineering-type thermoplastics.

TFE exhibits the lowest dielectric constant and lowest dissipation factors of all solid materials. Because of its strong chemical linkage, TFE shows very little attraction for dissimilar molecules. This results in a coefficient of friction as low as 0.05.

Although PTFE has a low coefficient of friction, it is *not* suitable for use in load-bearing orthopedic applications, because of its low creep resistance and poor wear. This issue was discovered in a classic case by Sir John Charnley in the late 1950s in his pioneering work on total hip arthroplasty.[*]

Note: Fluoropolymers (TFE and PTFE) are sensitive to radiation sterilization. PTFE is obviously very difficult to bond; however, chemical or plasma etching may be used to produce a bondable surface.

Polysulfone and Polyphenylsulfone

Polysulfone was originally developed by BP Amoco and is currently manufactured by Solvay Advanced Polymers, S.A. (Brussels, Belgium), under the trade name Udel®. Polyphenylsulfone is sold under the trade name Radel®.

Polysulfone is a tough, rigid, high-strength transparent (light amber) thermoplastic that maintains its properties over a wide temperature range from $-150°F$ to above $300°F$. Designed for use in FDA-recognized devices, it also passed all tests of the USP Class VI (biological). It complies with the National Sanitation Foundation's potable water standard up to $180°F$.

Polysulfone has very high dimensional stability. The changes in linear dimensions after exposure to boiling water or air at $300°F$ are generally one-tenth of 1% or less.

Polysulfone has very high resistance to mineral acids, alkali, and salt solutions; resistance to detergents and hydrocarbon oils is good, even at elevated temperatures

---

[*] S. A. Brown, "Let's Not Repeat History: Good Examples of Bad Ideas" (paper presented at Proceedings of the Materials and Processes for Medical Devices Conference, ASM International, 2003).

under moderate stress levels. Polysulfone is not resistant to polar organic solvents, such as ketones, chlorinated hydrocarbons, and aromatic hydrocarbons.

Radel is used in instrument trays that require high heat resistance and high impact strength for hospital autoclave tray applications.

Polysulfone engineering resins combine high strength with long-term resistance to repeated steam sterilization. These polymers have proven successful as alternatives to stainless steel and glass. Medical-grade polysulfones are biologically inert, display unique long life under sterilization procedures, can be transparent or opaque, and are resistant to most common hospital chemicals.[*]

Polyimide Rod and Sheet (Vespel®, Kapton®)

Vespel is a graphite-filled polyimide material for extreme service bearings. It is *not* an FDA-compliant material.

Ryton (polyphenyl sulfide), unmodified or modified with glass fibers or other modifiers such as PTFE, molybdenum sulfide (MoS), or graphite, is used primarily in structural components. Characteristics are high stiffness, extremely high-use temperature (up to 600°F), excellent chemical resistance, and excellent electrical properties.

In both modified and unmodified forms, Ryton exhibits excellent machineability, with optical finishes possible by grinding and lapping.

Note: These types of filled and fiber-reinforced plastics are generally *not* FDA compliant.

INJECTION-MOLDED AND EXTRUDED PLASTICS

Injection-molded and extruded plastics are available in the widest array of materials and properties. They can be custom compounded in almost endless combinations. When choosing a material, a good rule is to use a plastic that is readily available with proven biocompatibility appropriate for its use and that meets the mechanical design and assembly requirements. Most mechanical plastics available in shapes for machining that are thermoplastics are available in injection-molding pellet form.

The injection-molding process will accommodate virtually any thermoplastic. Extrusion for catheters is usually done from the more flexible plastics such as Pebax®, polyurethane, PVC nylon, thermoplastic elastomers (TPEs), and FEP. Extrusion from rigid plastics, such as PEEK, is available in cases in which more pushability and torqueability of a catheter is required. Flexibility in these stiffer plastics in extrusions is achieved by use of thinner wall sections.

Considerations

One of the issues with injection-molded plastics is that plastics manufacturers tend to sell their material in large minimum quantities. For example, a minimum quantity order of Magnum® ABS from Dow is 760 kg (1,600 lb). This can be difficult to manage in an R&D environment, especially if you are molding a relatively low quantity of small-shot-size parts. One way to manage this is to request 20 or 50 lb samples, which most manufacturers will provide. Another is to deal with an injection-molding vendor

---

[*] B. L. Dickinson, UDEL polysulfone for medical applications. *J. Biomater. Appl.*, 3, 605–634, 1989.

that specializes in medical molding. They may keep cartons of common stock materials on hand that they can subdivide for customers with smaller material requirements.

When choosing a material for injection molding, it is important to have a material that meets the design requirements but is not overengineered. Selecting a material with more properties than you need may result in higher material costs, longer cycle times, and possibly a less cosmetically pleasing part. This can drive up costs and erode margins, especially for single-use disposables. It is also important to choose a material carefully because different materials have different shrink factors and will produce slightly different size parts from the same mold if materials are changed.

A way to work with plastics available only in injection-molding pellets is to have a custom extrusion made from the material that you want to use. A number of feet of extrusion can be made from a material sample. This allows the use of a material that may be machined into prototypes.

When evaluating candidates for a plastic material, be sure to look at the example applications of a manufacturer's material used in a medical application. Not only will this help you determine whether the material is suitable for your application, but also you may find innovative ways to use these materials that you had not considered before.

In the following section some of the more common medical plastics for molding are described.

COMMODITY PLASTICS

ABS

ABS (acrylonitrile–butadiene–styrene) is the most common plastic for injection molding. ABS is a two-phase polymer blend. A continuous phase of SAN gives the materials rigidity, hardness, and heat resistance. The toughness of ABS is the result of submicroscopically fine polybutadiene rubber particles uniformly distributed in the SAN matrix.

ABS is a versatile, less expensive plastic with a combination of high processability, excellent surface finish, and toughness. It resists the formation of blemishes from flow marks and knit lines, even with more difficult part geometries.

Medical grade ABS is sold under the Magnum® name by Dow Chemical,[*] and Lustran® by Bayer Plastics,[†] and Cycolac® by GE.

PC/ABS

PC/ABS is a versatile blend of ABS and PC. It is especially suitable for molded housings and parts that require high impact strength. The ABS component makes the material more moldable, and the PC provides high toughness.

PC/ABS is more expensive than ABS, and while highly moldable, it is not as moldable as plain ABS. More care needs to be taken in part design to avoid flow and knit lines.

---

[*] http://www.dow.com/engineeringplastics/bus/na/med/#magnum.
[†] http://www.bayerus.com/new/2000/01.21.00plas.html.

Introduction to Medical Plastics

PC/ABS is available from Bayer Plastics in its Bayblend® material, from GE in its Cycoloy® blend, and from Dow as Emerge®.

Acrylic

Acrylic for injection molding is available in a wide range of properties, depending on the modifiers, copolymerization, and alloying of the base PMMA.

Acrylic can be an attractive and cost-effective alternative to PC in less demanding applications. It has lower heat deflection performance; however, this means that it also molds at lower temperatures, allowing better fill of thin walls and intricate parts. Acrylic is water clear and has excellent optical properties, as well as alcohol and lipid resistance. Unlike PC, which discolors yellow under gamma sterilization, acrylic takes on a blue-green tint.

Acrylic for injection molding of medical devices is marketed by the Cyro Corporation under the trade name Cyrolite® acrylic-based multipolymers and Cyrex® acrylic–polycarbonate alloys.

Polycarbonate

PC is one of the workhorse materials in medical devices. It is clear, tough, and tolerates a variety of sterilization methods. Because it is clear, it is especially suited to assembly with UV cure adhesives. PC is a popular material for molding smaller devices, such as luer fittings and stopcock bodies.

PC tends to yellow under radiation sterilization. Radiation-stable grades of PC are available for these applications.

PC is sold under the trade names of Markolon® and Apec® from Bayer, Dow Calibre®, Zelux® from Westlake, and GE Lexan®.

Polyethelene

PE is an easy-to-mold plastic with excellent surface lubricity and flexibility. High-density polyethylene (HDPE) and low-density polyethylene (LDPE) are used in fluid fittings, stopcock valves, and syringe bodies. It is excellent for snap fits, but it does not bond easily.

Polyolefin

Polyolefin is a plastic commonly found in blow molding applications. It is very flexible under a wide range of temperatures. It is also a popular material for molding toys, especially rotationally molded (e.g., Little Tikes). It is a low-surface-energy plastic and can be difficult to bond.

Polyolefin is also used in a majority of heat-shrink tubing used in the electronics industry. Texloc Corporation (Ft. Worth, TX) produces a medical-grade polyolefin heat-shrink tubing.

Styrene

Styrene is an economical commodity plastic. It has low heat resistance and is readily attacked by many aromatic solvents. It is useful in such items as cups and trays and other low-cost applications. One common application of styrene is insulated foam beverage containers (styrofoam cups).

ELASTOMERS

Elastomeric Plastics

When specifying an elastomer, a balance of properties is needed. For example, in extruded catheters there is a balance between pushability, flexibility, torqueability, and lubriciousness. In general, the softer the plastic, the higher the surface tackiness will be, and the catheter will be softer and more flexible, but less lubricious and harder to push. Fillers such as barium, in addition to providing radiopacity, can improve the lubricity of an elastomeric catheter.

TPEs are useful when molding rubber-like parts. Some TPEs have excellent properties, making them candidates for replacement of thermoset silicones in some applications. Following are some of the more common TPEs.

Polyurethane

Polyurethane (PU) is a material that may exist as either a thermoplastic or a thermoset. PU is a product of diisocyanates and diamines, and was invented by Otto Bayer and his associates in 1937. Thermoplastic PU is used in film applications, such as heat seal bags, and is a common material for extrusion of soft catheters. PU is highly versatile, in molded and extruded solid plastic, as well as polyurethane foams, both open cell and self-skinning. PUs are some of the most commonly used plastics in catheter manufacturing.

PUs are common rigid casting materials for model-making applications, as well as two-part mixes for dip molding and casting prototype rubber parts.

An innovative use of PU is the Synbone® (Switzerland), an injection-molded bone model for training orthopedic surgeons, made from Bayer Baydur 60®.

Medical thermoplastic PUs are sold under trade names, including Pellethane® (Dow Chemical); Baydur® (Bayer); Tecoflex®, Tecothane®, Tecophillic®, and Carbothane® (Noveon Thermedics, Wilmington, MA); and Chronoflex® (Cardiotech Inc.). PUs such as Pellethane are not plasticized to achieve their flexibility, making them suitable for situations in which leaching of extractable plasticizers can cause biocompatibility problems.

Kraton®

Kraton is a styrenic block copolymer made by the Kraton Corporation of Houston, TX. Kraton is a very moldable TPE plastic in a very wide range of hardness and properties.

Kraton styrenic TPEs are compounded for medical and consumer applications by the GLS Corporation (McHenry, IL) under the Versaflex®, Versaloy®, and Dynaflex® trade names. These are a family of materials based on Kraton styrenic TPE, and they are offered in a wide range of durometers and surface tackiness from 3 Shore A to 80 Shore A. These materials are especially suited to overmolding applications, with grades specified for many medical applications. GLS Kratons are particularly suited to overmolding to difficult-to-bond olefinic substrates.

K-Resin®

K-Resin is a family of styrene–butadiene rubber copolymers (SBCs) made by Chevron-Phillips Chemical. It is used in numerous disposable medical devices, toys, and food-packaging applications.

Introduction to Medical Plastics

Monoprene®
Monoprene is manufactured by the Teknor Apex Company, a privately held company founded in 1924 and headquartered in Pawtucket, RI. Monoprene TPEs are a versatile family of TPEs composed of saturated styrene block copolymer rubbers and thermoplastic olefin resins. Monoprene is available in softness ranging from gel to 90 Shore A. Monoprene is used in applications such as resuscitator bags and other applications requiring a rubbery material that is FDA compliant.

Pebax®
Pebax is a highly versatile family of polyether block amides that are plasticizer-free thermoplastic elastomers. Pebax has been utilized in high-performance industrial articles, medical textiles, and sporting goods. It is manufactured by the Arkema Group (France).

It is one of the more common materials in catheter extrusion. It is easy to bond, is readily formed in secondary operations, such as flaring and tipping, and releases easily from glass molds that are pretreated with mold release.

Polyvinylchloride
PVC[*] is used in rigid (nonplasticized) and flexible (plasticized) forms. It is a common commodity plastic for disposable medical devices, especially tubing. One common type of PVC tubing is Tygon®, made by Norton Performance Plastics, a subsidiary of Saint-Gobain (France). PVC was once found in nearly 60 percent of all disposable medical devices until concern over phthalate plasticizers[†] (diethylhexyl phthalate [DEHP]) was raised by the European Union and activist groups. A concern over DEHP-plasticized PVC in medical use is its potential release of chlorine when incinerated, as well as alleged health issues. Another potential drawback of some PVCs is their corrosiveness to P-20 steel injection molds.

Saint-Gobain has removed DEHP from its PVC tubing, and other manufacturers have sought alternatives to PVC in their devices. However, PVC has a set of desirable properties, such as clarity, sterilizability, and economy. Vendors now offer DEHP-free PVCs for medical use.

Non-DEHP-plasticized PVCs for molding are available from Colorite Polymers under the name Flexchem®. Solmed® and Solcare® are available from Solvay-Draka.

Ethylene Vinyl Acetate
Ethylene vinyl acetate (EVA) is used as an alternative to PVC in film applications in which plasticizers need to be avoided. EVA film is made by Solvay-Draka in its Solmed® film line.

---

[*] For more information on medical molding of PVCs, see Mario Bertora, *Injection Moulding of PVC for Medical Use* (Sandretto Industries, 2000), http://www.thecannongroup.com/immaginigruppo/papers/MedicalMouldingPVC.pdf.
[†] Benjamin Lichtman, "Flexible PVC Faces Stiff Competition."

THERMOSETS

Santoprene®

Santoprene is a thermoset rubber material that is processable by injection molding and manufactured by Exxon-Mobil.* Santoprene is especially useful where abrasion resistance is important. It is known as a thermoplastic vulcanizate (TPV).

Santoprene and other vulcanized rubbers are often black. This is due to the addition of carbon black, a material that blocks UV and protects the rubber from degradation. Santoprene is commonly used in automotive interiors, grips, and rubber covers and bumpers.

Silicone

Silicone is a polymer of silicon and carbon first successfully commercialized in a joint venture between Corning and General Electric in the 1940s. It is very stable, very heat resistant, virtually inert, and well tolerated by the body (despite bad press from litigation over its use in certain cosmetic surgery applications). Silicone is cured with one of two catalyst systems, peroxide cure or platinum cure.

Silicone is used in tubing, seals, and prosthetics. In RTV (room temperature vulcanized) form, it is a popular material for producing rubber molds for short-run prototypes and production.

Silicone is provided to the medical industry mostly by smaller suppliers. NuSil (Carpenteria, CA) is a major supplier of silicones to the medical device industry.

Polyisoprene

Polyisoprene is a synthetic version of the natural rubber originally harvested by the Mayans and Aztecs from the hevea tree.† It is polymerized by the Ziegler–Natta vinyl polymerization reaction. Polyisoprene is used in balloons, syringe bulbs, and other dip-molded devices.

Nitrile

Nitrile is a popular substitute for latex in rubber gloves. It does not have the elongation of latex, but is free from potentially allergenic latex protein monomers. Nitrile is a terpolymer made up of acrylonitrile, butadiene, and carboxylic acid. It is processed as an emulsion, much like latex rubber. Nitrile has a superior resistance to oils and fats compared with latex or polyisoprene.‡

Latex

Latex is a natural protein from the sap of the hevea tree grown in rainy, elevated areas of Southeast Asia. It is useful in thin-film applications, such as surgical gloves,

---

* http://www.santoprene.com/home.html.
† See website maintained at the University of Southern Mississippi, Department of Polymer Science, for a detailed and entertaining description of the Ziegler–Natta reaction.
‡ For more information on the barrier properties of nitrile, see Jeffrey L. Welker, "Nitrile as a Synthetic Barrier," *Source to Surgery* 6, no. 2 (December 1998), accessed August 6, 2012, http://www.ansellhealthcare.com/temps/products/gloveevaluation/10Step.cfm.

condoms, and other barrier devices. Concerns over latex allergies have led to the elimination of natural rubber latex in many medical devices, and many manufacturers will certify products containing elastomers as latex-free.

Latex is used as a film, usually in dip molding. This is how gloves and condoms are produced. Latex is often coated with cornstarch powder to prevent self-adhesion. When used, this powder becomes a further source of potential contamination in surgical applications. Latex has exceptional tear resistance, elongation, and elastic recovery.*

Liquid latex is a water-based colloid of latex monomer micelles that polymerizes as it dries. Liquid latex is available in forms for glove-type mold making and dip molding from TAP Plastics and Douglas and Sturgess, an artists' and sculptors' supply house in San Francisco.†

Although problematic for use in medical devices, easily available natural latex is a very useful material for prototyping dip-molded membranes, balloons, and rubber tips and bumpers. The results obtained in testing should approximate what can be achieved with synthetic polyisoprene.

HIGH-PERFORMANCE ENGINEERING PLASTICS FOR MOLDING

POLYETHERIMIDE (PEI), ULTEM®, PEEK®, POLYSULFONE

These materials are available in pellet form for injection molding when exceptional strength and heat resistance are required. The trade names, properties, and manufacturers of these materials are described earlier in the chapter.

Keep in mind that some engineering plastics can also be quite expensive per pound of material. When designing a cost-effective disposable device, it is important not to overspecify the plastic and not to have a part that is more expensive than it needs to be, which also may be more difficult to mold.

If a product is to be reused and withstand high-temperature sterilization, or has other high-performance requirements, engineering plastics can be a very attractive alternative to formed or machined metal parts.

USEFUL SPECIALTY PLASTIC MATERIAL FORMS

EXTRUDED PTFE (ZEUS, TEXLOC)

Extrusion of PTFE is a specialty process because of the high heat required and the difficult rheology of the fluoropolymer material. Teflon tubing is commonly available as a sheath for electronics wiring. Some vendors for medical-grade PTFE tubing are Zeus (Orange, NJ) and Texloc (Shiner, TX).

---

* Latex has exceptional tear resistance and elongation to break in thin films. In fact, in a fraternity house trick, a latex rubber condom can be made to expand and hold nearly 1 gallon of water without breaking.
† Douglas and Sturgess, http://www.artstuf.com, is a great resource for a wide range of hard-to-find sculpting, modeling, and casting materials.

Expanded PTFE

A special form of PTFE is a stretched or expanded PTFE (EPTFE). This material was originally developed by W. L. Gore & Associates and sold under the trade name Gore-Tex. This produces a PTFE that is flexible, hemocompatible, and can act as a scaffold for ingrowth of intimal tissue.* EPTFE is available from W. L. Gore (Newark, DE), Zeus (Orange, NJ), Impra, a division of C.R. Bard (Phoenix, AZ), and International Polymer Engineering (Tempe, AZ). EPTFE is used as highly lubricious liners for catheters, lubricious and flexible heat-resistant liners for thermal ablation devices, seals and gaskets, low-friction catheter liners, and vascular graft material, which allows for ingrowth of endothelium, and cycles with the pulsatile expansion and contraction of blood flow. EPTFE is highly heat resistant. EPTFE for vascular grafts is available from Impra and Atrium (divisions of C. R. Bard) and W. L. Gore. Other EPTFE shapes are available from Zeus Corporation and International Polymer Engineering.

SHEET AND FILM AND FOAM PLASTICS

Polyethylene Terephthalate (PET) and Polyethylene Terephthalate Glycol (PETG)

PET and PETG are popular film and sheet material for vacuum-formed medical blister packs and trays that are closed with heat-sealed Tyvek® lids. PETG film is often treated with a silicone coating to prevent sticking while tray parts are nested together during shipment.

PETG film is sold under the Klöckner Pentaplast name and BP Chemical Barex®.

Tyvek®

Tyvek is a nonwoven olefin fiber fabric developed by DuPont. It is especially useful in medical packaging, as the mesh of the material is breathable and allows the passage of gas molecules, such as ethylene oxide sterilizing gas, but is a barrier against larger-size microbes. Tyvek is thin, waterproof, and very tear resistant.[6]

PVC and Polyethelene Film

Polyvinyl and polyethelene films are widely used in bagging and packaging applications, especially heat-sealed bags and enclosures.

Polyester Film (Mylar®)

Polyester film was the material used on the first successful high-pressure angioplasty balloons. Polyester has the property of being extrudable into very thin tubing and being noncompliant, meaning it did not stretch into a sphere, as would a latex balloon, for example. This allowed a device that would expand to slightly larger than a blood vessel, and no more, while holding high pressure to remold arterial plaque and

---

* For more information on EPTFE and medical textiles, see Bhupender S. Gupta, "Medical Textile Structures: An Overview," *Medical Plastics and Biomaterials* (January 1998), http://www.mddionline.com/article/medical-textile-structuresan-overview.

restore blood flow by dilatation. Thin polyester tubing is used to blow a wide variety of medical balloons. It may also be irradiated to modify its properties.

Mylar was originally developed by DuPont. Polyester tubing is also very useful in medical devices, as very thin wall shrink tube as well as balloon stock tubing. This polyester tubing is manufactured by Advanced Polymers (Salem, NH).

Polyimide

Polyimide is a unique thermoset material that is both an exceptional insulator and very heat resistant. It is also resistant to attack from most chemicals. It is most commonly available in tubing form, which can be made in exceptionally thin walls. It can also be made into extremely small diameter tubing. Polyimide in thin films is very flexible and fatigue resistant. It is commonly used in flex circuit applications and in very thin and strong catheter tubing. Polyimide tube is supplied by the Microlumen Company (Tampa, FL) and in custom coextrusions from Putnam Plastics (Dayville, CT).

Styrene Butadiene Rubber Foam and Elastic Fabric (Wetsuit Material)

A common material in braces and wraps is wetsuit material, which is a layer of rubber or TPE foam with an outer layer of Spandex® nylon stretch fabric. This foam comes in two basic forms, one a neoprene thermoset rubber foam material for UV-resistant durable wetsuits, and the other a styrene butadiene rubber (SBR) blend for lower cost consumable and disposable applications, as well as padded bags and covers. One useful form of SBR foam material has a stretch nylon fabric side and a hook-compatible plush side. This allows the construction of bands and wraps closable with hooked Velcro® tabs.

Foam Sheet Material

Another type of plastic foam material is polyolefin foam. This is a popular material in the construction of backings for conductive hydrogel on several types of electrical conducting pads, such as adhesive electrode pads for radio frequency (RF) electro-surgery, electrocardiogram (EKG), and defibrillator pads.

RESOURCES

REFERENCES: RADIATION EFFECTS ON PLASTICS

An important consideration with medical plastics is their tolerance of sterilization, especially by ionizing radiation such as electron beam or gamma radiation.

Bennett, Jeff. *Irradiation Processing*. Oak Brook, IL: Sterigenics Corporation. A detailed article and chart on this subject is available at http://www.sterigenics.com/services/medical_sterilization/contract_sterilization/material_consideration_irradiation_processing.pdf.

Davis, J. R., ed. *Handbook of Materials for Medical Devices*. Materials Park, OH: ASM International Press, 2003. This book covers both plastics and metals, with an emphasis on orthopedic and dental applications.

Harper, Charles A., ed. *Handbook of Materials for Product Design* New York: McGraw-Hill, 2001. A comprehensive overview of industrial materials used in product design.

Kurtz, Steven. *The UHMWPE Handbook*. New York: Elsevier Academic Press, 2004. Covers the use of ultra-high-molecular-weight polyethylene in orthopedic applications.

Ratner, Buddy D. et al., eds. *Biomaterials Science: An Introduction to Materials in Medicine*, 2nd ed. New York: Elsevier Academic Press, 2004. This comprehensive and definitive source of information is completely updated and revised from the first edition. Highly recommended.

ACKNOWLEDGMENT

The assistance of Larry Stock of Polymer Plastics Corporation (Mountain View, CA) is gratefully acknowledged in the preparation of this chapter.

ENDNOTES

1. Jay P. Mayesh and Mary F. Scranton, "Legal Aspects of Biomaterials," in *Biomaterials Science: An Introduction to Materials in Medicine*, 2nd ed., ed. Buddy D. Ratner et al. (New York: Elsevier Academic Press, 2004): 797–804; and Joan Sylvain Baughan, "Limiting Liability of Medical Device Materials Suppliers" (March 2003; accessed August 6, 2012), http://www.packaginglaw.com/2581_.shtml. The most well known of these cases are those involving Dow Corning and silicone breast implants. Despite scientific evidence to the contrary, Dow Corning was driven into bankruptcy, and billions of dollars paid out to plaintiffs and trial lawyers over alleged autoimmune disorders from silicone gel-filled implants. Other well-known cases involved the Dalkon Shield intrauterine device (IUD) made by A. H. Robins, several cases involving pacemaker leads, and suits against Vitek for its temporomandibular joint (TMJ) implant product. In the Vitek case, DuPont found itself spending millions of dollars to extricate itself from deep-pocket liability over the use of a few cents' worth of material by a small company. This case led DuPont to embargo the sale of its Teflon material for medical use.
2. "The United States Pharmacopeia (USP) is a nongovernmental, standards-setting organization that advances public health by ensuring the quality and consistency of medicines, promoting the safe and proper use of medications, and verifying ingredients in dietary supplements. USP standards are developed by a unique process of public involvement and are accepted worldwide. In addition to standards development, USP's other public health programs focus on promoting optimal health care delivery and are listed below. USP is a nonprofit organization that achieves its goals through the contributions of volunteers representing pharmacy, medicine, and other health care professions, as well as science, academia, the U.S. government, the pharmaceutical industry, and consumer organizations." See http://www.usp.org/about-usp (accessed August 6, 2012).
3. "The best starting point for understanding biocompatibility requirements is ANSI/AAMI/ISO Standard 10993, *Biological Evaluation of Medical Devices*. Part 1 of the standard is the guidance on selection of tests, Part 2 covers animal welfare requirements, and Parts 3 through 17 are guidelines for specific test procedures or other testing-related issues. Testing strategies that comply with the ISO 10993-1 are acceptable in Europe and Asia. In 1995, the FDA issued a Blue Book Memorandum G95-1, which replaced the Tripartite Guidance (the previous biocompatibility testing standard). The FDA substantially adopted the ANSI/AAMI/ISO guideline, although in some areas FDA's testing requirements go beyond those of ISO. The specific test procedures spelled out in the ISO standard vary slightly from the USP procedures historically used for FDA submissions. The ISO procedures tend to be more stringent, so companies planning to register their product in Europe and the U.S. should follow ISO test methods. FDA requirements should be verified since additional testing may be needed. Japanese procedures

for sample preparation and testing are slightly different from either USP or ISO tests. Pacific BioLabs highly recommends discussing your proposed biocompatibility testing plan with a FDA reviewer before initiating testing." Pacific BioLabs, Inc., *Assessing Biocompatibility: A Guide for Medical Device Manufacturers* Hercules, CA, chapter 4 of this book.
4. "PMMA was introduced to dentistry in 1937. During World War II shards of PMMA from shattered gun turrets unintentionally implanted in the eyes of aviators, suggested that some materials might evoke only a mild foreign body reaction." Buddy D. Ratner et al., *Biomaterials Science: An Introduction to Materials in Medicine* (New York: Academic Press, 1996): 1. PMMA was developed and marketed in the 1930s by the Rohm and Haas Company under the name Plexiglas®, and with lesser success by DuPont under the name Lucite®.
5. Nylon was a discovery of Dr. Wallace Carrothers, who also discovered neoprene. Nylon was not trademarked, with the hopes that it would become a generic term and popularize use of the fiber. Neoprene was likewise a name coined at DuPont and allowed to go generic. DuPont has been the source of many of the most important materials used in medical devices, such as PTFE (Teflon®), polyimide, Mylar, Tyvek, nylon, and Delrin.
6. "Tyvek® is a classic case of a slow starter. It grew out of a research into nonwoven fabrics begun by William Hale Charch in 1944, took 15 years to develop, and required another 15 years to become profitable. Today Tyvek® building wrap can be seen in nearly every housing development, and it has gained a firm foothold in the envelope market. Tyvek® is also popular as a sterile packaging and protective clothing in the medical field." http://www2.dupont.com/Phoenix_Heritage/en_US /1966_a_detail.html (accessed August 6, 2012).

2 Getting Stuck in a Good Way
Basics of Medical Device Adhesives

Theodore R. Kucklick

CONTENTS

Medical Device Adhesives: An Overview	30
Major Categories of Adhesive Systems	33
Solvent Adhesives	33
Epoxy Adhesives	34
Epoxy, Chemistry Systems	34
Two-Part, Mixed, and One-Part Epoxies	34
Prepackaged Epoxy	34
Thermally and Electrically Conductive Epoxy	35
CA Adhesives	35
Specialty Formulations	36
CA Surface Primers and Accelerators	36
CA Adhesives: Process Considerations	36
UV and Light-Cure Adhesives	36
Chemistry System	37
Cure Lights	37
Light-Cure Cyanoacrylates	37
Process Considerations	37
Silicone Adhesives	38
Surface Preparation	38
Silicone Dermal Adhesives	38
Urethane Adhesives	38
Adhesive Joint Design	39
Mechanical Testing of Adhesive Bonds: Quality and Consistency	39
Conclusion	40
Resources	40
Vendors: General Information	40
Vendors: Medical Device Adhesives Distributors	41
Endnote	41

It is hard to imagine the modern medical device industry without all of the stuff that holds most of these devices together: modern medical device adhesives. Without these adhesives, the mass production of advanced catheters and disposables would be impossible. Adhesives manufacturers have made huge advances allowing simple and consistent joining of materials once thought impossible to glue. What are the adhesive systems that are applicable to medical devices, and how do you get the best results from them?

There are several ways to hold parts together. Fasteners, snap fits, press fits, welding, and adhesives. For disposable medical devices welding (ultrasonic or thermal) and adhesives are the most common.

MEDICAL DEVICE ADHESIVES: AN OVERVIEW

The basic adhesive systems for disposable medical devices are epoxy, cyanoacrylate (CA), acrylic-based light (UV) cure, and solvent bonding. The most widely used for disposable plastic medical device assembly are CA and UV cure (UVC). Epoxy is often used for metal-to-metal bonding and potting. Solvent bonding (SB) with solvents such as cyclohexanone are used in the assembly of low-cost tubing sets. Solvent bonding can be cheap and efficient; however, the flammability and toxicity of these solvents, and venting of volatile organic compounds (VOCs) can be a significant problem. CA and UVC are one part, easy to use, and highly versatile, and they work at room temperature and do not require solvents or catalysts, making them the most popular adhesives in medical device assembly. Each system has its own set of capabilities, so it is important to become familiar with the range of adhesive systems available to the medical device designer and to have a toolkit of capabilities from which you can knowledgably choose the best adhesive system for your application.

Medical-grade epoxy is available from several suppliers, such as Epotek, Master-Bond, and Loctite. CA is popularly known by the consumer trade name Krazy Glue®. CA was originally developed by Eastman Chemical, then a division of Kodak, and is now made and marketed in a wide range of commercial and medical versions by Loctite (a division of Henkel). Medical-grade UVC adhesives are manufactured by Dymax and Loctite. Contact the manufacturer for the name of your local distributor of medical device adhesives. The local distributor will have a knowledgeable sales representative who can be a valuable resource in obtaining samples and recommending appropriate product solutions. The manufacturers will have technical specialists that can help you solve any of your specific bonding challenges.

CA and epoxy are readily available for nonclinical research and development (R&D) use in hardware-store grades. UVC and light-cure adhesives are typically available only from industrial adhesives suppliers.

There are numerous and specialized formulations of these adhesives. There are special formulations for joining nearly every plastic, in a wide range of viscosities, and surface treatments for difficult-to-bond substrates. Loctite offers an excellent and comprehensive course in the use of their CA adhesives, which I highly recommend to any device designer. Dymax also offers a seminar in the use of their UVCs. Contact these vendors for a schedule of courses in your area.

To understand how best to bond parts, it helps to know the basic potential failure modes of a bond. These are cohesive, adhesive, and substrate failure. Cohesive failure occurs when the adhesive fails to bond to one surface or the other. Adhesive failure occurs when there is a bond to both surfaces, but the adhesive takes the load and fails. Substrate failure occurs when the adhesive bond is stronger than what is being bonded, and it fails. The goal is to have two materials, for which the adhesive forms a molecular bond to the substrates, and the two parts that are joined act as one material. Substrate failure is the ideal failure mode, in which case the substrate of the part being joined fails before the adhesive joint. Adhesives join parts in one of two basic ways, either a molecular bond, in which the adhesive joins chemically to the substrates, or mechanically, in which the adhesive grabs into a substrate's surface without bonding chemically. Sometimes secondary operations, such as grit-blasting metal or etching nonreactive substrate materials, such as polytetrafluoroethylene (PTFE; Teflon) or silicone, are required to achieve a successful mechanical bond.

Recommendations for a successful union include the use of fresh adhesive, clean parts, and compatible materials. One way to avoid adhesive bonding problems is to choose materials that bond more easily when possible, such as styrenes, acrylonitrile–butadiene–styrene (ABS), polycarbonates, acrylics, and urethanes. "Blocked" polymers, such as Pebax, and low-surface energy plastics, such as polypropylene, may be bonded with proper surface preparation. These surface preparation "primers" are available from the adhesive manufacturer. Low-durometer materials with high levels of plasticizer can be problematic. Difficult-to-bond materials include the fluorinated polymers (PTFE, fluorinated ethylene propylene [FEP], Teflon) and Delrin (acetal). Another difficult-to-bond material is silicone, a nonstick thermoset rubber (which cannot be thermally bonded) that typically requires a silicone-based adhesive and, possibly, coronal etching mechanical surface preparation. Some of the materials that are attractive in terms of their nonstick surface and nonreactivity to the body become a problem to bond because of their nonreactivity to adhesives.

Because CAs are moisture-cured, the humidity on the production floor and bonding of hygroscopic materials (water absorbing, such as nylon) can affect bond consistency. Some epoxy systems require heating to cure. It is important that the materials being bonded can tolerate this. If room-temperature epoxies are used, the exothermic reaction during curing may warp and distort thin-walled parts.

Clean parts are essential, as is fresh adhesive. Other tips for a successful bond include allowing a sufficient "glue gap." Mating parts sometimes are made to too close a fit, which wipes the glue off the parts during assembly and "starves" the joint. For example, a glue gap, or diametrical gap 0.00 inches between a cylindrical object in a bore is common.[*]

Use the right viscosity as measured in centipoise (cP). For reference, water has a cP of 1 and the viscosity of honey is about 5000 cP. Use a thinner, or lower cP adhesive when bonding smaller glue gaps, and a higher viscosity when closing larger gaps.

---

[*] Henkel Technologies, *Loctite Needle Bonding Design Guide* (Rocky Hill, CT: Henkel Technologies, 2004): 3.

Another useful rheological property is "thixotropic." This is a material that becomes less viscous in response to shear stress (e.g., shaking or mixing) and becomes more viscous when the shear stress is removed. A familiar example of a thixotropic material is tomato ketchup. When the ketchup is in the bottle, it is resistant to flow. Shaking the ketchup helps it to flow, and once it flows, and is applied to a surface, it tends to stay put. Think of how ketchup stays put on a hot dog. A thixotropic or gel-like adhesive is useful when you want the glue to "stay put," particularly on vertical surfaces. A thixotropic material is also less prone to be absorbed into a porous substrate.

The other important property of an adhesive is "wettability."[*] Wetting depends on both the adhesive and the substrate. Some materials are "low surface energy" and resist wetting. Examples of these materials include polyolefins, polyethylenes, and fluorocarbons. When a material and adhesive combination wet poorly, the liquid adhesive beads up on the surface of the substrate. This is not desirable, and this will lead to a poor bond. When an adhesive "wets" the surface, it spreads evenly without beading up, and causes a better bond. Surface treatments such as mechanical or chemical etching or plasma etching can help to increase wettability.

When using UVCs, some visually transparent materials block UV, such as amber-colored polyimide tubing, and prevent curing. This is because the amber or orange colored material absorbs light in the blue part of the spectrum, and does not allow enough UV light to penetrate to activate the photoinitiator in the UVC adhesive.

When scaling a process from R&D to production an often-overlooked, but necessary, piece of equipment is a controlled application system. Sometimes products are taken to production scale with adhesive still being dispensed out of squeeze bottles. This is great for R&D but not for production. Invest in a controlled dispensing system (e.g., from Nordson EFD, see Figure 2.1) to help achieve consistent results. A well-controlled production environment should have a Cpk (Process Capability) of 1.3 or better, and this is hard to do with squeeze bottles.[†]

Other issues to consider as a prototype makes its way to a production device include biocompatibility and sterilization. Adhesives are a material just like any other material in your finished device and thus must be tested in its "as-built" and "as-sterilized" condition. This will take into account any interactions between your materials and the adhesives that might affect biocompatibility. There are "medical-grade," International Organization of Standardization (ISO)-10993 or U.S. Pharmacopeia (USP) Class VI adhesives; however, this does not imply that they are Food and Drug Administration (FDA) approved because the FDA does not "approve" materials. It simply means that the materials are produced under controlled conditions, and there are no materials or by-products that are likely to fail biocompatibility testing. For more information on biocompatibility testing see Chapter 4, "Assessing Biocompatibility."

---

[*] Wetting: the physics behind wetting, accessed August 6, 2012, http://www.adhesives.org/Training Education/StudentResources/Wetting.aspx.
[†] For a definition of Cpk see: "What Is Process Capability?" *The NIST/SEMATECH e-Handbook of Statistical Methods*, last modified April 1, 2012, accessed May 29, 2012, http://www.itl.nist.gov/div898/handbook/pmc/section1/pmc16.htm.

Getting Stuck in a Good Way

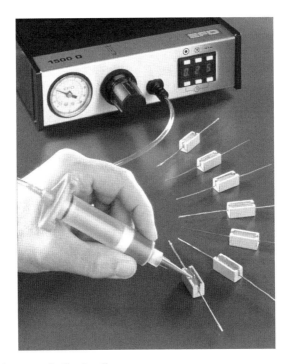

FIGURE 2.1 Automated adhesive dispenser.

Mechanical testing after sterilization is critical as well to ensure that the adhesive joints in the device perform consistently and to specification after being subjected to EtO, E-beam, gamma, or other production sterilization method.

MAJOR CATEGORIES OF ADHESIVE SYSTEMS

This section discusses the major categories of adhesive systems in more detail.

SOLVENT ADHESIVES

Two common solvent adhesives are methylene chloride and cyclohexanone. Methylene chloride is the watery solvent used to bond acrylic and is available at plastics hobby shops. Cyclohexanone is a somewhat-oily fluid that is good for bonding vinyl and styrenic materials (e.g., styrene and ABS). Other solvent bonding materials include toluene and methyl ethyl ketone (KET).

Solvent bonding is a quick and inexpensive method to bond low-cost items, such as drain tube sets. If you have ever assembled polyvinylchloride (PVC) plumbing pipe you are familiar with solvent bonding. Concerns and regulatory restrictions over the release of volatile organic compounds (VOCs), flammability, and exposure of assemblers to volatile and toxic solvents has made solvent bonding less popular. Solvent bonding may not be used on thermoset plastics.

To solvent bond an assembly, such as a tubing set, dip the tube in the solvent, and wet about 0.25 inches of the tube. Allow the solvent to soften the tube slightly and press it into the mating fitting (if a male-female junction) or over a male luer or barb fitting (if a female-male junction) and allow the assembly to dry in a well-ventilated area.

EPOXY ADHESIVES[*]

Epoxies were one of the original medical device adhesives, and they were used in some of the original cardiac pacemakers. Epoxies have the advantage of being "gap filling" and are used for "potting" or encapsulating an object, such as an electrical circuit with epoxy adhesive. Epoxies can glue nearly any bondable material. Epoxies are suitable for use in wide range of temperatures up to 500° F, which makes them suitable for reusable devices that will be steam or autoclave sterilized, to extreme cold cryogenic applications.[†]

Epoxy, Chemistry Systems

Epoxies, generally speaking, are polymers consisting of epoxide groups or oxirane rings. They are cured using a variety of chemistry systems, including amines, anhydrides, phenols, and amino resins.[‡] Epoxies are generally thermoset (cross-linked) when cured.

Two-Part, Mixed, and One-Part Epoxies

Epoxies generally include two components: a part A and a part B. These parts must be mixed according to the volume or weight ratios specified by the manufacturer. Maintaining the correct epoxy mixing ratios is essential. I have watched technicians mix epoxy, and remove and re-add mixed material to hit a target overall weight for the mixture in the work instructions, and then wonder why the epoxy will not cure (after the mixing ratios have gone out the window). These process errors are some of the places to look when you have seemingly "voodoo" adhesive failures.

One-part epoxies are a premixed system that are shipped refrigerated and cure when the epoxy warms up, or they have one component that is activated only when heated.

Prepackaged Epoxy

Prepackaged epoxies are convenient to use. Parts A and B are contained in a pouch and are separated by a clip or a barrier. The clip is removed, or one side of the pouch

---

[*] For more information on standards for the use of epoxies in medical devices, see *ASTM F602-09 Standard Criteria for Implantable Thermoset Epoxy Plastics*, ASTM International, http://www.astm.org/Standards/F602.htm. Other standards, F641, F624, F665, D883, and F639 for medical device and implantable epoxies are available for purchase as well.

[†] Walter Brenner, "Designers Intro to Advanced Medical Adhesives," *Medical Design Magazine* (November 2008), http://medicaldesign.com/materials/adhesives/designers_intro_advanced_1108/index.html.

[‡] Henkel Technologies, *Loctite Design Guide for Bonding Plastics*, vol. 4 (Rocky Hill, CT: Henkel Technologies, 2004): 26.

is squeezed to break the barrier, and the mixture is kneaded until mixed completely. Then, the pouch is opened and the adhesive is dispensed.

Thermally and Electrically Conductive Epoxy

Epoxies can be loaded with powders, such as sliver, alumina, ceramics, and boron nitride. Silver-filled conductive epoxies are sometimes used as a replacement for solder in electronics assemblies.[*]

CA Adhesives

CA was originally developed in the 1940s by Dr. Harry Coover when working on an improved transparent acrylic plastic for gunsights and aircraft canopies. Like many important discoveries, its practical use was not immediately apparent. Dr. Coover and Fred Joyner of Kodak Laboratories and Tennessee Eastman later discovered its exceptional adhesive properties nearly a decade after its initial discovery when they accidentally glued two refractometer prisms together with it. The original commercial version was Eastman 910, first sold in 1958. Its adhesive properties were so revolutionary that the glue sold slowly. Because it was so different from any glue ever seen before, customers did not believe that it could set nearly instantaneously and actually could have such remarkable strength, with a very small amount of glue. Clever marketing demonstrations helped to tell the story.[†]

CA has developed into an especially versatile adhesive system with very high strength. It has the ability to glue nearly any substrate and is highly biocompatible. CA is an acrylic resin adhesive. The CA monomers polymerize in the presence of the hydroxyl ions in water through anionic polymerization. Trace amounts of moisture on most surfaces will initiate the reaction. Acids tend to inhibit the reaction, as do dry surfaces with insufficient moisture to initiate curing. Newer surface-insensitive formulations help to bond dry or acidic substrates such as paper. CAs tend to bond best when used in a thin film. This allows the polymerization to propagate between the substrate surfaces and form a molecular bond to the substrates. CA adhesives are suitable for heat resistance up to about 212° F (100° C).

Because CA adhesives are initiated by moisture, having a consistent humidity in a production environment is important to achieving consistent glue bonds. CA adhesives will harden from moisture in the air, so it is important to keep the adhesive container closed when not in use. Refrigeration can help to extend the shelf life of CA adhesives as well. It is especially important to use fresh adhesive in a production environment. Stale adhesive that has been allowed to partially polymerize can result in bond failures.

Needless to say, CA will bond skin instantly and will bond aggressively to clothing fabrics, especially cotton. Be careful, especially with the water-thin grades of CA,

---

[*] Michael Hodgin and Richard Estes, "Advanced Boron Nitride Epoxy Formulations Excel in Thermal Management Applications" (paper from proceedings of the Technical Programs NEPCON WEST, Anaheim, CA, February 23–25), http://www.epotek.com/SSCDocs/whitepapers/Tech%20Paper%2042.pdf.

[†] "SUPER GLUE: The Amazing Story of CA Glue," *SAMTalk: SAM 600 of Australia Newsletter* (January 2004), http://www.tpbweb.com/media/catalog/354.pdf.

as they can run along a part, unnoticed, until you find your fingers glued to the part. Acetone solvent can help dissolve these accidental CA glue bonds.

CA for industrial use are of the methyl-2 and ethyl-2 CA variety. Industrial CA glues are not suitable for medical use as surgical tissue adhesives. Methyl and ethyl CA glues tend to break down into toxic byproducts and are inflammatory to tissue. Longer chain n-butyl and 2-octyl CAs that break down more slowly, with fewer toxic by-products are now available for surgical uses, such as topical wound closure, sealing sutures, and hemostasis. These are sold under the trade names Vetbond®, Dermabond®,* and others.†

Specialty Formulations

CA adhesives are available in a wide variety of viscosities and with other properties, such as heat resistance, toughness, and flexibility. Plain CA is hard and brittle. Formulations are available to glue nearly any substrate, including polyolefins, polypropylene, and PTFE fluorocarbons.

CA Surface Primers and Accelerators

Bonding problems with difficult-to-bond substrates often can be solved with the right combination of surface preparation primer. There are a number of different primers, some that help to generate molecular bonding sites on substrates such as polyolefin for the CA to bond to, some to neutralize bond inhibitors, and some to mechanically etch surface such as fluorocarbons (e.g., Teflon). Depending on the combination of materials to be glued, a number of candidate CA adhesives and primers might work. Get samples of these, test sample assemblies, and test for strength and consistency. Your adhesives vendor can be helpful in getting samples and suggesting products to solve your particular bonding challenge. Be sure to look at all the possible options of adhesive systems (CA, UVC, etc.) to determine the optimal solution.

CA Adhesives: Process Considerations

One issue with CA adhesives is "bloom" or "frosting." This occurs in situations in which the CA adhesive will outgas monomers and leave a frosted film on the part that may be cosmetically unacceptable. This outgas may be due to excessive humidity or to the formulation of adhesive used. CAs cure rapidly; however, they still take a few hours to cure completely and will continue to outgas during that time. Solutions to bloom and frosting are as follows: chose a "lower bloom" formulation, control the humidity in the assembly area, or allow the parts to cure completely in a well-ventilated area before stacking or bagging.

UV and Light-Cure Adhesives

UV and light-cure adhesives are exceptionally versatile. They come in a wide variety of viscosities and special formulations to bond nearly any material, including hard-to-bond substrates like highly plasticized PVC.

---

* Ethicon Dermabond, accessed August 6, 2012, http://www.dermabond.com.
† Nathan D. Schwade, *2-Octyl Cyanoacrylate Wound Adhesives*, accessed August 6, 2012, http://emedicine.medscape.com/article/874047-overview.

Chemistry System

UV and light-cure systems typically rely on an acrylic resin chemistry. Light-cure silicones and CAs are also available. Another advantage of UVC adhesives is that some change color or fluoresce. This can help to determine that sufficient adhesive was used and that the adhesive cured completely.

Cure Lights

UVCs can require a relatively expensive mercury lamp light source to cure. For R&D, an inexpensive dental UV light source or light-emitting diode (LED) pens from your vendor can be used for prototyping. When using any UV source, use UV-blocking eye protection. UV exposure can cause permanent eye damage. Safety glasses are available from your vendor. If a UVC system is used in a production environment, it must be calibrated regularly to ensure that the light is completely curing the adhesive, because the UV lamps wear out over time and decrease output. These calibration devices are available from light source manufacturers (e.g., Efos, Dymax, Loctite). Light output from UV lights is in the 254–470 nm range. The shorter wavelengths promote surface curing and the longer wavelengths penetrate deeper for depth of cure. It is especially important that the cure light reaches all of the adhesive and hardens it completely and that there is no unhardened adhesive. When designing parts, be sure that the parts are transparent to UV where the bond is to occur. Any adhesive in opaque shadow areas, where the light does not reach, will not cure.

Some UVCs have the capability of secondary thermal cure (at about 2 hours at 80° C). Check with your manufacturer to see whether the adhesive you have chosen has this capability.

Visible light-cure (VLC) systems cure in the 400–650 nm range. VLC adhesives must be dispensed through light-proof dispensers and nozzles. Advantages of VLC adhesives are safety (no UV light) and less infrared (IR) heat transmitted to the part.

Light-Cure Cyanoacrylates

A special type of CA adhesive cures with UV light. This system has the advantage of "shadow curing"—that is, once the polymerization is initiated, it will continue to propagate into areas where there is adhesive but the light does not reach.

Process Considerations

One problem with UVCs is that some will exhibit surface tackiness even when given enough light to fully cure. This is known as "oxygen inhibition," in which oxygen in the air prevents the exposed surface of the UVC adhesive from curing completely. The surface will remain tacky as atmospheric oxygen will continuously inhibit the polymerization process. One way to avoid this is to design the glue joint with little or no UVC exposed to air. If a large surface of adhesive must be exposed to air, and surface tackiness is unacceptable, the part may be cured under a nitrogen gas blanket.*

---

* Derek Wyatt, "Processing Guidelines for UV Curable Adhesives," *Lasers and Optronics* (February 2000), http://www.henkelna.com/us/content_data/113819_lcproc.pdf.

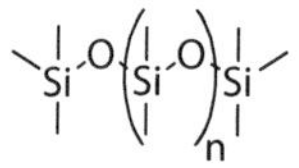

$$\text{-Si-O-(Si-O)}_n\text{-Si-}$$

FIGURE 2.2 General structure of silicone.

SILICONE ADHESIVES

Silicone is a truly amazing material. It is literally a glass rubber (polydimethylsiloxane), as it is a thermoset polymerization of silicon, oxygen, carbon, and hydrogen (see Figure 2.2). The strongly bound silicon-oxygen siloxane backbone is what gives silicone its exceptional flexibility and chemical resistance. It took the efforts of a number of pioneering chemists and teams of assistants a period of 40 years to turn silicones from the original useless "sticky messes" to a useful and versatile material that revolutionized industry.[1] Silicones are used in everything from adhesives, to implants, to lubricants, to antifoaming agents, including simethecone, for pharmaceutical production and over-the-counter antigas medications.

Silicone adhesives are useful for bonding silicone parts and also for forming seals and gaskets. There are two basic types of silicones, two-part "addition cure" and one- or two-part "condensation cure." Addition cure uses either a tin or platinum catalyst. One-part condensation cure silicones are known as room temperature vulcanized (RTVs). Free radical systems rely on peroxide to cure. One-part condensation cure rubbers require atmospheric moisture to cure and a substantial exposed surface area. Adhesives used for medical devices typically are two-part platinum catalyzed addition cure types, because they react and cure completely and do not leave residual by-products.[*]

Surface Preparation

Silicones typically require mechanical abrasion or coronal etching to bond. This is because the silicone substrate is highly nonreactive and does not offer molecular bonding sites to an adhesive.

Silicone Dermal Adhesives

Think of the sticking and releasing qualities of a 3M Post-it-Note®. This ability to adhere and release, without damaging the substrate or leaving adhesive residue, combined with the inertness and biocompatibility of silicone make for a useful dermal adhesive, as well as an effective transdermal drug delivery platform. Silicone dermal adhesives are available as pressure sensitive adhesives (PSAs) and soft skin adhesives (SSAs) in films and gels, and they can be loaded with a variety of materials.[†]

URETHANE ADHESIVES

Polyurethane adhesives are a thermoset polymer system. They are useful for bonding polyurethane parts and fittings and to bond metals to plastics. Polyurethane adhesives

---

[*] Regina M. Malczewski, Donald A. Jahn, and William J. Schoenherr, *Peroxide or Platinum? Cure System Considerations for Silicone Tubing Applications* (Midland, MI: Dow Corning Healthcare, 2003), http://www.dowcorning.com/content/publishedlit/52-1077-01.pdf.

[†] Xavier Thomas, *Silicone Adhesives in Healthcare Applications* (Midland, MI: Dow Corning Healthcare, 2003), http://www.dowcorning.com/content/publishedlit/52-1057-01.pdf.

Getting Stuck in a Good Way

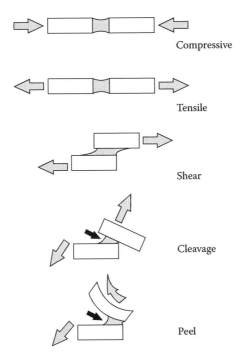

FIGURE 2.3 Basic types of stresses on an adhesive joint.

have the advantages of being tough, flexible, and low exotherm, but they have a potential disadvantage of requiring long cure times.

ADHESIVE JOINT DESIGN

When designing assemblies, consider alternatives to adhesives, such as thermal bonding ultrasonic welding, one-way snap fits, press fits, crimping, and insert molding. These methods may be more consistent and require less labor than assembly with adhesives. Sometimes, adhesives are the best approach. Have an open mind to all of the available assembly methods and choose the best method for your device.

There are five basic types of stresses on an adhesive joint: compressive, tensile, shear, cleavage, and peel (see Figure 2.3). Compressive, tensile, and shear are good. Cleavage and peel are bad. Look for ways to design out cleavage and peel. These conditions concentrate stress at the bondline and make the joint more prone to failure. The length of the glue joint under tension or shear contributes more to the strength of the joint given an equal glue joint surface area.

MECHANICAL TESTING OF ADHESIVE BONDS: QUALITY AND CONSISTENCY

For one-off R&D prototypes, it is probably not necessary to do a lot of testing. For pilot preclinical and clinical builds, however, testing for bond consistency may be advisable. When scaling up to production, testing for bond consistency is essential. The goal is to have bonds that test consistently, without a wide variation. A wide variation indicates a process that is not under statistical control and an unacceptable risk of field failures.

CONCLUSION

Medical device adhesives offer a powerful toolkit of capabilities for assembling advanced and reliable medical devices. Adhesives can join together nearly any material and a variety of dissimilar substrates. One of the challenges is sorting through the large variety of available adhesives to find the optimal solution for the assembly. Once a candidate has been selected, the material and adhesive combination needs to be tested for function, quality, and consistency before scaling up to production. The adhesive should have USP Class VI and ISO 10993 certification to ensure biocompatibility. The adhesive and materials also need to be tested after sterilization and aging to ensure their reliable performance. Adhesives manufacturers are an important resource for information, samples, and design guides for working with medical device adhesives. Understanding the basic types of forces that act on an adhesive joint, and the types of designed adhesive joints available to the designer, will help to produce a successful, cost-effective, and reliable assembly.

RESOURCES

VENDORS: GENERAL INFORMATION

Dow Corning Corporation
Corporate Center
P.O. Box 994
Midland, MI 48686-0994
Phone: 989-496-7875
Toll Free: 800-248-2481
http://www.dowcorning.com

Dymax Corporation, USA
318 Industrial Lane
Torrington, CT 06790
Phone: 860-482-1010 or 877-396-2988 or 877-396-2963
Customer Support Fax: 800-482-1012
Corporate Fax: 860-496-0608
Email: info@dymax.com
http://www.dymax.com

Henkel Corporation
Industrial Assembly
Phone (United States): 800-562-8483

Phone (Canada): 800-263-5043
Brands: Adhesin, Bonderite, Frekote, Hysol, Loctite, Macroplast, P3
Tapes, Labels, Graphics
Phone: 866-443-6535
Brands: Derma-Tak, Duro-Tak, Nacor, Technomelt

Henkel Transdermal, Drug Delivery
Phone: 866-443-6535
Brands: Duro-Tak, Proloc, Velox
http://www.henkelna.com
Henkel offers an excellent medical device adhesives seminar. Contact Henkel Corporation for more information.

NuSil Technology LLC
1050 Cindy Lane
Carpinteria, CA 93013 Phone: 805-684-8780
Fax: 805-566-9905
http://www.nusil.com

Shin-Etsu Silicones of America
1150 Damar Drive
Akron, OH 44305-1201
Phone: 800-544-1745
Fax: 330-630-9855
http://www.shinetsusilicones.com

Vendors: Medical Device Adhesives Distributors

Ellsworth Adhesives
W129 N10825 Washington Drive
Germantown, WI 53022
Phone: 262-253-8600 or 800-888-0698
Fax: 262-253-8619
http://www.ellsworth.com

R. S. Hughes Inc.
1162 Sonora Court
Sunnyvale, CA 94086.
Phone: 408-739-3211
www.rshughes.com

ENDNOTE

1. Silicones were originally discovered by F. S. Kipping in England in 1904. He originally deemed them useless "sticky messes" and coined the word "silicone." Kipping is incidentally the father of silicon chemistry, the basis for the modern semiconductor

industry. James F. Hyde developed the first commercially successful silicones in 1942, which led to a joint venture with the Dow Corning Corporation. Hyde also invented the process for producing fused silica fibers, the basis of modern fiber optics, and a major business for Corning in the 21st century. Eugene Rochow, working at a parallel time at General Electric, developed the first methylsilicones or RTV rubbers, common in caulking and sealing applications. Silicones were essential to the World War II effort. Silicone wire insulation helped make high-altitude flight possible without arcing and shorting of the wiring in aircraft, a common hazard of high-altitude flight during that time, which helped make possible the nonstop ferrying of aircraft over the Atlantic, and silicone supercharger seals helped make possible the high-altitude and long-range performance of the Boeing B-29. One of the first commercially sold items made of silicone was Silly Putty™ made from a mixture of silicone oil and boric acid.

3 Introduction to Needles and Cannulae

Theodore R. Kucklick

CONTENTS

Needle Gauges and Sizes 44
    Gauge Size 44
    French Catheter Size 45
Metric and English 45
Working with Hypodermic Tube 45
Common Hypodermic Tubing Materials 47
R&D Needle Grinding 47
Simple Compound Needle Grinding Fixture 48
Suture Needles 49
Basic Types of Suture Needle Tips 52
    Conventional Cutting 52
    Reverse Cutting 52
    Side Cutting 52
    Taper Point 52
    Blunt Point 52
Suture Attachment Methods 52
    Swaging Sutures to Needles 52
    Drill 53
    Channel 53
    Nonswaged, Closed Eye, French Eye, Slit, Spring 53
Suture Sizes 53
Suture Types 53
    Natural Absorbable 54
    Natural Nonabsorbable 54
    Synthetic Absorbable 54
    Synthetic Nonabsorbable 55
Trocars and Dilators 55
    Trocars 55
    Blunt Dilators 55
    Plastic Sharps and Trocars for Disposables 55
Glossary of Needles and Related Terms 57
Resources 61
    Reference: Phlebotomy 61

Vendors: Hypodermic Tubes, Needles, and Sharps 61
Vendor: Sharps Disposal (Mail Order) 63
Acknowledgments 63
Endnotes 63

One of the most common materials used in medical devices is small-diameter (hypodermic) stainless steel tubing. One of the most common medical devices is the hypodermic needle. Another is the suturing needle, and others include trocars and cannulae. Needles and cannulae have been used in medicine since the dawn of recorded history. The ancient Egyptians used metal tubes to gain access to the bladder and other structures. Needles are used for a wide variety of functions, such as injection, suturing, biopsy, gaining access to a surgical space, delivery of radio frequency (RF) energy for tissue ablation, delivery of electrical impulses for evoked potential tests, holding thermocouples for temperature measurement, guiding other devices such as guidewires and catheters, and numerous other applications.

A typical needle works by piercing tissue with its sharp point and then smoothly slicing through tissue with its sharpened edges. The needle is usually designed to penetrate tissue with the least amount of resistance, thus causing minimal disruption to tissue. The sharpness of the needle as well as the polish of the tubing and freedom from burrs and roughness contribute to the effectiveness of the needle to penetrate tissue with the least resistance and to cause a minimum of tissue damage and discomfort.

NEEDLE GAUGES AND SIZES

There are several (confusing and mutually incompatible) ways to measure hypodermic needle diameter. The first is needle gauge. This is based on the Stubs wire gauge. Other methods include the French catheter gauge, metric sizes in millimeters, or decimal or fractional English units.

GAUGE SIZE

Hypodermic tubing is commonly sized according to the English Birmingham or *Stubs iron wire gauge*.[1] Note that this is *not* the same as the Brown and Sharpe or the W&M music wire gauge.

In the Stubs wire gauge world, as the gauge number goes up, the size goes down. This is because the gauge number was originally based on a 19th-century standard of approximately how many times the wire was drawn to get smaller sizes. The more draws, the smaller the wire and the higher the gauge number. This means that there is no number that adds up to a gauge. In most cases, the gauge became based on a geometric constant, and each manufacturer had its own. In the Stubs iron wire system, which is used to measure hypodermic tubing, a 10-gauge is 0.134 inch, and a 20-gauge is 0.035 inch. The Stubs gauge was originally developed in the late 1800s[2] and continues to be used as a matter of convenience and convention.

Introduction to Needles and Cannulae

Obtaining a reference chart of gauge and decimal needle sizes from your tubing vendor is very helpful. Certain gauge sizes have become commonly used in medicine (e.g., the 22-gauge needle for venipuncture). It has become a convenient way for practitioners to remember needle sizes as opposed to a fractional or decimal measurement, but otherwise it is quite counterintuitive.

The other thing to remember about gauge size is that this measurement refers to *outside diameter* (OD). Inner diameter (ID) is measured in English or metric diameter.

FRENCH CATHETER SIZE

A French is a unit of linear measure; 1 French is equal to one-third of a millimeter (making it somewhat incompatible with the base 10 metric system). French size is abbreviated Fr. French size measures the circumference, not the diameter, of a catheter; 3 Fr = 3 mm circumference and approximately 1 mm diameter. The French size, for example, is not the diameter of a catheter with an oval cross section at its widest point. The name and the symbol Ch refer to the Charrière gauge scale, which is often called the French scale.[3]

This makes the French scale useful for measuring catheters that are not round. Think of it as the way you measure around your waist to get your pant size. Because most catheters are round, the French size in diameter is fairly consistent, even though this is not really what is being measured.

French is usually used when describing the diameter of flexible catheters, or larger tubes. On medical packaging French is often abbreviated F (e.g., 10F).

METRIC AND ENGLISH

In Europe and Asia, needle sizes and catheter sizes tend to be described in metric units, according to the diameter, either OD or ID. Engineers tend to describe diameters in either decimal English or metric units, according to their preference, and then translate these sizes into the units used by the medical professionals with whom they are dealing (see Table 3.1).

WORKING WITH HYPODERMIC TUBE

When working with hypodermic medical tubing, it is especially important to know how the tubing is made, especially if an assembly is being designed for which an obturator, stylet, catheter, wire, tube, or rod is being designed to fit into the tube's ID.

The first consideration is this: tubing is made by reducing the OD of the tube through a die. This means that the OD is controllable. The ID of the tube then becomes a function of the OD minus the nominal wall thickness of the tube after forming. This means that the ID is not absolutely controlled. The ID is a theoretical number. This can be seen in the accompanying illustration (see Figure 3.1). This must be taken into account when calculating tolerances between the ID of the tube and whatever you are designing to slide into the tube.

TABLE 3.1
Units Conversion Chart

Gauge Number	Metric (mm)	French Catheter (Fr.) (mm × 3)	Stubs Gauge	American (A.W.G.) or Brown and Sharpe (inch)
6	5.16	15.5	0.203	0.1620
7	4.57	13.7	0.180	0.1442
8	4.19	12.6	0.165	0.1284
9	3.76	11.3	0.148	0.1144
10	3.40	10.2	0.134	0.1018
11	3.05	9.2	0.120	0.0907
12	2.77	8.3	0.109	0.0808
13	2.41	7.2	0.095	0.0719
14	2.11	6.3	0.083	0.0640
15	1.83	5.5	0.072	0.0570
16	1.65	5	0.065	0.0508
17	1.47	4.4	0.058	0.0452
18	1.27	3.8	0.049	0.0403
19	1.07	3.2	0.042	0.0358
20	0.91	2.7	0.035	0.0319
21	0.82	2.4	0.032	0.0284
22	0.72	2.2	0.028	0.0253
23	0.64	1.9	0.025	0.0225
24	0.57	1.7	0.022	0.0201
25	0.51	1.5	0.020	0.0179
26	0.46	1.3	0.018	0.0159
27	0.41	1.2	0.016	0.0141
28	0.36	1	0.014	0.0126
29	0.34	—	0.013	0.0112
30	0.31	—	0.012	0.0100
31	0.26	—	0.010	0.0089
32	0.23	—	0.009	0.0079

It is possible to draw tubing over a mandrel of a precise size or hone the ID; however, this is more expensive than using readily available standard-size hypotube.

Also, when designing a part to fit in to the inner lumen of a hypotube, remember that tubes are never perfectly round, perfectly straight, or perfectly smooth on the inside. All of these factors will affect how much tolerance to allow in order to fit a part into the hypotube lumen.

If you are planning to insert a long part into a long hypotube, remember to allow enough tolerance. Even if a part fits easily into a short section of tube, frictions and tolerance stack-ups rapidly accumulate. In this situation, a part may fit initially, but then become jammed as the part is advanced through the full length of the tube.

Introduction to Needles and Cannulae

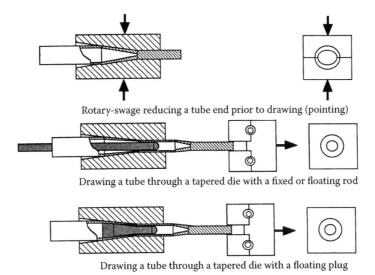

FIGURE 3.1 Typical metal tube drawing methods. (Courtesy of Microgroup, Inc., Medway, MA.)

When measuring tubing with a pin gauge, be sure that the end of the tube is free from burrs. Deburring the end of the tube with a 60-degree cone burr held in a pin vise is a convenient way to clean up a tube before measuring. Also, remember that a gauge pin the exact diameter of the tube will not fit in the tube. For example, a 0.125 inch pin will not fit in a 0.125 inch lumen.

COMMON HYPODERMIC TUBING MATERIALS

The most common hypodermic tubing material is 300 series stainless; 400 series stainless is required for heat treating. Nickel–titanium tubing is also now readily available from vendors, such as Memry Corporation (Bethel, CT) and Nitinol Devices Corporation (NDC; Fremont, CA). Tubing of other alloys, such as titanium, is available for use in magnetic resonance imaging (MRI) radiology applications.

If you look at a hypodermic needle, you will notice that the end is not ground to a simple bevel. Hypodermic needles are usually ground with a compound bevel, typically called a lancet point, and the angles of these bevels give the needle its characteristics (see Figure 3.2). Some needles are designed to pierce veins and arteries, others to penetrate into muscle, and yet others to penetrate tough fascia and joint capsule tissue (see Table 3.2).

R&D NEEDLE GRINDING

Glendo Corporation (Emporia, KS) makes a versatile grinder that works very well for grinding prototype sharps. It is a low-heat slow–resolution per minute (slow-rpm) diamond grinder originally designed to sharpen carbide tools (see Figure 3.3).

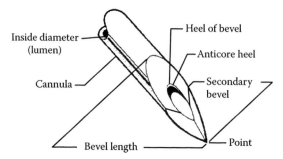

FIGURE 3.2 Typical hypodermic needle features. (Courtesy of Popper and Sons, Inc., New Hyde Park, NY.)

SIMPLE COMPOUND NEEDLE GRINDING FIXTURE

A simple fixture can be made for grinding prototype lancet sharps. Here are the general specifications:

> Take a block of Delrin or other abrasion-resistant plastic and mill two surfaces as shown. These establish the angle of the first main bevel and the secondary bevels. Next, drill two holes through the block perpendicular to these planes. Note: The length of these holes needs to be equal so that when the second bevels are ground, they form a point and do not obliterate the first bevel. The grinds need to meet at the point. The angle of the secondary bevel must be steeper than the first bevel to form a lancet point.
>
> Next, drill holes for the index pin. It will be at the 12:00 position, as shown in Figure 3.4, for the primary bevel, and at approximately the 11:00 and 1:00 positions for the secondary bevels, depending on the desired angle of rotation for the secondary bevels. Next make an index pin holding collar and mount it to a pin vise. Insert an index pin as shown in Figure 3.4. When the hypotube is held in the pin vise, this will index the angles of rotation for the bevels.
>
> To grind a needle, place the pin vise in the index hole for the first bevel, and slide the hypotube through the pin vise and the fixture block for the first bevel. With just enough tube sticking out to grind the bevel, tighten the pin vise and grind the first bevel. The Glendo™ grinder works well for this application. Next, move the tube to the secondary bevel grinding position. The tip of the first bevel should sit right at the edge of the hole for the second bevel, with a slight overlap to ensure a complete sharp-tip grind. Insert the index pin into the 11:00 position and grind the first secondary bevel; then move the pin to the 1:00 position and grind the next secondary bevel. The heel of the needle should then be dulled with a small fine-grained grindstone if tissue coring is to be prevented.

With this fixture setup, it is simple to make a set of blocks for a variety of combinations of first bevel angle, second bevel angle, and angle of rotation for the secondary bevels. Once proof of concept is achieved, one of the vendors listed in the Resources section at the end of this chapter can produce your needles in volume under good manufacturing practice (GMP) guidelines or can supply an off-the-shelf version.

TABLE 3.2
Basic Types of Needles and Typical Applications

Bevel Type	Gauge Range	Bevel Angle (approximate degrees)	Mean Bevel Angle (degrees)	Typical Use
Regular	7–12	15–17	12	Subcutaneous and intramuscular injection
	13–16	13–14		
	17–21	12		
	22–27	12		
	28–33	13–14		
Intravenous	15–18	12–14	13	Disposable IVs
Medium	13–16	16–17	15	Subcutaneous IV and intramuscular injection
	17–21	15		
	22–27	13–15		
Short	10–12	23–25	19	Nerve block, IV intra-arterial
	13–16	19–22		
	17–21	18–19		
	22–27	15–18		
Arterial	15–17	21–22	20	Intra-arterial injection
	18–20	18–19		
Spinal	7–12	26–31	22	Spinal anesthesia
	13–16	23–25		
	17–21	18–22		
	22–30	15–17		
Intradermal	26	23.5	23.5	Intradermal
Regular Quincke	—	22	—	—
Short Quincke	—	30	—	—
Pitkin	—	45	—	—

Source: Courtesy of Popper and Sons, Inc., New Hyde Park, NY.

SUTURE NEEDLES

Curved suture needles,[*] very similar to needles used in the 21st century, were first used in ancient India.[†] Other shapes of needles are straight needles, which are less commonly used for suturing, the common curved needle, the half-curved ski needle, and the compound curved needle for specialty applications, such as microvascular surgery (see Table 3.3).

---

[*] For an introductory article on sutures and needles, see Steven Lai and Daniel Becker, "Sutures and Needles," Medscape Reference, http://www.emedicine.com /ent/topic38.htm, which provides a detailed overview describing many of the important parameters in needle and suture selection.

[†] Albert S. Lyons and R. J. Petrucelli, *Medicine: An Illustrated History* (New York: Abradale Press, 1997): 115.

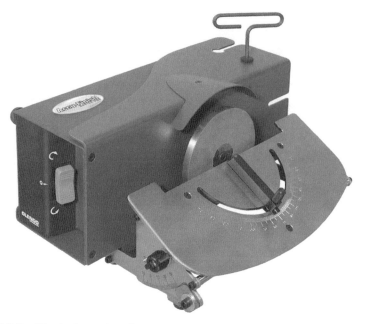

FIGURE 3.3 Glendo Accu-Finish® grinder. (Glendo, Inc., Emporia, KS.)

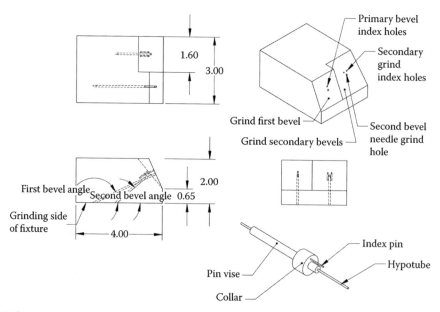

FIGURE 3.4 Prototype needle grinding fixture.

TABLE 3.3
Suture Needle Identification Chart

Needle Type	Description	Point Shape(s)
Regular trocar point	A round bodied needle with triangle cutting edges	
Regular taper point	A round-tapered point needle	
Regular taper cutting	A round-tapered point needle with short cutting edges	
Regular reverse cutting edge	A triangle cutting edge needle	
Regular diamond point	A side cutting needle	
Regular conventional cutting edge	An inside apex triangle cutting edge needle	
Regular blunt taper point	A blunt-tapered point needle	
Regular ball point	A blunt point needle	
Premium lancet point	A hand-honed side cutting needle	
Premium diamond point	A hand-honed side cutting needle	
Premium cutting edge	A hand-honed triangle cutting edge needle	
Cardiovascular (CV)	A round-tapered point, square bodied needle	

Source: Courtesy of BG Sulzle, Inc., N. Syracuse, NY.

The most important feature of a suture needle is that it passes through tissue, causing the least amount of trauma. It is also important that the needle pass through smoothly. Some needles are coated with silicone or other lubricious coating. The needle must be of a material that will hold its shape while being passed through tissue, hold a sharp point or edge, and not be so hard that the needle becomes brittle and prone to breakage. Suture needles are driven through tissue with needle holders. Some needle holders have special carbide inserts in the jaws to provide extra grip on the needle while driving the needle through tough tissue.[4]

BASIC TYPES OF SUTURE NEEDLE TIPS

Conventional Cutting

In a conventional cutting configuration, there are three cutting edges, with one cutting edge facing the inside of the needle arc. This is known as a surface-seeking needle.

Reverse Cutting

Reverse-cutting needles cut on two sides and have the third cutting edge on the outside of the needle arc. This is known as a depth-seeking needle.

Side Cutting

Side-cutting needles, or spatula needles, have two cutting edges perpendicular to the arc of the needle. These are used for ophthalmic procedures.

Taper Point

A taper point is similar to a regular sewing needle. The sharpness is determined by taper ratio and tip angle. The needle is sharper if it has a higher taper ratio and lower tip angle. The taper-point needle is used for easily penetrated tissues, such as abdominal viscera and subcutaneous tissue, and minimizes potential tearing of tissue.

Blunt Point

Blunt needles dissect, rather than cut, tissue. Blunt needles are used to suture friable tissue, such as liver.

SUTURE ATTACHMENT METHODS

Swaging Sutures to Needles

A swaging suture is usually permanently swaged to the needle. Needles with sewing needle-style eyelets require two strands of suture, which causes more tissue damage as the double strand is passed through tissue.

Introduction to Needles and Cannulae

DRILL

In a drill suture the proximal end of the needle is drilled with a hole, and the needle is swaged to retain the suture. This makes the proximal end smaller than the needle body.

CHANNEL

In the channel method, the end of the needle is formed into a channel, and the needle is crimped to retain the suture. In this case, the proximal end becomes larger than the needle body.

NONSWAGED, CLOSED EYE, FRENCH EYE, SLIT, SPRING

Various methods to retain the suture include nonswaged, closed eye, French eye, slit, and spring sutures. These methods have the disadvantage of pulling a double strand of suture through the tissue.

SUTURE SIZES

Sutures are sized in the United States according to a system from the U.S. Pharmacopoeia (USP). Sutures are gauged not only by diameter, but also by tensile strength and knot security. Sutures sizes are measured on two scales:

1. A whole number system for larger sutures, from 5 (largest) to 0 (smallest).
2. A composite number system for smaller sutures (smaller than 0), from 1–0 (largest) to 12–0 (smallest). These are the "aught" sizes (e.g., 12–0 is pronounced 12-aught or 12-oh).

The following chart of suture sizes lists the largest sizes on the left and the smallest microsurgery sizes on the right:

Larger																Smaller
5	4	3	2	1	0	1–0	2–0	3–0	4–0	5–0	6–0	7–0	8–0	9–0	10–0	11–0	12–0

Various types and sizes of suture needles are illustrated in Figure 3.5.

Although European suture is measured in diameter, two sutures of the same size can be very different in tensile strength. The USP system tries to rank suture gauge so that two sutures of the same gauge will have similar tensile strength.

SUTURE TYPES

There are two basic categories of suture material, natural and synthetic. There are two basic types of performance characteristics, absorbable and nonabsorbable. Suture is constructed in either braided or monofilament forms.

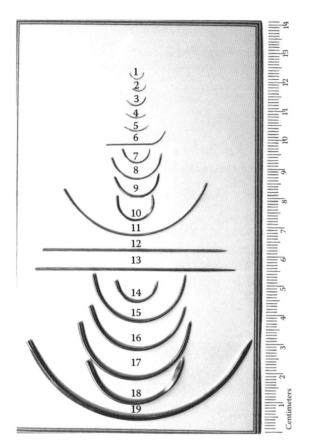

FIGURE 3.5 Assorted suture needles. (Courtesy of BG Sulzle, Inc., N. Syracuse, NY.) For a complete chart of sizes, see http://www.bgsulzle.com/products.

Natural Absorbable

Natural absorbable sutures include gut (made from sheep or beef intestine), which is available in fast and slow absorbing types. Chromic gut is treated with chromium salts to slow absorption.

Natural Nonabsorbable

Natural nonabsorbable sutures include surgical silk, surgical stainless steel (for suturing bone, e.g., a sternotomy), and cotton. Note: Surgical steel wire is specified according to the Brown and Sharpe wire gauge, *not* the Stubs needle gauge.

Synthetic Absorbable

Examples of synthetic absorbable sutures include Polygalactin 910 (Vicryl™), poliglecaprone 25 (Monocryl™), polydioxanone (PDS II™), and polytrimethylene carbonate (Maxon™).

Introduction to Needles and Cannulae

SYNTHETIC NONABSORBABLE

Synthetics nonabsorbable sutures include Nylon (Ethilon™, Dermilaon™, monofilament Nurlon™, Surgilon™ braided), polybutester (Novofil™), polyester fiber (Mersilene™/Dacron [uncoated] and Ethibond™/Ti-cron™ [coated]), and polypropylene (Prolene™).*

TROCARS AND DILATORS

TROCARS

Trocars are usually larger diameter devices used to make a surgical entry into the body. Trocars are common features of laparoscopic and arthroscopic surgical ports.

BLUNT DILATORS

A blunt dilator is used to dissect rather than cut tissue (see Figures 3.6–3.9). A blunt dilator is used to minimize a tissue defect from cutting, or to protect sensitive tissues distal to the axis of penetration (e.g., bowel in laparoscopy or articular cartilage in arthroscopy).

PLASTIC SHARPS AND TROCARS FOR DISPOSABLES

Plastic sharps, as well as dilators, are commonly used in single-use disposable medical devices. When properly designed, plastic parts have sufficient penetration acuity. Plastic sharps are common in disposable intravenous (IV) bag spikes. There are

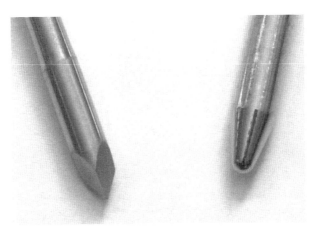

FIGURE 3.6 Metal trocar and blunt dilator.

---

* For detailed engineering information on sutures, see C. C. Chu, J. A. von Fraunhofer, and H. Greisler, *Wound Closure Biomaterials and Devices* (Boca Raton, FL: CRC Press, 1997).

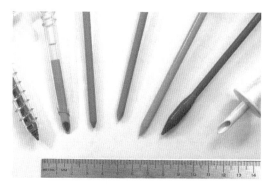

FIGURE 3.7 Assorted plastic sharp and blunt devices.

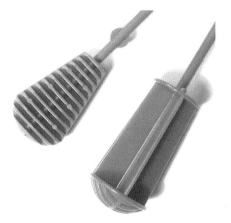

FIGURE 3.8 Plastic dilator and trocar handles showing coring out of thick sections.

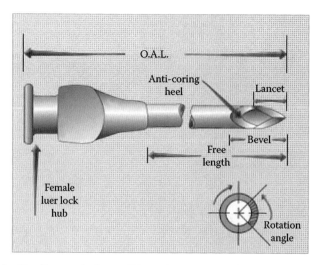

FIGURE 3.9 Needle terminology. (Illustration courtesy of Connecticut Hypodermic, Yalesville, CT.)

Introduction to Needles and Cannulae 57

numerous designs for laparoscopic trocars that incorporate a combination of plastic and metal components.

An important design consideration in plastics is to minimize thick sections of material. Excessively thick sections make for long molding cycle times as well as potential voids and molded in stress.

GLOSSARY OF NEEDLES AND RELATED TERMS

Abrams' needle: A biopsy needle designed to reduce the danger of introducing air into tissues; used in pleural biopsy.

Acuity: The sharpness of a surgical needle.[5]

Agar cutting needle: A needle with a sharpened punch end and an obturator to pick up and transfer a sample of agar media.

Aneurysm needle: A needle with a handle, used in ligating blood vessels.

Angle of rotation: The amount of rotation performed on secondary grinds (lancets) of a cannula. This is an important variable for needle-point sharpness.

Anneal: A heat-treating process is performed on metal to make it more malleable. This can aid many small-diameter stainless steel tube components that are bent, flared, or swaged to prevent cracking or splitting.

Anticoring heel blast: The heel of a bevel is blasted with media to dull it in order to reduce coring. It is the heel of a needle that tends to produce coring. (See Figure 3.8 for location of needle heel.)

Aspirating needle: A long, hollow needle for removing fluid from a cavity.

ASTM A 96796: Chemical passivation standard for treating stainless steel parts. Replaces QQP-35C.

Back bevels: Bevels that are ground on the side of a flat bevel. This provides a greater cutting edge on a short-bevel needle.

Bevel: Ground surface of a cannula or needle point. There are many styles, including but not limited to A-bevel, B-bevel, C-bevel, bias, Chiba, Crawford, deflected tip, Francine, Hustead, Huber, trocar, and Tuohy.

Bevel length: Length measured from tip of needle point to farthest distance of heel.

Bias: Angle grind.

Blunt end: Tube with square-cut (90-degree) end.

Brockenbrough needle: A curved steel transseptal needle within a Brockenbrough transseptal catheter; used to puncture the interatrial septum.

Burr: Deflection of the point. Usually considered unacceptable when perceptible to feel or greater than 0.001.

Cannula: A hollow tube meant to be inserted into a body cavity, sometimes with the assistance of an inner sharp trocar or blunt obturator.

Cataract needle: A needle used in removing a cataract.

Chiba needle: A common type of thin, flexible biopsy needle with a small-diameter needle and a stylet in the needle lumen.

Cope's needle: A blunt-ended hook-like needle with a concealed cutting edge and snare, used in biopsy of the pleura, pericardium, peritoneum, and synovium.

Deschamps' needle: A needle with the eye near the point, and a long handle attached; used in ligating deep-seated arteries.

Discission needle: A special form of cataract needle.

Echotip: Creates an enhanced visualization of the needle tip when used with ultrasonic imaging equipment. This is where the tip is roughened or knurled or coated with an acoustic reflective material to increase echogenicity.

Emulsifying needle: A small tube with luer fittings at each end for mixing a liquid and an emulsifying agent by pushing the liquids through the tubing into opposing syringes. A simple type of static mixer.

Flared end: End of tube is spread out, increasing the diameter. Typically, flare diameter can be a maximum of 1.3 times the tube diameter.

Free length: On a needle assembly, free length is the length from the end of the part to the point at which it protrudes from the hub.

Gauge: Stub gauge number referring to hypodermic tube size. For hypodermic tubing, the gauge number increases as the tube diameter gets smaller.

GG-N-196: U.S. government specifications for hypodermic needles dating back to 1947.

Grit blast: Refers to roughened surface added to components by means of pressure blasting with media. This may provide a better bonding surface for hypodermic needles or tubing or wire components.

Hagedorn's needles: Surgical needles that are flat from side to side and have a straight cutting edge near the point and a large eye.

Hasson cannula: A cannula made for laparoscopy with a blunt dilating obturator and an anchoring balloon at the distal end.

Hasson trocar: A blunt trocar inserted into the peritoneal cavity after a celiotomy. Used for insufflation and introduction of a laparoscope.

Hook burr: Burr on needle point that exceeds 0.002 inch.

Hub: Fitting at the end of a needle that can connect to a syringe or other component.

ID: Inside diameter of tubing, usually measured with pin gauges to determine proper size.

ISO 9626: International standard for stainless steel needle tubing for the manufacture of medical devices.

Knife needle: A slender knife with a needle like point, used in discission of a cataract and other ophthalmic operations, as in goniotomy and goniopuncture.

Lancets: These are the two secondary bevels on a triple-ground point. Other common terms for lancets are side grinds and diamond points.

Ligature needle: A slender steel needle with a long handle and an eye in its curved end, used for passing a ligature underneath an artery.

Luer: Male or female taper on the end of hub or syringe to connect a needle to a syringe or other Luer fitting. Hubs can be Luer Slip or Luer Lock, conforming to ISO 594-2.

Eponym for Otto Luer, who, in the 1880s, in Germany came up with the idea of a 6 percent taper as a way of putting a stopper in a bottle, keeping it there, and then getting it out again. Many years later, Luer's taper was used by hospital equipment manufacturers to ensure that one piece of IV set tubing would fit into another.*

In 1925 Fairleigh S. Dickinson, cofounder of Becton-Dickinson, patented what became known as the Luer-Lok™ fitting, which added to the Luer's tapered fluid fitting a locking sleeve by incorporating a lead screw that prevented a hypodermic syringe from slipping off of a hypodermic syringe.† This made a hypodermic safer to use when dispensing viscous fluids, which tended to force the needle hub off of the luer slip fit. The luer lock fitting described in Dickinson's 1930 patent‡ is virtually identical to locking luer fittings used in the 21st century.

After plastic medical disposable devices were introduced in the 1950s, the Luer-Lok fitting and variations of it were incorporated into a wide range of plastic medical fluid fittings.

Lumen: This is the open space inside a tube.

Magnetic permeability: The property of stainless steel tubing that determines its relative influence in a magnetic field. Work hardening of 300 series stainless can affect the magnetic permeability.

Malleable: Easily bendable without breaking or cracking. Small-diameter stainless steel tubing can be drawn to less-than-full-hard conditions to make it more malleable. Another method is to have the hypodermic tube size parts bright annealed through heat treating.

Menghini needle: A needle that does not require rotation to cut loose the tissue specimen in a biopsy of the liver. This represented a significant advance in the previously slow and hazardous methods of liver biopsy. "Menghini introduced modern liver biopsy in 1958. He used a new, very thin suction needle. His original article was entitled 'One-Second Needle Biopsy of the Liver' in the journal *Gastroenterology*."§

Obturator: A blunt rod that fills the inner lumen of a cannula. A removable plug of a tubular instrument. From Latin *obturo*, "to close up."

Overall length (OAL): Entire length measured from one end to opposite end.

Passivate: To treat stainless steel with acid to prevent corrosion per ASTM A 96796.

Pencil point: Tubing is swaged to conical point.

Pitkin bevel: A 45-degree bevel without a secondary lancet bevel.

Proximal end: Hub end of a needle; the end closest to you.

Quincke bevel: A type of needle grind named for Heinrich Irenaeus Quincke (1842–1922), a German, who pioneered the lumbar puncture technique for aspirating cerebral spinal fluid (CSF) to diagnose neurological disorders. A regular Quincke bevel is 22 degrees and a short Quincke bevel is 30 degrees.

---

* British Standards Institution, *Conical Fittings with 6% (Luer) Taper for Syringes, Needles, and Certain Other Medical Equipment: Lock Fittings* (London: BSI, 1997), http://biotech.law.lsu.edu/cases/devices/hanson_v_baxter_app.htm.
† "Timeline," Becton Dickinson, http://www.bd.com/aboutbd/history/timeline.asp.
‡ U.S. patents 1,742,497 and 1,793,068.
§ Menghini, G. "One-Second Needle Biopsy of the Liver," *Gastroenterology*, 1958(35):190–99, http://www.vh.org/adult/patient/internalmedicine/aba30/2001/liverbiopsy.html.

Reverdin's needle: A surgical needle having an eye that can be opened and closed by means of a slide.

Seldinger needle: A needle with a blunt, tapered external cannula with a sharp obturator; used for the initial percutaneous insertion characteristic of the Seldinger technique for arterial or venous access. The Seldinger technique is the common method for placing a guidewire into a vessel (e.g., into the femoral artery for cardiovascular access), to allow the placement of catheters over the guidewire. Named for Sven-Ivar Seldinger (1921–1999), radiologist, born in Mora, Sweden. Dr. Seldinger published the description of a percutaneous-entry technique in the journal *Acta Radiologica*.[*]

Side port: Opening on the side of a tube. It can be a slot or hole.

Silverman needle: An instrument for taking tissue specimens, consisting of an outer cannula, an obturator, and an inner split needle with longitudinal grooves in which the tissue is retained when the needle and cannula are withdrawn.

Stop needle: A needle with a shoulder that prevents it from being inserted beyond a certain distance.

Stylet: A rod that fills the inner lumen of a hypodermic needle or trocar and is ground to match the sharp end of the needle or trocar.

Swaged needle: One permanently attached to the suture material. Curved needles for suturing tissue normally have the suture swaged to the proximal end of the needle.

Swaging: Forming process to reduce tube outside diameter (OD) and shape to die configuration. Also a method to crimp together.

Transseptal needle: A needle used to puncture the interatrial septum in transseptal catheterization.

Trephine: A saw-type end on a needle or cylindrical tube that allows cutting of tissue as the needle or cannula is rotated, similar to a hole saw. Often used to cut a disc-shaped piece of bone or other firm tissue.

Triple grind: Typical three-sided grind of hypodermic needle.

Trocar: A cannula with a three-pointed obturator stylet. Sometimes refers to the sharp obturator alone. From French *trois* (three) and *carré* (the edge of a sword).

Trocar point: Three-sided point ground on stylet. Each grind is approximately 120 degrees apart, usually to the center of the diameter.

Tuohy needle: One in which the opening at the end is angled so that a catheter exits at an angle. The end of the Tuohy needle provides controlled penetration during the administering of spinal anesthesia and placement of an epidural spinal catheter. Named after Edward B. Tuohy, an American anesthesiologist. Sometimes called the Huber needle, as it was designed jointly by Tuohy and Ralph Huber.[†] A pioneering development that made continuous epidural anesthesia in obstetrics possible.

Veress needle: Named for Janos Veress, a German doctor. A spring-loaded needle originally used to drain ascites and evacuate fluid and air from the chest. Was later

---

[*] History and Innovators, accessed August 6, 2012, http://www.cookgroup.com/history/seldinger.html.

[†] Tuohy, E. "The Man, His Needle, and Its Place in Obstetric Analgesia." *Regional Anesthesia and Pain Medicine* 27(5) (2002): 520–523.

adapted to use in laparoscopy. A hollow needle consisting of a sharp trocar with a slanted end surrounding an inner cylinder with a blunt end. After the trocar is introduced into a body cavity, the blunt cylinder is advanced outward so that internal organs are not injured by the sharp edge. Used for insufflation of a body cavity, such as for pneumoperitoneum in minimally invasive surgery.

RESOURCES

REFERENCE: PHLEBOTOMY*

McCall, R. E., and Tankersley, C. M. *Phlebotomy Essentials*, 3rd ed. Baltimore: Lippincott, Williams & Willkins, 2002.

VENDORS: HYPODERMIC TUBES, NEEDLES, AND SHARPS

Avid Medical
9000 Westmont Drive
Stonehouse Commerce Park
Toano, VA 23168
Toll Free: 800-886-0584
Fax: 757-566-8707

BG Sulzle
1 Needle Lane
N. Syracuse, NY 13212
Phone: 315-454-3221
Largest independent manufacturer of drilled end-suture needles.

Connecticut Hypodermics
519 Main Street
Yalesville, CT 06492
Phone: 203-265-4881
Fax: 203-284-1520

Disposable Instrument Company
P.O. Box 14248
Shawnee Mission, KS 66285-4248
Phone: 913-492-6492
Fax: 913-888-1762

Eagle Stainless
10 Discovery Way
Franklin, MA 02038
Toll Free: 800-528-8650
Fax: 800-520-1954

---

* Phlebotomy is the art of drawing blood with a needle.

Electron Microscopy Services
P.O. Box 550
1560 Industry Road
Hatfield, PA 19440
Phone: 215-412-8400
Fax: 215-412-8450
EMS supplies, microminiature needles, and sharps.

K-Tube
13400 Kirkham Way
Poway, CA 92064
Phone: 858-513-9229
Fax: 800-705-8823

Medical Sterile Products
P.O. Box 338
Rincon, PR 00743
Phone: 800-292-2887
Fax: 787-823-8665
Manufactures sharps of all kinds.

Microgroup
7 Industrial Park Road
Medway, MA 02053
Phone: 800-255-8823
Fax: 508-533-5691

Point Technologies
6859 N. Foothills Highway
Boulder, CO 80302
Phone: 303-415-9865
Fax: 303-415-9866
Point Technologies provides electrochemical sharpening of microwires.

Popper and Sons
300 Denton Avenue
New Hyde Park, NY 11040
Phone: 516-248-0300
Fax: 516-747-1188

Vita Needle Company
919 Great Plain Avenue
Needham, MA 02492
Phone: 909-699-8790
Fax: 909-699-7490
Specialize in small minimum lot manufacturing.

Vendor: Sharps Disposal (Mail Order)

GRP & Associates, Inc.
P.O. Box 94
Clear Lake, IA 50428
Phone: 888-346-6037

ACKNOWLEDGMENTS

The assistance of Bob Lamson of Microgroup, Zev Asch of Popper and Sons, Connecticut Hypodermics, and BG Sulzle, Inc., is gratefully acknowledged.

ENDNOTES

1. "The gauge system for sizing medical catheters and equipment is used widely around the world. Yet both its origins and its interpretation, in terms of conventional measurements, have long been obscure. The gauge, formally known as the Stubs Iron Wire Gauge, was developed in early 19th century England. Developed initially for use in wire manufacture, each gauge size arbitrarily correlates to multiples of .001 inches. This sizing system was the first wire gauge recognized as a standard by any country (Great Britain, 1884). It was first used to measure needle sizes in the early 20th century. Today it is used in medicine to measure not only needles, but also catheters and suture wires. However, owing to the potential confusion inherent in using a gauge system, the iron wire gauge is rarely used in manufacture of nonmedical equipment." K. V. Iserson, "The Origins of the Gauge System for Medical Equipment," *Journal of Emergency Medicine* 5 (1987): 45–48. See also J. S. Poll, "The Story of the Gauge," *Anaesthesia* 54 (1999): 575–581.
2. For further reference, see http://www.sizes.com/materls/wire.htm. It is interesting to note that the Morse drill bit gauge system used today was copied from the Lancashire wire gauge system (yet another system), as this is the wire the Morse company apparently imported from England to manufacture its twist drills.
3. "Joseph-Frederic-Benoit Charriere, a 19th century Parisian maker of surgical instruments, has by virtue of his ingenuity and advanced thinking, continued to have his presence felt in medicine throughout the 20th century. His most significant accomplishment was the development of a uniform, standard gauge specifically designed for use in medical equipment such as catheters and probes. Unlike the gauge system adopted by the British for measurement of needles and intravenous catheters, Charriere's system has uniform increments between gauge sizes (one-third of a millimeter), is easily calculated in terms of its metric equivalent, and has no arbitrary upper end point. Today, in the United States, this system is commonly referred to as French (Fr) sizing. In addition to the development of the French gauge, Charriere made significant advances in ether administration, urologic, and other surgical instruments, and the development of the modern syringe." K. V. Iserson, "J.-F.-B. Charriere: The Man behind the French Scale," *Journal of Emergency Medicine* 5 (1987): 545–548.
4. "During the last two decades, major advances in surgical needle and needle holder technology have markedly improved surgical wound repair. These advances include quantitative tests for surgical needle and needle holders performance, high nickel stainless steels, compound curved needles, needle sharpening methods, laser-drilled holes for swages, needle: suture ratios of 1:1, and the atraumatic needle holder." R. F. Edlich et al., "Past, Present, and Future for Surgical Needles and Needle Holders," *American Journal of Surgery* 166 (1993): 522–532.

5. "The acuity (sharpness) of surgical needle points was assessed by measuring the force required for repeat needle penetrations through a medium-gauge latex sheet glued to a perforated Plexiglas frame. The data on the variation in the applied force with repeat penetrations showed that needles obeyed the general relation: $P = A + B \cdot n$; where P is the applied penetration force in grams, n is the number of penetrations, and A and B are constants. Constant A characterized the needle-point acuity and B the maintenance of acuity. This relationship indicated both needle acuity and acuity maintenance with repeated passes through a reproducible target material. Determining the microhardness of needles provided data on their strength, which helped to account for differences in the acuity of apparently similar needles. The tensile strength of the union between suture and needle was determined to evaluate the security of suture attachment." J. A. von Fraunhofer, R. J. Storey, and B. J. Masterson, "Characterization of Surgical Needles," *Biomaterials* 9 (1988): 281–284. See also T. B. Frick, et al., "Resistance Forces Acting on Suture Needles," *Journal of Biomechanics* 34 (2001): 1335–1340.

4 Assessing Biocompatibility
A Guide for Medical Device Manufacturers[*]

Tom Spalding[†‡]

CONTENTS

Executive Summary 66
   Purpose of Biocompatibility Testing 66
   Biocompatibility Test Planning 66
   Conducting Tests 67
   Evaluating the Data 67
Introduction to Biocompatibility Testing 67
   What Is Device Biocompatibility? 67
   What Are the Food and Drug Administration and European Union/
   International Organization for Standardization Requirements for
   Biocompatibility Testing? 68
   Do I Need Biocompatibility Data? 69
   How Do I Determine Which Tests I Need? 70
   Should I Test Device Materials, or Only a Composite of the Finished
   Device? 70
   Is GLP Treatment Required for Biocompatibility Testing? 73
Planning Biocompatibility Testing 74
   Choosing Extraction Media 74
   Sample Preparation 76
      Noncontact Devices 79
Biological Test Methods 79
   Cytotoxicity (Tissue Culture) 79
   Sensitization Assays 81
   Irritation Tests 81

---

[*] To view this booklet online, go to http://www.PacificBioLabs.com (Rev. 1.7, 5-2012).
[†] This chapter, "Assessing Biocompatibility," is a revised and updated version of the chapter that appeared in the first edition of *The Medical Device R&D Handbook* (2005). The editor thanks Tom Spalding, President of Pacific Biolabs (Hercules, CA), and the entire biocompatibility department for the contribution of this chapter.
[‡] Roger O'Meara and Aaron Burke contributed to this chapter.

  Acute Systemic Toxicity..82
  Subchronic Toxicity..82
  Genotoxicity 83
  Implantation Tests 83
  Hemocompatibility...84
  Carcinogenesis Bioassays...84
  Reproductive and Developmental Toxicity 84
  Pharmacokinetics..86
  Preclinical Safety Testing...86
  Histopathology Services...87
 Materials Characterization and Analytical Testing of Biomaterials 87
  Traditional Extractable Material Characterization............................88
  Tests Procedures for Extractable Material 88
  Bulk Material Characterization 89
  Surface Characterization 89
 About the Author..89
 Resources 89
  Contact Information 90

EXECUTIVE SUMMARY

PURPOSE OF BIOCOMPATIBILITY TESTING

Biocompatibility is, by definition, a measurement of how *compatible* a device is with a *bio*logical system. The purpose of performing biocompatibility testing is to determine the fitness of a device for human use, and to see whether use of the device can have any potentially harmful physiological effects. As stated by the International Organization of Standards, "The primary aim of this part of ISO 10993 is the protection of humans from potential biological risks arising from the use of medical devices" (ISO 10993-1, 2009).

 The overall process of determining the biocompatibility of any medical device involves several stages. One should begin by collecting data on the materials the make up the device, and then perform in vitro screening (often only on components of the device), and finally conduct confirmatory in vivo testing on the finished device. It is essential to make sure that the finished device is challenged to ensure that human use of the device does not result in any harmful effects.

BIOCOMPATIBILITY TEST PLANNING

The primary goal of a biocompatibility screening program is the protection of humans. Because animal testing is necessary for many biocompatibility tests, a secondary goal is to eliminate unnecessary testing and minimize the number and exposure of test animals. With this in mind, it is important to conduct research beforehand to document all relevant data on the component materials of the device and on similar devices with an established clinical history. Existing data may be sufficient to demonstrate biological safety of parts or of the entire device, thus precluding the need to conduct certain tests.

Assessing Biocompatibility

The required tests also will depend on the use of the device and the manner and duration in which it will interact with the body. In test planning, it is important to note whether the device is a surface device, an external communicating device, or an implant device, and what tissues the device will contact. (Implant devices interacting with the blood, for instance, will require more thorough testing than a surface device with an expected contact time of only a few days.)

When planning, it is also important to note that Good Laboratory Practice (GLP) compliance is required for certain biocompatibility regulatory submissions. Because of this, it is generally a good idea to conduct biocompatibility testing according to GLP to allow for the maximum regulatory flexibility and compliance.

CONDUCTING TESTS

Typically, material characterization and analysis of the device's components are conducted before any biological testing. This involves extracting leachable materials from the device or components at an elevated temperature, and analyzing the leachable extracts for potentially harmful chemicals or cytotoxicity.

Once in vitro testing has been completed, in vivo biological testing can be done based on the device's intended use. This testing can range from skin irritation testing to hemocompatibility and implantation testing. Turnaround time for tests can range from three weeks to greater than several months, depending on the specific test data needed. Subchronic or chronic implantation testing can last even longer.

EVALUATING THE DATA

After tests are completed and all data have been collected, it is recommended that an expert assessor interpret the data and test results. This expert will be able to provide insight as to whether additional tests need to be conducted or whether the existing data provide enough information for an overall biological safety assessment of the device.

INTRODUCTION TO BIOCOMPATIBILITY TESTING

WHAT IS DEVICE BIOCOMPATIBILITY?

The word biocompatibility refers to the interaction between a medical device and the tissues and physiological systems of the patient treated with the device. An evaluation of biocompatibility is one part of the overall safety assessment of a device. Biocompatibility of devices is investigated using analytical chemistry, in vitro tests, and animal models, in vivo tests. The biocompatibility of a device depends on several factors, including the following:

- Chemical and physical nature of its component materials
- Types of patient tissue that will be exposed to the device
- Duration of that exposure

Of course, the primary purpose of a device biocompatibility assessment is to protect patient safety. Manufacturers will want to consider corporate regulatory goals and compliance risks in planning a biocompatibility testing program. Inevitably, evaluating the biocompatibility of a device is a risk assessment exercise. There is no risk-free device or device material. The goal of device designers is to minimize risk while maximizing benefit to patients.

What Are the Food and Drug Administration and European Union/International Organization for Standardization Requirements for Biocompatibility Testing?

The best starting point for understanding biocompatibility requirements is International Organization for Standardization (ISO) Standard 10993, Biological Evaluation of Medical Devices. Part 1 of the standard is the Guidance on Selection of Tests, Part 2 covers animal welfare requirements, and Parts 3 through 19 are guidelines for specific test procedures or other testing-related issues. (A list of the individual sections of ISO 10993 can be found below.)

Testing strategies that comply with the ISO 10993 family of documents are acceptable in Europe and Asia. In 1995, the Food and Drug Administration (FDA) issued a Blue Book Memorandum G95-1, which replaced the *Tripartite Guidance* (the previous biocompatibility testing standard). FDA has substantially adopted the ISO guideline, although in some areas, FDA's testing requirements go beyond those of ISO.

The specific ISO test procedures vary slightly from the U.S. Pharmacopeia (USP) procedures historically used for FDA submissions. The ISO procedures tend to be more stringent, so companies planning to register their product in both Europe and the United States should follow ISO test methods. FDA requirements should be verified because additional testing may be needed. Japanese procedures for sample preparation and testing are slightly different from either USP or ISO tests.

ISO 10993: Biological Evaluation of Medical Devices, Listing of Individual Parts

Part	Topic
1	Evaluation and Testing
2	Animal Welfare Requirements
3	Tests for Genotoxicity, Carcinogenicity, and Reproductive Toxicity
4	Selection of Tests for Interactions with Blood
5	Tests for Cytotoxicity – in vitro Methods
6	Tests for Local Effects after Implantation
7	Ethylene Oxide Sterilization Residuals
8	Selection and Qualification of Reference Materials for Biological Test
9	Framework for Identification & Quantification of Potential Degradation Products
10	Test for Irritation and Sensitization
11	Test for Systemic Toxicity
12	Sample Preparation and Reference Materials
13	Identification and Quantification of Degradation Products from Polymers
14	Identification and Quantification of Degradation Products from Ceramics

ISO 10993: Biological Evaluation of Medical Devices, Listing of Individual Parts *(Continued)*

Part	Topic
15	Identification and Quantification of Degradation Products from Coated and Uncoated Metals and Alloys
16	Toxicokinetic Study Design for Degradation Products and Leachables
17	Establishment of Allowable Limits for Leachable Substances
18	Chemical Characterization of Materials*
19	Physicochemical, Mechanical, and Morphological Characterization (Draft)
20	Principles and Methods for Immunotoxicology Testing of Medical Devices (Draft)

* The U.S. ISO Member Body, ANSI/AAMI, is considering a version of this document for use in the United States.

DO I NEED BIOCOMPATIBILITY DATA?

Biocompatibility data of one kind or another is almost always required for devices that have significant tissue contact. Most commonly, companies arrange for their own biocompatibility studies. You may be able to reduce the amount of testing you will need on a specific device if you have some or all of the following types of biocompatibility data.

1. *Data from previous submissions:* If data are available from a previous submission, consider the following points as you apply it to your current device. You will need to perform confirmatory testing if there are significant changes in any of these areas.
   a. Materials selection
   b. Manufacturing processes
   c. Chemical composition of materials
   d. Nature of patient contact
   e. Sterilization methods
2. *Data from suppliers of materials or components:* If vendor data are used, manufacturers should obtain copies of the original study reports. It is important that the laboratory that generated the reports had an experienced staff, a strong track record of current Good Manufacturing Practice (cGMP) and GLP) compliance, and an animal science program accredited by the Association for Assessment and Accreditation of Laboratory Animal Care International (AAALAC). Usually, manufacturers will want to conduct at least some confirmatory testing of their own (e.g., cytotoxicity and hemocompatibility studies).
3. *Analytical data:* Manufacturers may use analytical data to help demonstrate that a device has a low overall risk or a low risk of producing a given biological effect. Section 18 of ISO 10993, Chemical Characterization of Materials, gives some guidance on this process.

4. *Clinical data:* Clinical data can be used to satisfy some biological effects categories from the ISO 10993-1 test selection matrix. The data may come from clinical trials of the device in question or from clinical experience with predicate devices or devices containing similar components or materials.

How Do I Determine Which Tests I Need?

The core of the ISO standard is confirmation of the fitness of the device for its intended use. The first step in this process is chemical characterization of device components.

Biological testing is probably the most critical step in a biocompatibility evaluation. The ISO materials biocompatibility matrix on the next page categorizes devices based on the type and duration of body contact. It also presents a list of potential biological effects. For each device category, certain effects must be considered and addressed in the regulatory submission for that device. ISO 10993-1 does not prescribe a specific battery of tests for any particular medical device. Rather, it provides a framework that can be used to design a biocompatibility testing program.

Device designers should generally consult with an experienced device toxicologist and their clinical investigators to determine how best to meet the requirements of the materials biocompatibility matrix. For each biological effect category, the rationale for the testing strategy should be documented. This is especially true when a manufacturer decides not to perform testing for an effect specified by the matrix for their category of devices.

Should I Test Device Materials, or Only a Composite of the Finished Device?

As a manufacturer, you should gather safety data on every component and material used in a device. In addition, you should definitely conduct testing on the finished device as specified by ISO 10993-1. Generally, the best approach is as follows:

1. Assemble vendor data on candidate materials.
2. Conduct analytical and in vitro screening of materials.
3. Conduct confirmatory testing on a composite sample from the finished device.

There is a risk in testing the finished device without developing data on component materials. If an adverse result occurs, it can be difficult to track down the component that is causing the problem. You may end up delaying your regulatory submission while you repeat testing on the individual components.

Screening device materials minimizes this risk. The initial chemical characterization should detect leachable materials that could compromise device safety. Inexpensive nonanimal studies (such as cytotoxicity and hemocompatibility tests) provide an additional screen for material safety. Material screening tests also help ensure that you will not be forced to redesign your device because of biocompatibility test failures. Many manufacturers assemble data on a library of qualified materials used in their products.

ISO Materials Biocompatibility Matrix

Medical Device Categorization			Biological Effect — Initial Evaluation Tests								Supplementary Evaluation Tests			
Nature of Body Contact		Contact Duration: A - Limited (≤ 24 hours); B - Prolonged (24 hours–30 days); C - Permanent (> 30 days)	Cytotoxicity	Sensitization	Irritation or Intracutaneous Reactivity	Systemic Toxicity (acute)	Subchronic Toxicity (Subacute Toxicity)	Genotoxicity	Implantation	Hemocompatibility	Chronic Toxicity	Carcinogenicity	Reproductive/ Developmental[3]	Biodegradation[3]
Category	Contact													
Surface Device	Skin	A	•	•	•									
		B	•	•	•									
		C	•	•	•									
	Mucosal Membrane	A	•	•	•									
		B	•	•	•	F	F		F					
		C	•	•	•	F	•	•	F		F			
	Breached or Compromised Surface	A	•	•	•	F								
		B	•	•	•	F	F		F					
		C	•	•	•	F	F	•	F		F			
External Communicating Device	Blood Path, Indirect	A	•	•	•	•				•				
		B	•	•	F	•	F			•				
		C	•	•	•	•	•	•		•	•	•		
	Tissue/Bone/Dentin[1]	A	•	•	•	•								
		B	•	•	•	•	•	•	•					
		C	•	•	•	•	•	•	•		•	•		

(Continued)

ISO Materials Biocompatibility Matrix

Medical Device Categorization		Contact Duration	Biological Effect — Initial Evaluation Tests	Biological Effect — Supplementary Evaluation Tests
Implant Device	Circulating Blood	A	• • • • • • •	
		B	• • • • • • • F²	•
		C	• • • • • • • •	•
	Tissue/Bone	A	• • • F • • •	
		B	• • • • • • •	•
		C	• • • • • • • •	•
	Blood	A	• • • • • • •	
		B	• • • • • • • •	•
		C	• • • • • • • •	•

Sources: Adapted from ISO 10993-1 (2009) and FDA 510(k) Memorandum, #G95-1, Tables 1 and 2 (2009).

Note: This table is only a framework for the development of an assessment program for your device and is not a checklist. Consult with the FDA before performing any biocompatibility testing if you are submitting an IDE or if you have a device–drug combination.

• = ISO Evaluation Tests for Consideration
F = Additional tests may be required for U.S. submissions.

[1] Tissue includes tissue fluids and subcutaneous spaces.
[2] For all devices used in extracorporeal circuits.
[3] Depends on specific nature of the device and its component materials.

Some test procedures do not lend themselves to testing of composite samples. Because of physical limitations, agar overlay or direct contact cytotoxicity tests and implant studies require separate testing of each device component.

For all biocompatibility studies, test samples should be sterilized using the same method as will be used for the finished device.

Is GLP Treatment Required for Biocompatibility Testing?

As a general rule, all studies designed to assess the safety of a medical product in nonclinical models (including biocompatibility studies for medical devices) should be conducted according to GLP procedures. GLP treatment is explicitly required for Investigational Device Exemption (IDE) and Premarket Approval (PMA) submissions. FDA reviewers indicate they strongly prefer GLP treatment for studies supporting 510(k)s. In addition, manufacturers of device components and materials should have their biocompatibility studies done according to GLP so that their clients can use the data in any type of regulatory submission.

GLP procedures are similar across geographic boundaries and examples include the United States 21 *Code of Federal Regulations* (CFR) Part 58 and the Organisation for Economic Co-operation and Development's ENV/MC/CHEM(98)17 (OECD, 1998). A good review of GLP procedures can be found in the World Health Organization's *Handbook on Good Laboratory Practices* (WHO, 2009).

GLP procedures stress the importance of the following:

- *Resources:* organization, personnel, facilities, and equipment
- *Characterization:* test items and test systems
- *Rules:* protocols, standard operating procedures (SOPs)
- *Results:* raw data, final report and archives
- *Quality assurance:* independent monitoring of research processes

When implementing biocompatability testing for medical devices, certain GLP requirements should be kept in mind. Relative to the main points above:

1. *Resources:* The study director occupies a pivotal point of control for the study, is appointed by the test facility management, and assumes full responsibility for the GLP compliance of all activities within the study. The study director must therefore be aware of all events that may influence the quality and integrity of the study. Even when certain phases or parts of the study are delegated to other test sites, the study director retains overall responsibility for the entire study, including the parts delegated. This responsibility is reflected in a signed and dated GLP Compliance Statement, which is included in all study reports.
2. *Characterization:* For nonclinical studies, intended to evaluate safety, it is necessary that the study director have detailed knowledge about the properties of the test item. Characteristics, such as identity, potency, composition, stability, and impurity profile, as they apply to medical devices, should be known for the test item and should be provided to the study director. Documentation of test article characterization is often found in a

Certificate of Analysis, which should be included in the final report of study results. Additional information related to the requirement for characterization of test materials can be found in the section Materials Characterization and Analytical Testing of Biomaterials. The manufacturer's batch record for the lot from which test samples are pulled can be a good source of data on device characterization.

3. *Rules:* The principal steps of studies conducted in compliance with GLP are described in the study protocol. The protocol must be approved and signed by the study director before the study starts. Alterations to the study design can be made only through a formal amendment to the protocol. Adherence to a protocol ensures that the study can be reconstructed at a later point in time.
4. *Results:* GLP study results are interpreted by the study director based on the study design and actual conduct of the study. The GLP principles do not include allowance for the out-of-specification (OOS) process that is commonly employed in evaluation of study results for cGMP processes (e.g., manufacturing). Confounding or contributing factors that could result in misinterpretation of study results, however, can be noted by the study director.
5. *Quality assurance:* The Quality Assurance Unit (QAU) is charged with assuring management that GLP compliance has been attained in the test facility as a whole and in each individual study. For GLP studies in which various aspects of an individual study are conducted at multiple sites (e.g., test article characterization, clinical chemistry analysis, histopathology, etc.), it is required that the additional sites have a functioning QAU and that these off-site QAU units provide assurance in the form of a written report to the study director that these off-site aspects of the study have been conducted according to the protocol and that they are in compliance with GLP processes.

PLANNING BIOCOMPATIBILITY TESTING

When beginning a biocompatibility testing program, it is important to ensure that enough devices can be produced to complete testing, and to understand the length of time needed to generate test results. The following sections will help to determine the number of devices needed and time needed to complete testing.

CHOOSING EXTRACTION MEDIA

Medical device biocompatibility problems are most often caused by toxins that leach out of the device into the surrounding tissues or body fluids. Consequently, in the laboratory, extracts of device materials (leachables) are often used to assess biocompatibility. These extracts generally are prepared using exaggerated conditions of time and temperature to allow a margin of safety over normal physiological conditions.

Analytical extraction studies allow the chemist to identify and quantitate specific leachable moieties. This data, in turn, can help the device toxicologist or risk assessor determine the worst-case scenario for patient exposure and the risk to patient health.

TABLE 4.1
Extracting Media*

Sodium Chloride for Injection, USP (SCI)
Vegetable Oil
1:20 Alcohol in SCI
Polyethylene Glycol 400 (PEG)
Dimethyl sulfoxide (DMSO)
Clinically Relevant Solvents

* For most devices, only saline and vegetable oil extracts are needed.

Extracts are also used in many of the biological tests specified by ISO 10993. Table 4.1 lists the most commonly used extracting media.

Extracts are selected on the basis of the biological environment in which the test material is to be used. A saline (sodium chloride for injection [SCI]) extract approximates the aqueous, hydrophilic fluids in the body. It also permits the use of extreme temperatures in preparing the extracts, thus simulating certain sterilization conditions.

Tissue culture media may even more closely approximate aqueous body fluids, but it cannot be used for high-temperature extractions. Vegetable oils are nonpolar, hydrophobic solvents that simulate the lipid fluids in the body. For technical reasons, dimethyl sulfoxide (DMSO) extracts are often used in certain genotoxicity and sensitization tests. Two other common extracting media—alcohol in SCI and polyethylene glycol (PEG)—should be used only if they approximate the solvent properties of drugs or other materials that will contact the device during its normal use. For most devices, however, extracts using saline and vegetable oil are sufficient.

Extraction conditions (temperature and time) should be at least as extreme as any conditions the device or material will encounter during sterilization or clinical use. Generally, you will want to choose the highest extraction temperature that does not melt or fuse the material or cause chemical changes. To provide some margin of safety for use conditions, it is recommended that an extraction condition of at least 50°C for 72 hours be used. For devices that are susceptible to heat, an extraction condition of 37°C for 72 hours may be acceptable. Table 4.2 lists common extraction conditions.

TABLE 4.2
Extraction Conditions

37°C for 72 hours
50°C for 72 hours
70°C for 24 hours
121°C for 1 hour
Other Conditions (*justification required*)

Sample Preparation

Typically, the standard surface area of your device is used to determine the volume of extract needed for each test performed. This area includes the combined area of both sides of the device but excludes indeterminate surface irregularities. If the surface area cannot be determined because of the configuration of the device, a mass/volume of extracting fluid can be used. In either case, the device is cut into small pieces before extraction to enhance exposure to the extracting media. In some cases, it is not appropriate to cut the device; such devices are tested intact.

The simplest method for determining the surface area of a device is usually to use the computer-aided design (CAD) program from the design engineering group. Typically, the surface area can be calculated with just a few keystrokes. Alternatively, you can calculate the surface area using the equations below.

The table on the next page lists the amount of sample required for many procedures. Generally, we recommend using the ratio of sample to extracting media

Formulas for Surface Area Calculation

Device Shape	Formula
Square or Rectangle	$A = L \times W$
Hollow Cylinder	$A = (ID + OD) \pi \times L$
Disk	$A \text{ (one side)} = \pi r^2$
Ellipse	$A = (\pi \times X \times Y)/4$
Regular Polygon	$A = (b \times h \times n)/2$
Solid Cylinder (including ends)	$A = (OD \times \pi \times L) + (2 \pi r^2)$
Triangle	$A = (b \times h)/2$
Sphere	$A = 4 \times \pi r^2$
Trapezoid	$A = (h \times [p + q])/2$
Circular Ring	$4 \pi^2 R_r r_c$

Legend
A = surface area
OD = outer diameter
W = width
R_R = ring radius (circular ring)
X, Y = longest and shortest distances through the center of an ellipse
h = height
p, q = length of the parallel sides of a trapezoid
r_o = ½ OD
ID = inner diameter
L = length
R = radius
r_c = cross section radius (circular ring)
π = 3.14
b = base length
n = number of sides of a polygon
r_i = ½ ID

Assessing Biocompatibility

Test Turnaround Time and Sample Requirements

Requirement	Test Name	Sample Amount			Estimated turnaround (in weeks)
		Surface Area Double amounts for materials < 0.5 mm in thickness	Irregular, powders or liquids		
			Grams	mL	
Cytotoxicity	ISO Agar Overlay	1 × 3 pieces	4	20	4
	ISO MEM Elution	60 cm²			
	ISO Direct Contact	60 cm²			
	ISO MTT	60 cm²			
	ISO Colony Formation	60 cm²			
Sensitization	ASTM Murine Local Lymph Node Assay (LLNA)	N/A	16	30	5
	Maximization Test	60 cm² × 6 devices	24	60	7
	Closed Patch Test	1 in² × 130 devices	60	80	8
Irritation	ISO Intracutaneous Test	60 cm² × 2 devices	8	40	5
	ISO Dermal Irritation	60 cm² × 2 devices	4	10	5
	ISO Ocular Irritation	60 cm² × 2 devices	2	5	5
	Mucous Membrane Irritation	Varies	Varies	Varies	Varies
Systemic Toxicity	Material Mediated Pyrogen Test	60 cm² × 5 devices	24	120	5
	ISO Acute Systemic Test	60 cm² × 2 devices	8	40	5
	Subacute	Varies	Varies	Varies	Varies
	Subchronic	Varies	Varies	Varies	Varies
	Chronic	Varies	Varies	Varies	Varies
Genotoxicity	Ames Test	120 cm² × 2 devices	8	40	8–9
	Mouse Lymphoma Assay	240 cm² × 2 devices	16	80	15–17
	Mouse Micronucleus Assay	1200 cm² × 2 devices	40	200	15–17
	Chromosomal Aberration Test	120 cm² × 2 devices	8	40	12–14

(Continued)

Test Turnaround Time and Sample Requirements

Requirement	Test Name	Sample Amount — Surface Area Double amounts for materials < 0.5 mm in thickness	Sample Amount — Irregular, powders or liquids (Grams)	Sample Amount — Irregular, powders or liquids (mL)	Estimated turnaround (in weeks)
Implantation	Implantation Test (Local effects) (All ISO Implant Tests Include Histopathology) (7 days or greater)	12 strips 1 × 10 mm			Varies
Hemocompatibility	Hemolysis – ASTM Direct and Indirect Contact	6 devices/160 cm^2	12	20	4
	In Vivo Thrombogenicity	6 – 2 ½" long pieces			10–12
	In Vitro Platelet Aggregation Assay	120 cm^2 × 2 devices	20	Inquire	6–8
	Partial Thromboplastin Time (PTT)	60 cm^2	4	N/A	6–8
	Prothrombin Time (PT)	60 cm^2	4	N/A	6–8
	Complement Activation	60 cm^2 × 2 devices	8	Inquire	8–9
Carcinogenesis	Lifetime Toxicity	Inquire			Inquire
Analytical Tests	USP Physicochemical Tests	720 cm^2		N/A	6
	Other Procedures	Inquire			Inquire

specified in ISO 10993-12 (i.e., either 6 cm²/mL or 3 cm²/mL, depending on the thickness of the test material). For some types of materials, the ratio used for USP Elastomeric Closures for Injections (1.25 cm² per mL) is preferred.

Noncontact Devices

Noncontact devices are devices that do not contact the patient's body directly or indirectly. Examples include in vitro diagnostic devices. Regulatory agencies rarely require biocompatibility testing for such devices.

BIOLOGICAL TEST METHODS

The following pages describe some of the specific procedures recommended for biocompatibility testing. This listing does not imply that all procedures are necessary for any given material and it does not indicate that these are the only available tests.

CYTOTOXICITY (TISSUE CULTURE)

Cell culture assays are used to assess the biocompatibility of a material or extract through the use of isolated cells *in vitro*. These techniques are useful in evaluating the toxicity or irritancy potential of materials and chemicals. They provide an excellent way to screen materials before in vivo tests.

There are two categories of cytotoxicity evaluation: qualitative and quantitative. Quantitative cytotoxicity tests are preferred by regulatory agencies and institutions.

There are three cytotoxicity tests commonly used for medical devices. The *direct contact* procedure is recommended for low-density materials, such as contact lens polymers. In this method, a piece of test material is placed directly onto cells growing on culture medium. The cells are then incubated. During incubation, leachable chemicals in the test material can diffuse into the culture medium and contact the cell layer. Reactivity of the test sample is indicated by malformation, degeneration, and lysis of cells around the test material.

The *agar diffusion* assay is appropriate for high-density materials, such as elastomeric closures. In this method, a thin layer of nutrient-supplemented agar is placed over the cultured cells. The test material (or an extract of the test material dried on filter paper) is placed on top of the agar layer, and the cells are incubated. A zone of malformed, degenerative, or lysed cells under and around the test material indicates cytotoxicity.

The *MEM elution* assay uses different extracting media and extraction conditions to test devices according to actual use conditions or to exaggerate those conditions. Extracts can be titrated to yield a semiquantitative measurement of cytotoxicity. After preparation, the extracts are transferred onto a layer of cells and incubated. Following incubation, the cells are examined microscopically for malformation, degeneration, and lysis of the cells.

Two quantitative cytotoxicity tests have been internationally tested for chemicals and medical devices:

Device Categories: Definitions and Examples

Device Categories		Examples
Surface Device	Skin	Devices that contact intact skin surfaces only. Examples include electrodes, external prostheses, fixation tapes, compression bandages, and monitors of various types.
	Mucous membrane	Devices communicating with intact mucosal membranes. Examples include contact lenses, urinary catheters, intravaginal, and intraintestinal devices (stomach tubes, sigmoidoscopes, colonoscopes, gastroscopes), endotracheal tubes, bronchoscopes, dental prostheses, orthodontic devices, and intrauterine devices.
	Breached or compromised surfaces	Devices that contact breached or otherwise-compromised external body surfaces. Examples include ulcer, burn, and granulation tissue dressings or healing devices and occlusive patches.
External Communicating Device	Blood path indirect	Devices that contact the blood path at one point and serve as a conduit for entry into the vascular system. Examples include solution administration sets, extension sets, transfer sets, and blood administration sets.
	Tissue/bone/dentin communicating	Devices communicating with tissue, bone, and pulp/dentin system. Examples include laparoscopes, arthroscopes, draining systems, dental cements, dental filling materials, and skin staples. This category also includes devices that contact internal tissues (rather than blood contact devices). Examples include many surgical instruments and accessories.
	Circulating blood	Devices that contact circulating blood. Examples include intravascular catheters, temporary pacemaker electrodes, oxygenators, extracorporeal oxygenator tubing and accessories, hemoadsorbents and immunoabsorbents.
Implant Device	Tissue/bone	Devices principally contacting bone. Examples include orthopedic pins, plates, replacement joints, bone prostheses, cements, and intraosseous devices. Devices principally contacting tissue and tissues fluid. Examples include pacemakers, drug supply devices, neuromuscular sensors and stimulators, replacement tendons, breast implants, artificial larynxes, subperiosteal implants, and ligation clips.
	Blood	Devices principally contacting blood. Examples include pacemaker electrodes, artificial arteriovenous fistulae, heart valves, vascular grafts and stents, internal drug delivery catheters, and ventricular assist devices.

The *MTT cytotoxicity test* measures the viability of cells by spectrophotometric methods. This colorimetric method measures the reduction of the yellow, water-soluble MTT (3-4,5 dimethyl-thiazol-2-yl) – 2,5-diphenyl tetrazolium bromide by mitochondrial succinate dehydrogenase. A minimum of four concentrations of the test material are tested. This biochemical reaction is only catalyzed by living cells.

The *colony formation cytotoxicity test* enumerates the number of colonies formed after exposing them to the test material at different concentrations. This is a very sensitive test because the colony formation is assessed while the cells are in a state of proliferation (logarithmic phase), and thus it is more susceptible to toxic effects. A concentration-dependence curve evaluating the induced inhibition of the test material can be created, and the IC_{50} value (concentration of the test material that provides 50% inhibition) can be calculated. The quantitative tests can be performed on extracts and by direct contact.

At least one type of cytotoxicity test, qualitative or quantitative, should be performed on each component of any device.

SENSITIZATION ASSAYS

Sensitization studies help to determine whether a material contains chemicals that cause adverse local or systemic effects after repeated or prolonged exposure. These allergic or hypersensitivity reactions involve immunologic mechanisms. Studies to determine sensitization potential may be performed using either specific chemicals from the test material, the test material itself, or most often, extracts of the test material. The Materials Biocompatibility Matrix recommends sensitization testing for all classes of medical devices.

The *guinea pig maximization test* (Magnusson-Kligman Method) is recommended for devices that will have externally communicating or internal contact with the body or body fluids. In this study, the test material is mixed with complete Freund's adjuvant (CFA) to enhance the skin sensitization response.

The *closed patch* test involves multiple topical doses and is recommended for devices that will contact unbroken skin only.

The *murine local lymph node assay* (LLNA) determines the quantitative increase in lymphocytes in response to a sensitizer. If a molecule acts as a skin sensitizer, it will induce the epidermal Langherhans cells to transport the allergen to the draining lymph nodes, which in turn causes T-lymphocytes to proliferate and differentiate. This method may be used only for chemicals that come into direct contact with intact skin or are transported through the skin. Additionally, this method can only reliably detect moderate to strong sensitizers. *From an animal welfare perspective, this test is preferable to the guinea pig maximization or the closed patch test, and it allows for faster turnaround time. However, if a negative result is seen in the LLNA test, a guinea pig maximization test must be conducted.*

IRRITATION TESTS

These tests estimate the local irritation potential of devices, materials or extracts, using sites such as skin or mucous membranes, usually in an animal model. The route of exposure (skin, eye, mucosa) and duration of contact should be analogous to the anticipated clinical use of the device, but it is often prudent to exaggerate exposure conditions somewhat to establish a margin of safety for patients.

In the *intracutaneous test*, extracts of the test material and blanks are injected intradermally. The injection sites are scored for erythema and edema (redness and swelling). This procedure is recommended for devices that will have externally communicating or internal contact with the body or body fluids. It reliably detects the potential for local irritation because of chemicals that may be extracted from a biomaterial.

The *primary skin irritation* test should be considered for topical devices that have external contact with intact or breached skin. In this procedure, the test material or an extract is applied directly to intact and abraded sites on the skin of a rabbit. After a 24-hour exposure, the material is removed and the sites are scored for erythema and edema.

Mucous membrane irritation tests are recommended for devices that will have externally communicating contact with intact natural channels or tissues. These studies often use extracts rather than the material itself. Some common procedures include vaginal, cheek pouch, and eye irritation studies.

Acute Systemic Toxicity

By using extracts of the device or device material, the *acute systemic toxicity* test detects leachables that produce systemic (as opposed to local) toxic effects. The extracts of the test material and negative control blanks are injected into mice (intravenously or intraperitoneally, depending on the extracting media). The mice are observed for toxic signs just after injection and at four other time points. The Materials Biocompatibility Matrix recommends this test for all blood contact devices. It may also be appropriate for any other device that contacts internal tissues.

The *material-mediated pyrogen* test evaluates the potential of a material to cause a pyrogenic response, or fever, when introduced into the blood. Lot release testing for pyrogenicity is done in vitro using the *bacterial endotoxin (LAL)* test. It must be validated for each device or material. For assessing biocompatibility, however, the rabbit pyrogen test is preferred. The rabbit test, in addition to detecting bacterial endotoxins, is sensitive to material-mediated pyrogens that may be found in test materials or extracts.

Subchronic Toxicity

Tests for *subchronic toxicity* are used to determine potentially harmful effects from long-term or multiple exposures to test materials or extracts during a period of up to 10% of the total life span of the test animal (e.g., up to 90 days in rats). Actual use conditions of a medical device need to be taken into account when selecting an animal model for subchronic toxicity. Appropriate animal models are determined on a case-by-case basis.

Two protocols are typically used for subchronic testing that are appropriate for many devices. They may use *intraperitoneal* administration of an extract of the device or device material or an *intravenous* route of administration. Implant tests are often performed for different durations appropriate to assess subchronic toxicity of devices and device materials.

Subchronic tests are required for all permanent devices and should be considered for those with prolonged contact with internal tissues.

Genotoxicity

Genotoxicity evaluations use a set of in vitro and in vivo tests to detect mutagens, substances that can directly or indirectly induce genetic damage directly through a variety of mechanisms. This damage can occur in either somatic or germline cells, increasing the risk of cancer or inheritable defects. A strong correlation exists between mutagenicity and carcinogenicity.

Genotoxic effects fall into one of three categories: point mutations along a strand of DNA, damage to the overall structure of the DNA, or damage to the structure of the chromosome (which contains the DNA). A variety of tests have been developed to determine whether damage has occurred at any of these levels. These assays complement one another and are performed as a battery.

The most common test for mutagenicity, the Ames test, detects point mutations by employing several strains of the bacteria *Salmonella typhimurium*, which have been selected for their sensitivity to mutagens. The *mouse lymphoma* and the HGPRT assays are common procedures using mammalian cells to detect point mutations. The mouse lymphoma assay is also able to detect clastogenic lesions in genes (chromosome damage). Assays for DNA damage and repair include both in vitro and in vivo Unscheduled DNA Synthesis (UDS). Cytogenetic assays allow direct observation of chromosome damage. There are both in vitro and in vivo methods, including the *chromosomal aberration* and the *mouse micronucleus* assays.

ISO 10993-1 specifies an assessment of genotoxic potential for permanent devices and for those with prolonged contact (>24 hours) with internal tissues and blood. Extracorporeal devices with limited contact (<24 hours) may require a genotoxicity evaluation. Generally, devices with long-term exposure require an Ames test and two in vivo methods, usually the chromosomal aberration and mouse micronucleus tests. Devices with less critical body contact may be able to be tested using only the Ames test.

When selecting a battery of genotoxicity tests, you should consider the requirements of the specific regulatory agency where your submission will be made. *Because of the high cost of genotoxicity testing, it is recommended that an FDA reviewer be consulted before authorizing genotoxicity testing.*

Implantation Tests

Implant studies are used to determine the biocompatibility of medical devices or biomaterials that directly contact living tissue other than skin (e.g., sutures, surgical ligating clips, implantable devices, etc.). These tests can evaluate devices, which, in clinical use, are intended to be implanted for either short-term or long-term periods. Implantation techniques may be used to evaluate both absorbable and nonabsorbable materials. To provide a reasonable assessment of safety, the implant study should closely approximate the intended clinical use.

The dynamics of biochemical exchange and cellular and immunologic responses may be assessed in implantation studies, especially through the use of histopathology.

Histopathological analysis of implant sites greatly increases the amount of information obtained from these studies.

Hemocompatibility

Materials used in blood-contacting devices (e.g., intravenous catheters, hemodialysis sets, blood transfusion sets, vascular prostheses) must be assessed for blood compatibility to establish their safety. In practice, all materials are to some degree incompatible with blood because they can either disrupt the blood cells (hemolysis) or activate the coagulation pathways (*thrombogenicity*) or the complement system.

The *hemolysis assay* is recommended for all devices or device materials except those that contact only intact skin or mucous membranes. This test measures the damage to red blood cells when they are exposed to materials or their extracts and compares it to positive and negative controls.

Coagulation assays measure the effect of the test article on human blood coagulation time. They are recommended for all devices with blood contact. The *prothrombin time assay (PT)* is a general screening test for the detection of coagulation abnormalities in the **extrinsic** pathway.

The *partial thromboplastin time assay (PTT)* detects coagulation abnormalities in the **intrinsic** pathway.

The most common test for thrombogenicity is the in vivo method. For devices unsuited to this test method, ISO 10993-4 requires tests in each of four categories: coagulation, platelets, hematology, and complement system.

Complement activation testing is recommended for implant devices that contact circulatory blood. This in vitro assay measures complement activation in human plasma as a result of exposure of the plasma to the test article or an extract. The measure of complement actuation indicates whether a test article is capable of inducing a complement-induced inflammatory immune response in humans.

Other blood compatibility tests and specific in vivo studies may be required to complete the assessment of material-blood interactions, especially to meet ISO requirements.

Carcinogenesis Bioassays

These assays are used to determine the tumorigenic potential of test materials or extracts from either a single or multiple exposures, over a period consisting of the total life span of the test system (e.g., two years for rat, 18 months for mouse, or seven years for dog).

Carcinogenicity testing of devices is expensive, highly problematic, and controversial. Manufacturers can almost always negotiate an alternative to full-scale carcinogenicity testing of their devices.

Reproductive and Developmental Toxicity

These studies evaluate the potential effects of test materials or extracts on fertility, reproductive function, and prenatal and early postnatal development. They are often required for devices with permanent contact with internal tissues.

Devices or Components Which Contact Circulating Blood and the Categories of Appropriate Testing—External Communicating Devices

Device Examples	Test Category				
	Thrombosis	Coagulation	Platelets	Hematology	Complement System
Catheters in place for less than 24 hours (Atherectomy devices)	x[a]			x[b]	
Blood monitors	x[a]			x[b]	
Blood storage and administration equipment, blood collection devices, extension sets		x	x	x[b]	x[c]
Catheters in place for more than 24 hours: guidewires, intravascular endoscopes, Intravascular ultrasound, laser systems, Retrograde coronary perfusion catheters.	x[a]			x[b]	x
Cell savers		x	x	x[b]	
Devices for absorption of specific substances from blood		x	x	x	x
Donor and therapeutic apheresis equipment and cell separation systems		x	x	x	x
Extracorporeal membrane oxygenator systems, haemodialysis/haemofiltration equipment, percutaneous circulatory support devices	x[a]			x	x
Leukocyte removal filter		x	x	x[b]	x

[a] Thrombosis is an in-vivo or ex-vivo phemonenon. Coagulation and platelet response are involved in this process. The manufacturer must decide if testing in coagulation and platelet testing are appropriate.
[b] Hemolysis testing only. [c] Only for aphaeresis equipment.

Devices or Components Which Contact Circulating Blood and the Categories of Appropriate Testing—Implant Devices

Device examples	Test Category				
	Thrombosis	Coagulation	Platelets	Hematology	Complement System
Annuloplasty rings, mechanical heart valves	x[a]			x[b]	
Intra-aortic balloon pumps	x[a]			x	x
Total artificial hearts, ventricular-assist devices	x[a]			x	
Embolization devices	x[a]			x[b]	x
Endovascular grafts	x[a]			x[b]	
Implantable defibrillators and cardioverters	x[a]			x[b]	
Pacemaker leads	x[a]			x[b]	x
Prosthetic (synthetic) vascular grafts and patches, including arteriovenous shunts	x[a]			x[b]	
Stents	x[a]			x[b]	
Tissue heart valves	x[a]			x[b]	
Tissue vascular grafts and patches, including arteriovenous shunts	x[a]			x[b]	
Vena cava filters	x[a]			x[b]	

[a] Thrombosis is an in-vivo or ex-vivo phemonenon. Coagulation and platelet response are involved in this process. The manufacturer must decide if testing in coagulation and platelet testing are appropriate.
[b] Hemolysis testing only.

Pharmacokinetics

Pharmacokinetic (PK) or Absorption/Distribution/Metabolism/Excretion (ADME) studies are used to investigate the metabolic processes of absorption, distribution, biotransformation, and elimination of toxic leachables and potential degradation products from test materials or extracts. They are especially appropriate for bioabsorbable materials or for drug–device combinations.

Preclinical Safety Testing

The objectives of preclinical safety studies are to define pharmacological and toxicological effects not only before initiation of human studies but also throughout clinical development. Both in vitro and in vivo studies can contribute to this characterization.

Histopathology Services

Implant studies are often the most direct evaluation of device biocompatibility. The test material is placed in direct contact with living tissue. After an appropriate period, the implant site is recovered and examined microscopically for tissue reaction. The histopathologist can detect and describe many types of tissue and immune system reactions.

Similarly, in subchronic and chronic studies, various organs and tissues are harvested at necropsy and evaluated microscopically for toxic effects. Many of these studies also call for clinical chemistry analysis of specimens or serum samples from the test animals.

MATERIALS CHARACTERIZATION AND ANALYTICAL TESTING OF BIOMATERIALS

Analytical procedures provide the initial means for investigating the biocompatibility of medical device materials. Knowledge of device materials and their propensity for releasing leachable matter will help manufacturers assess the risks of in vivo reactivity and preclude subsequent toxicology problems with finished devices.

Increasingly, the FDA has been asking for analytical characterization of device materials and potential leachables per ISO 10993-17 and 10993-18. Many firms also use analytical procedures for routine quality control of raw materials or finished products.

The degree of chemical characterization required should reflect the nature and duration of the clinical exposure and should be determined based on the data necessary to evaluate the biological safety of the device. It will also depend on the nature of the materials used (e.g., liquids, gels, polymers, metals, ceramics, composites, or biologically sourced material).

The following strategy is suggested as a sound program for chemical characterization of a device material:

1. Determine the qualitative composition of each device component or material. This information should be available from the material vendor, or it can be determined through laboratory testing. The list of constituents should include
   a. The identity of the matrix (i.e., the major component such as the specific polymer, alloy, or metal);
   b. All plasticizers, colorants, antioxidants, fillers, and so on deliberately added during fabrication of the material;
   c. Impurities such as unreacted monomers and oligomers; and
   d. Manufacturing materials such as solvent residues, slip agents, and lubricants.

2. Estimate the potential for patient exposure for each item on the material constituent list. Use literature searches of toxicological databases to assess the likelihood of tissue reactivity. For potentially toxic constituents, design and conduct laboratory studies to determine the extractable levels of those constituents. Use exaggerated conditions of time and temperature, and consider appropriate detection limits. Additional studies may be needed to assess levels of extractables released in actual use conditions.
3. Data generated from this characterization process can be used to create a material data file. The information can then be used as a reference for continued testing of device materials to ensure consistency of future production lots. This may in turn reduce the need for routine biological testing.

Additional uses of analytical characterization data might include the following:

1. Use in an assessment of the overall biological safety of a medical device.
2. Measurement of the level of any leachable substance in a medical device to allow the assessment of compliance with the allowable limit derived for that substance from health-based risk assessment.
3. Judging equivalence of a proposed material to a clinically established material.
4. Judging equivalence of a final device to a prototype device to check the relevance of data on the latter to be used to support the assessment of the former.
5. Screening of potential new materials for suitability in a medical device for a proposed clinical application.

TRADITIONAL EXTRACTABLE MATERIAL CHARACTERIZATION

- USP Physicochemical Tests—Plastics
- USP Physicochemical Test Panel for Elastomeric Closures for Injections
- USP Polyethylene Containers Tests—Heavy Metals and Nonvolatile Residues
- Indirect Food Additives and Polymers Extractables (21 CFR Part 177)
- Sterilant Residues—Ethylene Oxide, Ethylene Chlorohydrin, Ethylene Glycol

TESTS PROCEDURES FOR EXTRACTABLE MATERIAL

- Ultraviolet/Visible Spectroscopy
- Gas Chromatography
- Liquid Chromatography
- Infrared Spectroscopy
- Mass Spectrometry
- Residual Solvents
- Atomic Absorption Spectroscopy
- Inductively Coupled Plasma Spectroscopy

Bulk Material Characterization

- Infrared Spectroscopy Analysis for Identity and Estimation of Gross Composition
  - Reflectance Spectroscopy
  - Transmission Spectroscopy
- Atomic Absorption Spectroscopy
- Inductively Coupled Plasma Spectroscopy
- Thermal Analysis

Surface Characterization

- Infrared Reflectance Spectroscopy
- Scanning Electron Microscopy
- Energy-Dispersive X-Ray Analysis

ABOUT THE AUTHOR

Tom Spalding is the president of Pacific BioLabs, a contract research organization supporting medical device, pharmaceutical, and biotech product development and innovation. For more than 25 years, Mr. Spalding and the staff at Pacific BioLabs have been performing biocompatibility testing, designing protocols, and gathering data to support hundreds of US FDA medical device submissions.

RESOURCES

Association for the Advancement of Medical Instrumentation. *Biological Evaluation of Medical Devices*. AAMI Standards and Recommended Practices, vol. 4. This includes AAMI/ANSI/ISO Standard 10993. Annex B of 10993-1 is an extensive bibliography of U.S. and international reference documents.

ASTM International. *ASTM F-748-98: Practice for Selecting Generic Biological Test Methods for Materials and Devices*. ASTM International, 2000, doi: 10.1520/FO748-98.

Food and Drug Administration. *Guidelines for the Intra-Articular Prosthetic Knee Ligament*. Rockville, MD: Food and Drug Administration, 1987.

———. *PTCA Catheter System Testing Guideline*. Rockville, MD: Food and Drug Administration, 2010.

Gad, Shayne Cox. *Safety Evaluation of Medical Devices*. New York: Marcel Dekker, Inc., 2002.

"Good Laboratory Practice for Nonclinical Laboratory Studies." 21 CFR § 58.

International Organization for Standardization. Parts 1–20. *ISO Standard 10993: Biological Evaluation of Medical Devices*.

Organisation for Economic Co-operation and Development. "ENV/MC/CHEM(98)17." In *OECD Principles on Good Laboratory Practice*, rev. 1997 ed. OECD Series on Principles of Good Laboratory Practice and Compliance Monitoring, no. 1. Paris: Environment Directorate, OECD, 1998.

Stark, Nancy J. *Biocompatibility Testing and Management*. Chicago: Clinical Design Group, 1994.

U.S. Pharmacopeia. "The Biocompatibility of Materials Used In Drug Containers, Medical Devices, and Implants." USP <1031>.

World Health Organization. *World Health Organization Handbook: Good Laboratory Practice (GLP): Quality Practices for Regulated Non-Clinical Research and Development*, 2nd ed., 2009.

CONTACT INFORMATION

Pacific BioLabs
551 Linus Pauling Drive
Hercules, CA 94547
Phone: 510-964-9000
http://www.pacificbiolabs.com

Section II

Processes for Medical Device R&D

5 Catheter-Forming Equipment and Operations

Theodore R. Kucklick

CONTENTS

Basic Forming Operations 94
Hot-Air Station... 95
Hot-Air Station Setup 95
Types of Compressors 96
Particle Filters 96
Moisture Filters 96
Safety 96
Features and User Controls 97
    Temperature Gauge 97
    Airflow Control and Airflow Gauge 97
    Thermal Nozzle 97
    Cooling Air Nozzle 98
Basic Forming Operations 98
    Mandrels... 98
        Glass Molds 98
    Balloon Blowing 99
History of the Development of Glass Catheter Molds 100
Hole Punching... 101
Slug Ejection 102
Automated Hole Punching 102
Balloon Dip Molds.. 104
Conclusion 105
Resources 105
    Vendors: Hot-Air Stations and Automated Catheter Manufacturing
    Equipment 105
Acknowledgments... 106

BASIC FORMING OPERATIONS

Charles Dotter, considered the father of catheter-based interventional radiology, once said:

> My favorite conceptual trademark is a sketch that I did years ago of a crossed pipe and wrench. It's a gross oversimplification, of course, but what it means to me is that if a plumber can do it to pipes, we can do it to blood vessels.*

Some of the basic forming operations to catheter tubing will be familiar to anyone who has worked with malleable copper water pipe. Much of catheter tubing—necking, flaring, joining, and so on—is very similar to small plumbing parts, with tubes, tees, valves, and stopcocks. The difference is that you are working with plastic tubing, and the tube usually goes into a human blood vessel, a duct, or a hollow organ.

The basic forming operations for catheter tubing are tipping, bonding and laminating, necking, expanding, flaring, and forming. Tipping is to form a shape, usually cone or bullet, on the end of a catheter. Bonding is the process of thermally welding two compatible plastic materials under finely controlled heat without melting and distorting the plastic catheter tube. Necking is to reduce the outer diameter of a tube, by pulling the tube through a heated-reducing die. Flaring is to form a flange on the end of a tube with a cone-shaped heated die, or to mold the material into a clamshell mold. This flange is usually to produce a mechanical anchor when assembling the tube into a fitting. Expanding is using a heated tapered die to expand the end of a tube. Forming is the process of expanding a tube, usually under air pressure. Two types of forming are free blowing, or heating a tube while applying controlled pressure into the tube, and clamping one end with a hemostat, similar to glass blowing. This free-blowing process takes a fair bit of skill and practice. Tubing may also be blown into a mold, where the balloon takes the shape of the tool. Examples of these molds are shown later in the chapter. Shrinking and laminating using a shrink tube is also a basic operation. In laminating, a fluoropolymer shrink tube is used as a tool to laminate a sandwich of an inner tubing, a reinforcing braid, and an outer layer. The shrink tube is used to squeeze this assembly together while it is heated, causing the plastic tubes to fuse together and flow around the braid, capturing it in the middle layer of the finished tubing. A shrink tube is also used to bond joints between different sections of catheter tubing, such as a higher durometer shaft and a softer durometer distal tip. This is handled in more detail in Chapter 6, "Basics of Catheter Assembly." The basic tool for performing these thermal forming operations is the hot-air station (see Figure 5.1).

Once catheter tubing has been formed, a common secondary operation is making holes in the tubing for aspiration, for a balloon inflation port, to inject medications, or any other function a fenestration may have. Typically these holes are

---

* Misty M. Payne, "Charles Theodore Dotter: The Father of Intervention," *Texas Heart Institute Journal* 28, no. 1 (2001), http://www.pubmedcentral.nih.gov/articlerender.fcgi?tool=pubmed&pubmedid=11330737.

Catheter-Forming Equipment and Operations

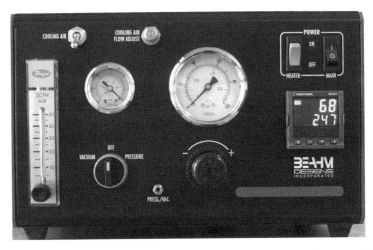

FIGURE 5.1 Control panel of prototype development hot-air station. (Courtesy of Beahm Designs, Campbell, CA.)

made with a small tube where the edge has been honed to a razor-sharp edge. Hole punches are not limited to round holes. Oval-shaped punches are also available to punch slots.

HOT-AIR STATION

A hot-air box is a basic piece of equipment for manufacturing catheters. It is used to perform forming and joining operations to extruded plastic catheter material. It is essentially a clean hot-air supply with fine air pressure and temperature control. The purpose is to bring the thermoplastic catheter material to its transition temperature, so that it may be formed into a desired shape, or melted and joined with another piece of catheter material. Another function of the hot-air box is balloon forming, where tubing is heated and compressed air is blown into the tube lumen. The balloon may be free blown, or blown into an exact shape into a heated glass mold. A hot-air box may also be used to form a conical tip on the end of a catheter, or to form a flare for mechanical assembly or a fluid fitting. Some of these operations require the use of nonsticking mandrels, which will be described in detail later in the chapter. Hot-air station forming is an evolution of the torch-forming methods used in early plastic catheter production.

HOT-AIR STATION SETUP

The first requirement in setting up the hot-air box is a supply of clean, dry compressed air. The requirements for the air supply are as follows:

- Clean and dry, free from water, particulates, and oil
- Minimum 1.2 cubic feet per minute (CFM) per hot-air station at 15 pounds per square inch (PSI)

An important consideration is to ensure that the air supply is free of contaminants. The three basic sources of these are dust, water, and oil from the compressor. The levels of compressed-air quality are commonly called shop air or plant air, which is basic unfiltered compressed air; instrument air for spray painting and laboratory use; and process air for food and pharmaceutical processing. International Organization of Standardization (ISO) 8573 gives more detailed specifications for the quality of compressed air.

TYPES OF COMPRESSORS

Most compressors that meet the basic air output requirements may be used. An oilless compressor will eliminate the need to filter out oil. Some compressors are made to produce an oil mist to lubricate pneumatic air tools and should be avoided when supplying a hot-air station. Compressors and systems to supply automotive finishing spray guns can be used, as they are designed to supply clean, dry air free of oil and particulates.

PARTICLE FILTERS

To filter out particulates, the use of a small mesh filter is recommended. The size of the filter should trap particles down to the size appropriate to the manufacturing environment where you are working. For example, if you are operating the hot-air station in a class 100,000 clean room, the mesh filter should trap particles of 100,000 microns and larger. Use the largest particle-size filter for your application. This will avoid line pressure drop and allow the compressor to operate most efficiently.

MOISTURE FILTERS

When air is compressed and decompressed, the water vapor in the atmosphere condenses, resulting in water in the compressed-air system. Removal of this water and water vapor is required. Most compressor systems have a basic in-line water trap. An in-line trap is *not* adequate for water removal in a hot-air station setup. To ensure dry air to the hot-air station, a point-of-use (at the hot-air station) dessicator is required. A common point-of-use dessicator is a pellet cartridge. A point-of-use filter will ensure that the air used by the hot air station is clean and dry. Consult your compressor dealer for information on filtering accessories.

SAFETY

Compressors generate noise and heat. Any compressed-air service must be handled carefully. Ensure that compressors are installed with proper ventilation and in a location that does not produce excessive environmental noise. Be sure to install the compressor according to local building and electrical codes and applicable Occupational Safety and Health Organization (OSHA) regulations. Lines and tanks should be properly labeled. Keep the user's manuals readily accessible and carefully follow the manufacturer's instructions for operation, safety, and regular maintenance.

Catheter-Forming Equipment and Operations

FEATURES AND USER CONTROLS

TEMPERATURE GAUGE

The temperature gauge is the most basic readout on the hot-air station. The temperature readout shows the air temperature at the thermal nozzle (see Figure 5.2)

The temperature should be set to the glass transition temperature of the plastic, or at the point at which the plastic begins to melt and becomes formable and weldable. Several factors can affect this temperature, such as ambient room temperature, the size of the thermal nozzle, and the nature of the material with which you are working. Consult the material data sheet for the melt temperature of the plastic you are forming for the temperature at which to set the hot-air box. Try a few test pieces of your material to fine-tune to the optimum setting for your process. Remember that the melt temperature of your plastic in the data sheet is an average under laboratory conditions. You will need to find the setting that works best for your material under your conditions.

AIRFLOW CONTROL AND AIRFLOW GAUGE

The airflow control knob regulates the velocity of airflow to the thermal nozzle. The airflow gauge shows the volume of airflow in cubic feet per minute (see Figure 5.1).

Airflow for welding and tipping operations should be set to 1.2 CFM. Airflow for other operations or balloon blowing should be set according to the material used and desired results.

THERMAL NOZZLE

Thermal nozzles are where the tubing material is heated. These nozzles come in several sizes according to your particular application (see Figure 5.2).

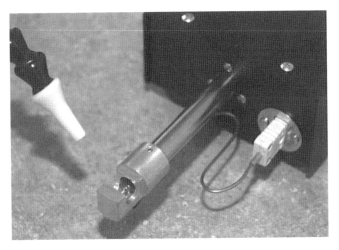

FIGURE 5.2 Temperature-controlled thermal nozzle and cooling air nozzle. (Courtesy of Beahm Designs, Campbell, CA.)

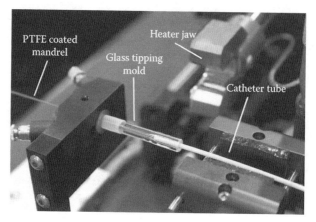

FIGURE 5.3 Parts of an automated tip-forming machine. Note how a mandrel is used to keep the guidewire lumen open. (Courtesy of Beahm Designs, Campbell, CA.)

COOLING AIR NOZZLE

The cooling air nozzle is used to cool off and set the plastic after melting and forming. The cooling air nozzle is typically foot-pedal controlled (see Figure 5.3).

BASIC FORMING OPERATIONS

MANDRELS

A basic accessory in forming catheter tubing is mandrels. These are metal wires or fluoropolymer rods that keep tubing lumens open while forming and joining tubing.

Metal wire mandrels are made of either 304 stainless or nickel–titanium alloy (superelastic nitinol.) These mandrels are coated with polytetrafluoroethylene (PTFE, Teflon) to keep them from sticking to the melted catheter tube plastic. Mandrels may be coated with paralyne polymer. Consult your mandrel vendor to determine which release material will best serve your needs.

While prototyping for bench testing, common piano wire may be used as a mandrel if a manufactured mandrel is not available. The wire may be polished, then sprayed with a PTFE mold release to keep it from sticking to the melted tubing plastic.

Note: Never use such a mandrel for a device intended for human use. Always use materials that conform to Food and Drug Administration (FDA) good manufacturing practice (GMP) guidelines for devices intended for human use.

Glass Molds

Glass molds are another important and versatile accessory for forming catheter tubing. Glass molds are used for blowing small balloons and tipping catheters, and glass tubes for performing joining operations (see Figure 5.4 and Figure 5.5).

Catheter-Forming Equipment and Operations

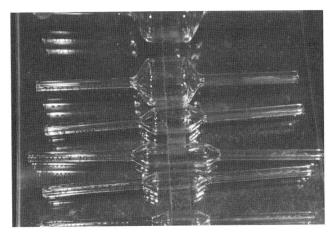

FIGURE 5.4 Assorted glass balloon blowing molds. (Courtesy of FSG, Inc., Grass Valley, CA.)

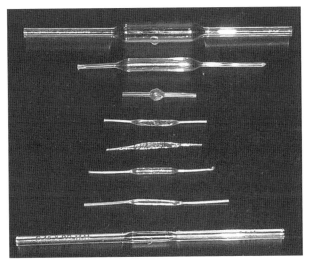

FIGURE 5.5 Balloon molds and blown plastic balloons. (Courtesy of FSG, Inc., Grass Valley, CA.)

BALLOON BLOWING

In this operation, a piece of thin-walled tubing is used, typically polyseter. One end of the tube is clamped with a hemostat. A glass mold that has the shape of the balloon inside is slipped over the tubing. The glass mold section is heated to the transition temperature of the plastic, and air pressure is blown into the open end of the tube. The result is that a balloon is blown into the shape of the inside of the glass mold. If you have never done this before, it may take some practice to get the desired results. Equipment is available from a number of vendors (e.g., Farlow's, Beahm Designs), including the hot-air station maker and glass mold maker to automate the process of balloon blowing. Also, a number of stock balloon sizes and shapes may be ordered from Advanced Polymer Corporation in Salem, NH, if you do not want to blow your own balloons.

HISTORY OF THE DEVELOPMENT OF GLASS CATHETER MOLDS

The following history of glass catheter molds is adapted from a history of Farlow's Scientific Glassblowing.*

Farlow's Scientific Glassblowing, Inc. (FSG), was established in 1980. The first shop was in a garage in Los Gatos, CA. In 1982, engineers from Advanced Cardiovascular Systems, Inc. (ACS) approached the company to develop the Glass Balloon Mold.

These molds were developed to form the plastic balloon catheters for the angioplasty industry. ACS at that time was forming their balloon in metal molds or by free blowing the plastic. The engineers discovered that using glass to form the balloons had some advantages. The glass allowed the engineer to see the balloon form and made the process of developing a program to blow the balloon much easier. When forming the plastic in the glass mold you could see how far to stretch the plastic. If the plastic separated or deformed, the engineer could quickly reprogram the machine to correct the problem. Another advantage of glass is that the inner surface is very smooth and would give the finished balloon a smooth surface with no flaws. Glass molds were able to hold very tight tolerances, ±.0002 on the inside dimensions of the glass molds.

As the Northern California medical device industry developed, engineers and doctors saw an opportunity to create their own niche and began leaving ACS to create new startup companies. These ACS engineers continued their development using the glass balloon technology with Farlow's. The engineers would bring glass mold technology and implement them into their new company's processes.

Along with the balloon molds Farlow's produces a part called capture tubes. This was needed for the attachment of the catheter to the balloons and dissimilar materials together.

Farlow's Glass and a medical company, Danforth Biomedical in Santa Clara, CA, entered into a joint venture in the medical mold business. They developed the BMM, a machine that uses glass molds to form catheter balloons for the medical industry.

Farlow's is currently producing and marketing a fourth generation of balloon-blowing machines, the BBM-5100 (see Figures 5.6 and 5.7).

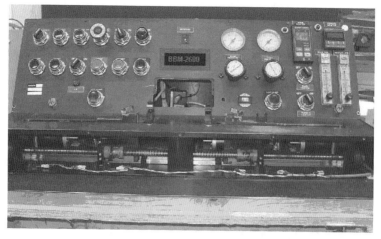

FIGURE 5.6 The original BMM-2600. (Courtesy FSG, Inc., Grass Valley, CA.)

---

* Courtesy of Gary Farlow and FSG, Inc., Grass Valley, CA, http://www.farlowsci.com.

Catheter-Forming Equipment and Operations

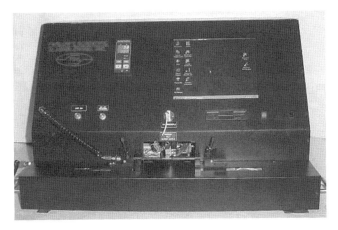

FIGURE 5.7 BBM-5100. (Courtesy FSG, Inc., Grass Valley, CA.)

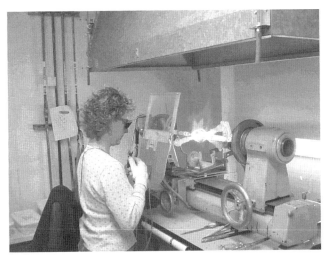

FIGURE 5.8 Producing a mold on a glass lathe. (Courtesy FSG, Inc., Grass Valley, CA.)

Farlow's now has many styles of molds, standard molds, and split molds; it has developed and is in the final stages of testing a clamshell mold (see Figure 5.8).

HOLE PUNCHING

As mentioned, holes are usually punched in catheter tubing with tubular cutting dies called catheter hole punches. A major supplier of these punches is Technical Innovations (Brazoria, TX). Types of hole-forming methods include punching, in which the hole punch tool is driven in perpendicular to the centerline of the tube, and skiving, where the tool cuts across the tube. Skived holes also may be made by making a notch with a sharp razor blade. Holes may be punched, where the die is

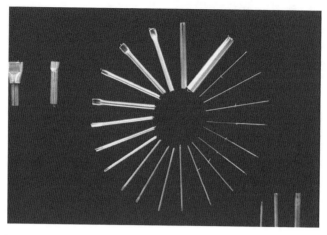

FIGURE 5.9 Assorted round and oval catheter hole punches. (Courtesy of Technical Innovations, Inc., Brazoria, TX.)

held stationary and pressed into the catheter tube, or drilled, where the die is spun and driven into the tubing. Obviously, a round punch may be used in either punching or drilling, and an oval hole punch must be used as a nonrotating punch tool (see Figure 5.9).

When punching holes, the durometer of the material has an effect on how easily and cleanly the hole can be punched. A thin, high-durometer tube will be more difficult to punch than a thicker, softer material.

SLUG EJECTION

When using a hole punch, it is important to clear the slugs or chads from the tool. If slugs build up in the tool, the cutter will have no clearance, and the tool will stop cutting. This can be done in a rudimentary way by pushing a gauge pin into the cutter, when doing a few prototypes by hand. Technical Innovations sells a pin vise with a spring-loaded ejection mechanism for low-volume hole punching by hand.

Figure 5.10 shows a hole-drilling and manual-indexing mandrel fixture. This punch holder fixture was sized to fit into a collet in a Bridgeport-style mill. The free-spinning disc allows the chads to be ejected without stopping the mill. One thing to note is the slow speed at which the punch rotates. Higher speeds tend to cause excessive friction and melt the plastic, making a rough hole. In this setup, the mill was run at about 850 to 1,000 revolutions per minute (rpm) to achieve good results.

AUTOMATED HOLE PUNCHING

Automated drilling and skiving setups are shown in Figures 5.11 to 5.13. Catheter tubing is held in a collet and rotated using programmable rotary and linear motion control. This allows the precise and repeatable punching of catheter tubes, even ones of very small diameter and hole size, as shown.

Catheter-Forming Equipment and Operations

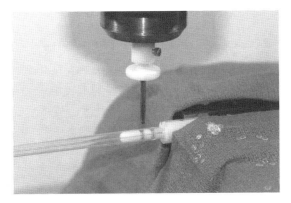

FIGURE 5.10 Hole-punching fixture with indexing and slug ejection mechanism. (T. Kucklick, Kucklick Design)

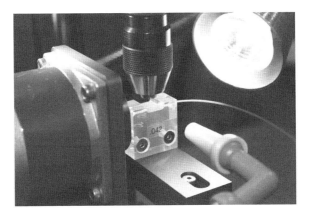

FIGURE 5.11 Small-hole (0.042-inch) automated hole-drilling setup. (Courtesy of Technical Innovations, Inc., Brazoria, TX.)

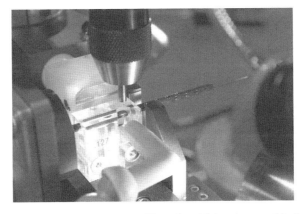

FIGURE 5.12 Automated skiving setup. Note the skiving support block. (Courtesy of Technical Innovations, Inc., Brazoria, TX.)

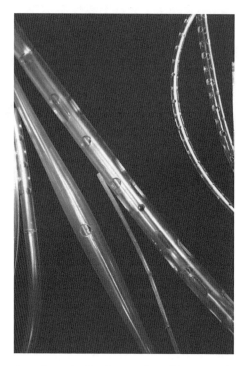

FIGURE 5.13 Examples of punched catheter tubes. (Courtesy of Technical Innovations, Inc., Brazoria, TX.)

BALLOON DIP MOLDS

Another way to form balloons and shapes is with dip molds. Bullet-shaped forms are quite simple to achieve with dip molds. One of the limitations for dip molding a double-necked balloon is the stretch factor of the material. For example, if the

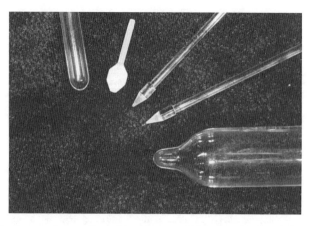

FIGURE 5.14 Assorted glass dip molds. (Courtesy FSG, Inc., Grass Valley, CA.)

material has a 300 percent stretch factor, or elongation to break, then the balloon cannot be more than 300 percent larger than the balloon necks. This can be overcome by building the balloon in two sections, and then bonding the halves together.

Dip molds are also simple to make from polished brass, aluminum, or stainless steel on a lathe (see Figure 5.14). When making a dip mold, ensure that there are no gaps in the mold, such as testing the mold made from a bulb-shaped part by inserting a rod. The seam where the rod goes into the bulb is a place for air bubbles to form. It is better to machine the mold of one piece of material. Dip-molding materials include latex, polyisoprene, nitrile, urethanes, silicones, and plastisol materials. Dip molds are useful for producing sheaths, condoms, gloves, balloons, bumpers, and numerous other elastomeric parts.

CONCLUSION

Catheter-making tools and equipment offer versatile capabilities to the medical device designer. Some of these pieces of equipment have only been widely available for a little over 10 years. Not that long ago, these types of capabilities had to be developed in-house from scratch, at significant expense, and some were closely guarded trade secrets. There is more capability and technology for developing innovative medical devices available off the shelf now than ever before. Processes that were once hand operations, and highly operator dependent, are being automated with programmable logic control, improving throughput, yield, and consistency. The tools and capabilities available to the imaginative engineer and designer to develop innovative medical devices have never been better.

RESOURCES

VENDORS: HOT-AIR STATIONS AND AUTOMATED CATHETER MANUFACTURING EQUIPMENT

Beahm Designs
568 Division Street
Campbell, CA 95008
Phone: 408-871-2351
Fax: 408-871-8295
http://www.beahmdesigns.com

Farlow's Scientific Glassblowing
200 Litton Drive #234
Grass Valley, CA 95945
Phone: 800-474-5513
http://www.farlowsci.com

Technical Innovations
20714 Highway 36
Brazoria, TX 77422

Phone: 979-798-9426
Fax: 979-798-9428
http://www.catheterholes.com

ACKNOWLEDGMENTS

The assistance of Brian and Anita Beahm (Beahm Designs); Gary Farlow, Ralph Joiner, and Bobbie O'Brien (Farlow's Scientific Glassblowing); and Gail Brinson and Scott Thompson (Technical Innovations) in the preparation of this chapter is gratefully acknowledged.

6 Basics of Catheter Assembly

Theodore R. Kucklick

CONTENTS

How This Catheter Is Built	108
Forming the Distal Tip Assembly	110
Other Ways to Tip a Catheter	111
Joining the Distal Tip Assembly and the Proximal Shaft	112
Punching the Air Hole for Balloon Inflation	112
Attaching the Proximal Luer Fitting	113
Attaching the Balloon to the Catheter Shaft Assembly	114
Assembling the Proximal Steering Hub	116
Glossary of Catheter Terms	118
Resources	123
References: Angioplasty	123
Vendors: Adhesives	123
Vendors: Luer Fittings	123
Vendors: Participating in the Relay Catheter	123
Vendors: Small-Gauge Wire for Pull Wires	124
Acknowledgments	124
Endnotes	124

Catheters are one of the more common medical devices. A catheter is a flexible tubular device inserted into a vessel, duct, body cavity, or hollow organ. This device is used in the introduction or withdrawal of fluids, delivery of energy, placement of a balloon, or placement of a device or biologic to the body. The device may be steerable to navigate through curved or branching structures. The catheter may also contain electronic sensors.

At a recent industry conference, an executive research and development (R&D) manager of a major medical device company outlined the company's vision for delivery therapies via the "vascular highway." He stated that nearly every structure in the body is accessible by this route. This means that there are significant future opportunities available for innovative catheter design in less invasive therapy.

Catheters have been at the foundation of the revolution in minimally invasive and less-invasive therapy. Advances in plastics, metals, electronics, sensors, and innovative construction techniques have produced catheters of unprecedented capability.

Some of the largest medical device companies (e.g., Boston Scientific and Guidant) were founded on catheter products.

This chapter will present an example study of building a generic deflectable balloon catheter. In this example, you will see some of the basic parts of a balloon catheter, manufacturing methods of the components, and basic assembly techniques and equipment. One of the most basic pieces of equipment is the hot-air station, which is described in Chapter 5. Common adhesive bonding materials will be described. The end of the chapter includes a glossary of common catheter types.

The example for this chapter will be a basic steerable catheter, the relay catheter, which was a demonstration piece for the annual Beahm Designs medical device technology open house, held in Santa Clara, CA. The device was named after the show at which it was built, in relay fashion from one vendor's booth to the other, while onlookers watched. *The Medical Device R&D Handbook* gratefully acknowledges the support of Venture Manufacturing, Santa Clara, CA, and all of the vendors who participated in the relay catheter for their assistance with this chapter.

This demonstration catheter serves as a valuable introduction to a number of catheter-building concepts. This demonstration includes examples of heat bonding of different durometer catheter shafts, tipping, and anchoring of a pull wire at the distal tip, and some basic principles of building a steerable catheter. Tools such as the hot-air box and tipping dies are demonstrated. Another important method in catheter building is also demonstrated: the use of shrink tubing to form heat-bonded joints.

Another feature of this demonstration piece is that many of the items to build this device are readily available, and some are even off-the-shelf components. Knowing what can be acquired quickly and inexpensively is a key skill of the R&D technician, as this will allow for the rapid iteration of prototypes, consume the least amount of scarce and expensive capital money, and quickly converge on a usable solution.

HOW THIS CATHETER IS BUILT

This catheter demonstrates some of the inner workings of a simple deflectable catheter that would not be obvious to someone who has not seen the device assembled. The distal catheter shaft is a soft 30 Shore D Pebax material, and the proximal shaft is a stiffer 72D Pebax (see Figure 6.1).

One of the things that is most notable about catheter building, especially when seeing it for the first time, is how much touch and art are involved. Some of the features of the device are rather small and tricky to get right the first time. In an R&D environment, it can be very helpful to have the assistance of an experienced medical device assembler. This technician can be a valuable resource and partner with the designer to build the device for assembly from the beginning. It is one thing to hand-build a one-off device; however, it is another matter to build 5 or 10 devices that are reliable and consistent, and yet another to scale up to make devices in the hundreds or thousands. Getting the input of a skilled and knowledgeable assembler will help the engineer design devices that are of higher quality, reliable, and consistent, with good yields and without unnecessary labor content. These assemblers often know efficient ways to put a device together that the engineer may not know.

Basics of Catheter Assembly

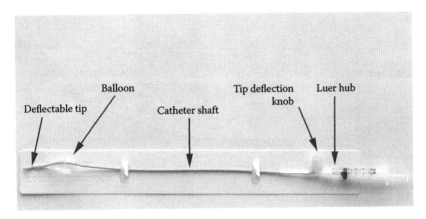

FIGURE 6.1 Parts of the relay catheter.

This catheter consists of a proximal luer fitting to inflate the balloon and an integrated screw mechanism to actuate a pull wire to deflect the tip section. In this demo unit this feature is insert molded to the catheter shaft, meaning that the catheter shaft is placed into an injection mold, and the hub is injection-molded around it. This allows the hub to be fused to the catheter shaft without adhesives. This is a useful method for higher production numbers; however, an off-the-shelf proximal hub may just as easily be bonded to the catheter shaft by either thermal bonding, cyanoacrylate, or ultraviolet (UV) cure adhesive.

The joint between the luer hub and the catheter shaft is covered with heat-shrink tubing. This is to provide a strain relief between the hub and the shaft, to prevent the shaft from kinking.

This deflectable catheter operates by having a proximal shaft that is relatively stiff, and a softer distal tip. A small-gauge stainless steel pull wire runs the length of the shaft to provide pulling force to the tip and deflect the catheter. The catheter shafts are a standard two-lumen design, with a small lumen for the pull wire and a larger lumen to pass air to inflate the balloon. Both the softer and stiffer shafts have the same extrusion profile. The catheter diameter is 8F (8 French, 2.7 mm, or 0.105 inches).

The method shown in the example makes a catheter tip that deflects in one direction. Other ways to make a steerable catheter are as follows. If the catheter is to steer in two or more axes, the extrusion profile will have two wire lumens 180 degrees apart, with the larger lumen in the center. These wires are anchored in the tip, and to get bidirectional steering, the wires are connected to a bell-crank mechanism in the handle (see Figure 6.2). A lever bends the tip in its two directions of deflection. This may be expanded to allow four axes of deflection, if wires are placed at the 12:00, 3:00, 6:00, and 9:00 positions in the catheter shaft, and connected to two bell-crank actuators at 90 degrees to one another. Gastroscopes and sigmoidoscopes have this type of four-way steering. This type of mechanism makes the catheter more versatile; however, it also makes it larger as well as more complex and expensive to build. This may be justified for a reusable endoscope costing thousands of dollars, but it is difficult to justify in a single-use device. It is often just as simple to torque a device to turn the catheter tip as to make a more complex four-way steering device.

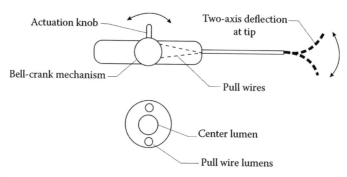

FIGURE 6.2 Two-axis steerable catheter and handle.

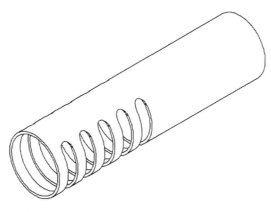

FIGURE 6.3 A vertebrated tube for flexibility.

Another way to make a flexible tip on a catheter is by means of a vertebrated section (see Figure 6.3). As the name implies, a tube of metal or plastic is notched to produce a series of rings, leaving a spine of material. This vertebrated tube is then covered with a flexible elastomeric sheath. The spine may be made of the remaining material in the tube, or it may be a piece of flat metal or wire spot-welded to a series of rings.

FORMING THE DISTAL TIP ASSEMBLY

The distal tip assembly is formed with a bullet-shaped glass mold. These molds are described in detail in Chapter 5 on the use of the hot-air station and glass molds.

First, a wire is cut to the length of the catheter. A piece of small-diameter polyethylene (PET) tube liner, cut to the length of the distal shaft plus about a 0.5 inch, is then slipped over the wire. This liner will allow the wire to operate freely, and provide a bridge piece between the soft distal shaft and the stiffer proximal shaft when they are heat bonded together.

To form the anchor for the pull wire, the wire is bent back 180 degrees in a hook, about 0.125 inch (see Figure 6.4). This is then pulled back until the wire hooks into the large lumen of the extruded tubing. Next, this assembly is pushed into a heated

Basics of Catheter Assembly

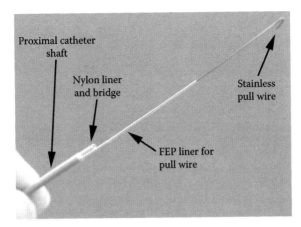

FIGURE 6.4 Pull wire and liver tubes of the catheter.

mold and heated to the melt temperature of the plastic. This forms a bullet tip on the end of the distal end of the catheter and melts the plastic around the wire, anchoring it in place. Fine stainless steel wire is available from Small Parts, Inc. (Miami Lakes, FL).

OTHER WAYS TO TIP A CATHETER

In this example, a custom-made glass mold is used to form the catheter tip. This was the best solution given the number of devices that needed to be built. You, however, may find yourself at the workbench late some afternoon or evening and need to put a tip on a catheter for an in vitro prototype. What do you do then?

One way to make a tipping die is to fabricate one out of brass or aluminum on a lathe. Drill out a metal rod to the diameter of the catheter tube with a plus tolerance for clearance. Grind a drill bit (hopefully an old dull one) to the shape of the tip you need and grind a cutting edge on this tool. You can do this with the shank end of the drill if you cannot afford to destroy the drill. Use this as a form tool to carefully bore out the tip shape in the metal rod. Machine the metal rod so that the wall thickness is about 0.125 inch for better heat transfer. Prime the tool with mold release, heat it to the transition temperature, push the catheter tube in until you feel that a tip has formed, cool the mold, and pull out your (hopefully) acceptably formed tip. One disadvantage over a glass mold is that you do not see the tip forming and need to do it more by feel. If you are really short on tools (you do not have a temperature-controlled hot-air station), an adjustable heat gun can work. With some trial and error and a barbeque thermometer that reads up to 500°F, you can calibrate your heat gun and get acceptable R&D or proof-of-concept-level results. Another way to form a tip is with a plastic tip die. A Teflon rod can make a tipping die; however, it can be difficult to heat.

A tip can also be formed with a piece of thick silicone tubing that is just large enough to stretch over your catheter tube. Heat the tip of the tube. The silicone will not melt; however, the plastic inside the tube will soften and melt. Work the catheter tubing until the silicone tube squeezes down and melts the end of the tube closed. No mold release is needed, as the catheter plastic will not stick to the silicone. The plastic will flow more as you heat the distal end of the tube, and the temperature gradient from the tip back will produce a taper. If you need to keep an open lumen, use a piece of clean piano wire coated with mold release as a mandrel. (Pam® no-stick cooking spray works in a pinch, again for in vitro prototype or bench testing only.) With some practice and the right size silicone tube, you can form an acceptable tapered tip with this method. One last way to form a rudimentary tip is to heat the plastic and (carefully, without burning your fingers) roll it between your thumb and forefinger until you get an acceptable tip.

JOINING THE DISTAL TIP ASSEMBLY AND THE PROXIMAL SHAFT

Once the pull wire and liner have been installed to the distal tip, and the tip has been formed, the distal tip assembly is ready to be joined to the catheter shaft. This is done with fluorinated ethylene propylene (FEP) shrink tubing. FEP tubing, being a fluoropolymer, is far more heat resistant than Pebax, and the melted catheter shaft material does not stick to it.

Purchase an FEP shrink tube that, when shrunk, recovers down to the diameter of the catheter shaft. The FEP shrink tube acts as a mold, allowing a butt weld between the distal and proximal catheter shafts, and pulls the shafts together as the tube shrinks lengthwise. As the FEP shrinks it squeezes the melted Pebax ends together to form a joint. Because the shrink tube recovers to the diameter of the catheter shaft, the joint is smooth and clean. Here you can see why the liner tubes are important. Without the liner tubes, the plastic would melt and close off the catheter lumens, and the catheter would not function. The FEP liner for the pull wire and the nylon liner and bridge are essential parts to make this device work. Once the joint is formed, the FEP tubing is carefully cut off.

Using the nylon liner is actually a shortcut in constructing this particular catheter. It is a way to perform this joining operation without special tooling. Normally, catheter lumens are held open during joining operations with wire mandrels, ground to size, and coated with nonsticking polytetrafluoroethylene (PTFE) or parylene. These wires are removed after the joining operation, leaving a clean open lumen at the joint. The mandrel acts as a mold core. Another way to form a butt joint is with a tubular glass mold instead of the FEP shrink. With the glass mold method, a closely fitted mold is heated, and the catheter shafts are pressed together inside to form the joint. One of the advantages to the FEP shrink tube method is that the tube clamps down evenly on the tube while welding and forms a very smooth and consistent joint (see Figures 6.5 and 6.6).

PUNCHING THE AIR HOLE FOR BALLOON INFLATION

Typically, holes are punched in catheter tubes with a sharpened tubular punch. These punches are available from Technical Innovations (Brazoria, TX). Another simple way to make a hole in catheter tubing is to skive a small notch into the tube with a sharp razor blade. (Drilling is punching a hole perpendicular to the tube; skiving is slicing off a notch at a 90-degree angle across the tube.) This is a simple way to get a hole in a catheter tube when prototyping.

Basics of Catheter Assembly

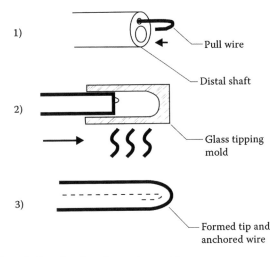

FIGURE 6.5 Steps in forming the wire anchor and tip.

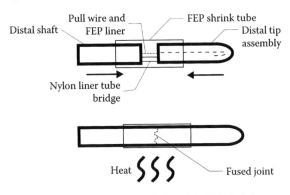

FIGURE 6.6 Fusing the proximal and distal shafts with FEP shrink.

Neither of these methods, however, was used to make the small air hole in the catheter to inflate the balloon. In this case, the hole was made with a clean, pointed, hot soldering iron tip. This method is a convenient way to make a small, clean hole in catheter tubing, quickly and consistently, without tooling.

ATTACHING THE PROXIMAL LUER FITTING

In this example, a custom luer fitting was insert molded to the proximal end of the catheter. Typically, an off-the-shelf Y connector or some other fitting is glued to the catheter shaft. Standard luer fittings are available from a number of vendors, including Quosina, Merit, Value Plastics, Brevet, B Braun, and several others. Quosina (http://www.quosina.com) is a handy resource for all types of medical fittings. It carries a wide variety of fittings and accessories from several manufacturers and has very reasonable minimum order requirements. Many times when building prototypes, a luer fitting with the exact diameter needed is not available off the shelf. In this case, these standard fittings are often drilled out or modified to meet the need at the moment.

Another trick to fit a larger tube to a smaller hole is this: Say you have a slightly oversize tube and a fitting that you cannot or do not want to drill out. If possible, heat the catheter tube until is slightly soft, and pull carefully, like taffy. This will stretch the tube, reducing the cross-sectional diameter. If you pull the tubing until it stretches and breaks, you now have a tapered tube; you can slice it off with a razor blade at the desired diameter. This may not work all the time, but it is a useful trick in a pinch.

Usually the adhesive of choice for this application is a UV cure adhesive (made by Loctite, Inc., or Dymax, Inc.). Other adhesives like cyanoacrylates and epoxy can be used, but in this application, UV cure is the most versatile.

To use UV cure adhesive, the fitting must be clear to allow the passage of UV light, and you must have a UV light source. These light sources can be expensive (around $1,000 for a low-end model), but they are very useful accessories to have if you are doing a lot of catheter prototyping and assembly. Newer light-emitting diode (LED)-based curing wands from Loctite may offer an economical alternative to lamp-based spot-curing wand systems. Another economical alternative is a used UV light source originally designed for curing dental composites.

UV adhesives are versatile and ubiquitous in medical device manufacturing. They are used for everything from gluing together oxygen masks to gluing hypodermic needles to luer hubs. UV cure adhesives are also used widely in the electronics industry. There are numerous types and grades of UV adhesives to bond nearly any material, where at least one is transparent to allow the passage of UV light. UV cure adhesives have excellent gap filling and solidify as soon as they are exposed to UV. The Dymax and Loctite websites have excellent information on how to choose the right adhesive for bonding your combination of materials.

It is important to design a part to be UV bonded so that UV light completely illuminates the adhesive. If any adhesive is in a shaded area, it will not cure. Also, even though a material may be transparent to visible light, this does not mean it is transparent to UV. Most clear materials are, such as acrylic, styrene, and polycarbonate. A notable exception is polyimide tubing, which is amber colored and transparent to visible light but opaque to UV. A glue joint that is under a polyimide tube will not cure under UV light.

It is important to use proper eye protection with UV cure systems. Use the eye protection provided by the manufacturer. *Exposure to high-intensity UV can cause permanent eye damage.*

Once the luer fitting is bonded to the catheter shaft, the joint is then covered with a length of standard polyolefin heat shrink tube. This is done to provide a strain relief between the catheter shaft and the luer fitting.

ATTACHING THE BALLOON TO THE CATHETER SHAFT ASSEMBLY

The catheter is now ready for the attachment of the balloon. The balloon in this example is an off-the-shelf item available from Advanced Polymers (Salem, NH). The balloon for this example is a polyurethane balloon that is heat bonded to the Pebax catheter shaft.

To accomplish the heat bonding of the balloon neck to the tube as shown in Figure 6.7, a close-fitting PET heat shrink tube from Advanced Polymers is used.

Basics of Catheter Assembly

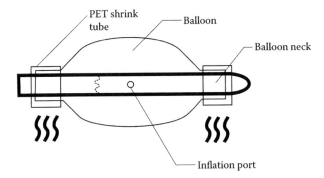

FIGURE 6.7 Balloon bonding with shrink tube schematic.

It is slipped over the balloon neck, and the assembly is heated. The shrink tube clamps down on the balloon neck, and the balloon neck fuses to the catheter shaft. When the balloon bonding is complete, the PET tubing is carefully cut away, as it does not bond to the materials used. A custom clamshell mold of this kind, as pictured in Figure 6.8, is not a necessity; however, if a hot-air box heater jaw is to be used, the operation must be done very carefully to prevent damage to the catheter assembly.

In this example, a special clamshell mold is used to localize the heat and prevent damage to the thin balloon material.

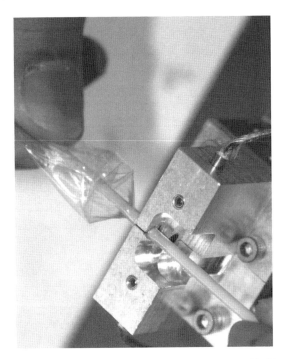

FIGURE 6.8 Balloon bonding using a custom-heated clamshell mold. (Courtesy of Venture Manufacturing, Santa Clara, CA.)

ASSEMBLING THE PROXIMAL STEERING HUB

In this example, a compact, simple, and effective steering mechanism is used. The steering mechanism is a lead screw that when unscrewed pulls on the stainless steel wire and bends the distal catheter tip. The actuation anchor on the wire is a small steel bearing, drilled with a hole, soldered to the pull wire with silver solder. This bead sits in a cone-shaped pocket at the top of the screw mechanism. Figures 6.9 to 6.12 show the construction and assembly of the steering hub.

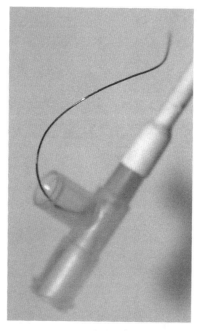

FIGURE 6.9 Pull wire and luer hub.

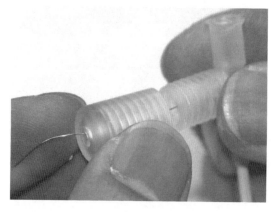

FIGURE 6.10 Assembling lead screw pull mechanism.

Basics of Catheter Assembly

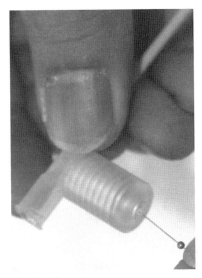

FIGURE 6.11 Fitting bearing bead to wire.

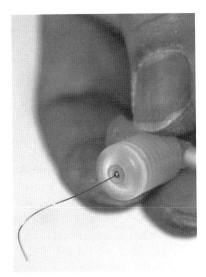

FIGURE 6.12 Soldering wire to bearing bead. Wire is trimmed, and cap glued over bearing.

This is an example of a generic catheter with rudimentary tip-steering and balloon capabilities. For the designer, several approaches are apparent to make the catheter easy to build.

This example shows how much may be done with simple tools and off-the-shelf components. The extrusions, both for the catheter shaft and for the liners and shrink tubes for assembly, must be custom ordered. For any particular catheter of this type, the sizes of the tubing must be carefully matched to produce a useable device.

Figure 6.13 shows is a fixture for trimming the shrink tube from the catheter when done.

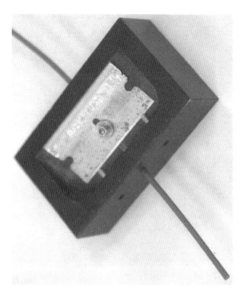

FIGURE 6.13 Fixture for slicing shrink tube from a catheter assembly. (Courtesy of Venture Manufacturing, Santa Clara, CA.)

GLOSSARY OF CATHETER TERMS

Acorn tip catheter: A catheter with a cone-shaped knob at the distal end to occlude the urethra when delivering contrast.

Amplatz catheter: A type of J-shaped guiding catheter to direct a cardiac catheter through the aortic arch and into a coronary artery. Also used in urology and other applications. Named for Kurt Amplatz, pioneer in radiology and development of guidewires.

Angiography catheter: A cardiac catheter for injecting contrast dye into the heart for an angiogram, a radiologic study of the blood flow in the heart that looks for blockages.

Atherectomy catheter: A device that cuts atherosclerotic plaque from the arteries, as opposed to squeezing it out of the way as with an angioplasty catheter.

Balloon catheter: A catheter with an expandable device affixed to a catheter for the purpose of either anchoring a catheter in place (Foley catheter), expanding and dilating a vessel (angioplasty catheter), occluding a vessel, or pulling out a thrombus (Fogarty catheter).

Bonding (heat): The method of assembling catheter parts together by welding or fusing, as opposed to bonding with adhesives.

Bougie tip: A soft, flexible tip at the end of a stiffer catheter to facilitate the passage of a catheter into a tubular structure. Usually cylindrical or conical. From the French word for a wax candle. Often used for dilating strictures. Specialized types are the Hurst and Maloney bougies. A wax bougie is used to detect calcific stones in the urethra, which scratch the surface of this bougie. A flexible bougie tip can help a device find its path through a passage without dissection, such as passing a stiff catheter tube into the esophagus.

Bozeman–Fritsch: A curved two-channel urinary catheter with fenestrations at the tip.

Braasch catheter: A bulb-tipped catheter for dilation.

Braid: A woven material thermally bonded to the surface of a catheter to increase its resistance to kinking and collapsing. A reinforcement structure to produce a composite structure with a plastic catheter. Braid is typically a woven tube of stainless steel wire.

Brush catheter: A catheter with a stiff bristled brush at the distal tip for collecting cell or biopsy samples.

Catheter: A tubular instrument. From Greek *katheter*, *kathemi*, to send down.

Catheter drill, punch: A sharpened tube for punching holes in catheter material.

Central venous catheter: A catheter inserted into a peripheral vein and placed into the thoracic vena cava.

Compliance: The tendency or resistance of a balloon to expand into a sphere. A compliant balloon is elastic and, when inflated, will eventually blow up into a sphere. A noncompliant balloon is not elastic and will inflate to a predetermined shape. An example of a compliant balloon is a latex Foley balloon. An example of a noncompliant balloon is an angioplasty balloon that is sized to expand only to the size of the vessel to be dilated, and no more, to prevent dissection of the vessel. Radiation cross-linking of balloon plastics is often used to produce a noncompliant balloon.

Coude: A bend in a catheter. A bicoudate catheter has two bends, or elbows.

Cyanoacrylate adhesive: A versatile fast-setting acrylic-based adhesive commonly used in medical device assembly (also known as Krazy Glue®).

dePezzer: A self-retaining catheter with a bulb on the end.

Dotter, Charles: Dotter is considered the father of interventional radiology. Brilliant, energetic, and unconventional, he was nicknamed Crazy Charlie by colleagues. He is credited with such far-reaching and fundamental innovations as the use of x-ray roll film for angiography and the first percutaneous transluminal angioplasty (nicknamed Dottering), in which stenoses were dilated with catheters. Dotter also developed the double-lumen balloon catheter, the safety guidewire, and the J-tipped guidewire. He was the first to experiment with self-expanding nitinol coiled stents. One of his students was Melvin P. Judkins, developer of the Judkins guiding catheters. He worked with Andreas Gruentzig and was instrumental in his success in developing balloon angioplasty. He also worked with Bill Cook to develop innovative new catheter designs.[1]

Drainage catheter: A tube for draining fluid from a body cavity.

Drew–Smythe catheter: A device for puncturing the amniotic sac for the purpose of inducing labor.

Electophysiology (EP) catheter: A device for delivering radio frequency energy to the heart for thermal ablation to interrupt aberrant cardiac heartbeat electrical signals.

Extrusion: A method of producing catheter tubing by squeezing melted plastic through a shaped die. Virtually any cross section and configuration of lumens is possible.

Fenestrations: Holes or openings. From Latin for "a window."

Flaring: Forming a flange on the end of a catheter tube with a heated cone-shaped die.

Fluorinated ethylene propylene (FEP): A fluoropolymer used in a type of heat shrink tubing, especially useful in catheter construction.

Fogarty catheter: The eponymously named embolectomy balloon catheter, which is advanced past a clot and inflated, then withdrawn to remove the clot. Invented by innovator, vascular surgeon, and noted medical device industry entrepreneur, Thomas J. Fogarty, MD.[2,3]

Foley catheter: A urinary catheter with a balloon at the distal tip to provide retention in the bladder.[4]

Forssmann, Werner: Forssmann was the first person to demonstrate cardiac catheterization in Eberswald, Germany, in 1929. Because the procedure was considered especially risky, he performed it on himself, injecting contrast into his own heart through a catheter inserted into his arm, while an assistant operated a fluoroscope. Despite his repeated demonstrations of the safety and usefulness of the method, Forssmann was scorned as an eccentric. He switched specialties to urology and became a country doctor. The importance of his work was at last recognized in a shared Nobel Prize in 1956.

French (catheter scale): Catheters are most often measured according to the French catheter scale. A French is a unit of linear measure: 1 French is equal to 0.33 millimeter. French size measures the circumference, not the diameter, of a catheter, for example, 3 Fr = 3 mm circumference and approximately 1 mm diameter. The French size, for example, is not the diameter of a catheter with an oval cross section at its widest point. The name and the symbol Ch refer to the Charrière gauge scale, which is often called the French scale.[5] This makes the French scale useful for measuring catheters that are not round. French size is abbreviated Fr. French is usually used when describing the diameter of flexible catheters, or larger tubes. On medical packaging French is often abbreviated F (e.g., 10F).

Gouley's catheter: A curved instrument with a groove on the lesser curvature to slide over a guidewire. Inserted into a urethra to dilate strictures.

Gruentzig, Andreas: Pioneering figure in balloon angioplasty. Born in Dresden, Germany, he worked at the University Hospital in Zurich, Switzerland. After learning of the work of Charles Dotter, he set out to expand on Charles's work by adding a balloon to a dilating catheter. He built many early prototypes in his own kitchen, building the first balloon catheter device in 1975.[6] Gruentzig performed the first coronary balloon angioplasty on a patient in 1976. His meticulous work and superior presentation skills helped to shepherd this new technology through the intense scrutiny and skepticism of practicing cardiologists. The technology of balloon angioplasty spawned a revolution in minimally invasive alternatives to open surgery, and a major Silicon Valley success story, Advanced Cardiovascular Systems (ACS, now a division of Guidant). Andreas Gruentzig died in a plane crash in 1985.

Guidewire: A flexible wire, usually of stainless steel. This wire often has a lubricious coating of PTFE fluoropolymer and an atraumatic soft-coiled wire tip.

Basics of Catheter Assembly

The guidewire is placed into a blood vessel; a catheter slides over this wire to the target location. This is called the over-the-wire technique, and was pioneered by John Simpson, MD.

Guiding catheter: A stiffer catheter tube that guides another, more flexible catheter into place. Examples of these are Judkins catheters and the Amplatz catheter.

Hemostasis valve: A type of valve that allows the passage of a guidewire through an elastomeric bushing. A screw mechanism squeezes the bushing against the guidewire, forming a blood-tight seal, while allowing advancement of the guidewire. A type of Tuohy–Borst valve.

Hub: Generally, the round proximal end of a catheter.

Hydrophillic: A coating or material that absorbs water.

Hydrophobic: A coating or material that repels water.

Indwelling catheter: A catheter left in place for a long period. It is specially designed to prevent infection and irritation. An old term for an indwelling urinary catheter is *catheter à demeure*.

Introducer: A shorter sheath that allows the easier entry of a longer catheter. A catheter that forms an entry port in tissue.

Judkins catheter: A preformed guiding catheter for accessing the coronary arteries. Named for Melvin P. Judkins, who developed the femoral artery access method of cardiac catheterization.[7]

Luer fitting: A 6-degree taper fluid fitting originally developed by Otto Luer. Later Fairleigh Dickinson added a lead screw sleeve, inventing the Luer-Lok™ fitting.

Manifold: A rack of stopcock valves to control a plurality of fluid sources.

Olive tipped: A catheter with a bulbous end in the form of a prolate spheroid (olive).

Pacing catheter: A cardiac catheter with electrical leads at the tip to provide a pacing signal to the heart.

Pebax: Polyether block amide. A versatile plastic common in catheter construction.

Pushability: The ability of a catheter to be pushed into a long vessel without excessive frictional resistance or without collapsing. Pushability is enhanced by the columnar strength of the catheter shaft and its lubricity, or slipperiness.

Seldinger technique: Named for Sven-Ivar Seldinger, Swedish radiologist, this is a method for percutaneous puncture and catheterization of the arterial system. This method involves puncturing the femoral artery with a needle and stylet set, and verifying location in the vessel from spurting blood. A guidewire is inserted through the needle, the needle is withdrawn, and a catheter is advanced over the guidewire. This method made possible quick and simple transfemoral arterial access, without the invasive cut-down techniques used previously. This is the access method used for nearly all vascular catheter interventions.

Simpson, John: Cardiologist, learned of balloon angioplasty from Andreas Gruentzig. Developed the over-the-wire angioplasty system. Helped to commercialize, develop, and improve the technology as a founder of Advanced Cardiovascular Systems (now Guidant).

Sones, Mason: Performed the first selective coronary angiography at the Cleveland Clinic, Cleveland, OH. Conventional wisdom taught that the insertion of a catheter into a coronary artery would result in immediate and fatal cardiac arrest. Sones accidentally slipped a catheter into a coronary artery, injected contrast, and was able to image the artery, without ill-effect to the patient. Sones then developed and perfected this technique. Selective angiography is now a routine and vital diagnostic procedure.

Steerable catheter: A catheter with a pull wire deflectable tip.

Stent: A metal mesh tube expanded to prop open a blood vessel or duct. Julio Palmaz and Richard Schatz are credited with the first modern, approved coronary stent. Drug-eluting stents (e.g., Boston Scientific Taxus™) have achieved blockbuster status.

Stent delivery catheter: A balloon catheter specifically designed to place and expand a stent.

Stopcock: A small valve for the control of fluids or gasses. Available in either reusable metal or disposable plastic versions. For medical use, the ports are configured with male or female luer fittings.

Swan–Ganz: H. J. C. Swan and William Ganz invented the balloon-tipped, flow-directed pulmonary artery catheter in 1970. The Swan–Ganz catheter made possible simplified right-heart catheterization.

Tipping: To form a tip on a plastic catheter tube by means of heat and glass-, metal-, or heat-resistant plastic mold.

Thermodilution catheter: A catheter device that measures cardiac output by means of either injecting cold saline into the right ventricle or heating a volume of blood and recording the volume of heated or cooled liquid at the pulmonary artery.

Torqueability: An important performance characteristic of a catheter. Torqueability is the ability of a catheter to transmit twisting forces without kinking or absorbing the torsion in the catheter. Torqueability is enhanced by braid reinforcement of the catheter shaft.

Trackability: The ability of a catheter to be pushed through tortuous vasculature. A way to test for the pushability, torqueability, and trackability of a catheter is with an anatomical glass tube bench model.

Tuohy–Borst valve: A valve device developed in part by Edward Tuohy. This valve has an elastomer grommet with a central lumen in a screw compression setup. As the grommet is squeezed, it closes the center lumen. This valve is often used to pass guidewires. *See* hemostasis valve.

Ultraviolet (UV) cure adhesive: A versatile cure-on-demand adhesive commonly used in medical device assembly. Significant advantages are the adhesive's lack of volatile solvents, fast curing times, and ability to join dissimilar materials.[*]

Vertebrated catheter: A flexible catheter consisting of a notched tube with a remaining spine of material, or a series of rings joined by a strip or wire spine, and covered with an elastomeric sheath.

---

[*] For a general white paper on the use of UV light curing systems, see Chris LeConte et al., "Application Note 089" (Vanier, Quebec: EXFO, 2005), http://documents.exfo.com/appnotes/anote089-ang.pdf.

RESOURCES

REFERENCES: ANGIOPLASTY

Cohen, Burt, ed., Angioplasty.org, http://www.ptca.org. This useful website is provides historic information and catheter industry news and chronicles the past, present, and future of angioplasty and interventional radiology. It is sponsored by Boston Scientific, originally underwritten by John Abele, and supported by Richard Myler, MD.

VENDORS: ADHESIVES

Dymax, Inc.
http://www.dymax.com
Loctite, Inc.
http://www.loctite.com
Both companies make a wide range of UV cure and cyanoacryate adhesives. Both offer extensive design guides and compatibility charts to help find the right adhesive for your combination of materials.

VENDORS: LUER FITTINGS

Merit Medical Systems, Inc.
1600 West Merit Parkway
South Jordan, UT 84095
Phone: 801-253-1600
Manufactures and carries a wide range of off-the-shelf accessories specific to angioplasty, cardiology, and radiology.

Quosina
http://www.quosina.com
Every R&D engineer working on catheters should have a Quosina catalog. Nearly every plastic fitting you might need is available from them, as well as Tyvek sterilization pouches and many other component supplies.

VENDORS: PARTICIPATING IN THE RELAY CATHETER

Advanced Polymers
Salem, NH
Shrink tube and balloon

Beahm Designs
Campbell, CA
Hot-air station

Centerline Precision
San Jose, CA
Steering hub insert molding

Extrusioneering, Inc.
Temecula, CA
Catheter tubing

Farlow's Glassblowing
Grass Valley, CA
Tip mold

Peridot
Pleasanton, CA
Wire mount

Vendors: Small-Gauge Wire for Pull Wires

Small Parts, Inc.
13980 NW 58th Court
P.O. Box 4650
Miami Lakes, FL 33014-0650
Phone: 800-220-4242
Every R&D engineer should have a copy of the Small Parts, Inc., catalog.

ACKNOWLEDGMENTS

The kind assistance of Eric Lowe, Karl Im, and Marlone Legaspi of Venture Manufacturing, Santa Clara, CA, is gratefully acknowledged.

ENDNOTES

1. Misty M. Payne of the Oregon Health Sciences University, Portland, OR, has written an excellent biography of Dotter. See Misty M. Payne, "Charles Theodore Dotter: The Father of Intervention," *Texas Heart Institute Journal* 28, no. 1 (2001): 28–38, http://www.pubmedcentral.nih.gov/articlerender.fcgi?tool=pubmed&pubmedid=11330737. This article gives a picture of this remarkable innovator, his visionary contributions, and the institutional inertia he had to overcome. This full text of this article is available free from PubMed.
2. "Before earning his MD in 1960 from the University of Cincinnati Medical School, Fogarty had designed his most significant invention. The Fogarty Balloon Embolectomy Catheter is, like many revolutionary inventions, simple in concept. It is a catheter (hollow tube) about the width of a pencil, with a small balloon at its tip: the catheter is inserted through an incision into a blood vessel, and pressed through an embolus (blood clot); then the balloon is inflated, so that when the catheter is extracted, the balloon drags the clot out with it. Fogarty built the prototype in his attic, attaching the fingertip of a latex surgical glove to a catheter using fly-tying techniques familiar to him from boyhood fishing expeditions. Dr. Fogarty was winner of the year 2000 Lemelson Prize for Innovation and is an inductee into the Inventor's Hall of Fame." "Inventor of the Week," Lemelson-MIT, http://web.mit.edu/invent/iow/fogarty.html, accessed August 6, 2012. Fogarty was also a resident at the University of Oregon.
3. Chapter 20, "Interview with Thomas Fogarty," November 2005, by Ted Kucklick.

4. "Ninety-five years ago, Charles Russell Bard began research for the treatment of urinary discomfort. This led to the development of the first balloon catheter in cooperation with Dr. Frederick E.B. Foley." C. R. Bard, Inc., http://www.crbard.com, accessed August 6, 2012. The first Foley catheters were sold in 1934.
5. "Joseph-Frederic-Benoit Charriere, a 19th-century Parisian maker of surgical instruments, has by virtue of his ingenuity and advanced thinking, continued to have his presence felt in medicine throughout the 20th century. His most significant accomplishment was the development of a uniform, standard gauge specifically designed for use in medical equipment such as catheters and probes. Unlike the gauge system adopted by the British for measurement of needles and intravenous catheters, Charriere's system has uniform increments between gauge sizes (one-third of a millimeter), is easily calculated in terms of its metric equivalent, and has no arbitrary upper end point. Today, in the United States, this system is commonly referred to as French (Fr) sizing. In addition to the development of the French gauge, Charriere made significant advances in ether administration, urologic and other surgical instruments, and the development of the modern syringe." K. V. Iserson, "J.-F.-B. Charriere: The Man behind the French Scale," *Journal of Emergency Medicine* 5 (1987): 545–548.
6. All of the pioneers of minimally invasive vascular interventions mentioned in this chapter: Fogarty, Sones, Judkins, and Dotter, were all skilled hands-on product developers: "And he [Andreas Gruentzig] showed me where he made his catheters in his kitchen, and I took one look at how he was making his catheters and you had to marvel at it, because he took single lumen tubing and in order to get two lumens into the catheter, he would put a sheath over the outside. The first lumen was on the inner tube and the second lumen was in that space in-between. The problem had been, if he applied suction, it would tend to collapse the outer sheath. In order to prevent that sheath from collapsing, he took a razor blade and went all the way down the catheter twice making a 'V' groove. Which is, if you've ever tried that, trickier to do than brain surgery, to say the least." John Abele, cofounder of Boston Scientific, on his memories of Andreas Gruentzig, http://www.ptca.org/videos.html Angioplasty.org, Video Library (accessed August 6, 2012).
7. "Equipped with a plastic-impregnated human heart, a roll of wire, a wire-cutter, and pliers, Dr. Judkins began creating shaping wires. When not scrubbed in his cath lab, he concentrated on bending shaping wires, using various pipes and faucets at the scrub sink to mold the wires," writes Mrs. Judkins. "He would scrutinize the shape, place the wire over a chest radiograph on the view box, contemplate, and make changes. If a shape seemed workable, he would thread a catheter over the shaping wire, immerse it in boiling water to set the shape, and experiment on the heart specimen." Society for Cardiovascular Angiography and Interventions, "Catheterization and Cardiovascular Interventions" 64:259–261 (2005) available at http://www.scai.org/SearchResults.aspx?q=judkins, accessed August 6, 2012. Notably, Judkins did not enter the cardiology specialty as a resident until he was almost 40, after a stint as a solo family physician. He went to the University of Oregon, the only program willing to take him, where he worked with Charles Dotter.

7 Rapid Prototyping for Medical Devices

Theodore R. Kucklick

CONTENTS

Overview	128
Rapid Prototype Technology	129
In-House RP versus Service Bureaus	132
RP Service Bureaus	132
Office-Based RP Machines	133
Types of Available RP Technologies	133
3D Systems: SLA®	133
Stereolithography Materials	134
Sony: SCS™	135
3D Systems: SLS™	136
Stratasys: FDM	136
Resolution and Surface Finish	137
Solidscape	138
LOM™	139
Z Corp.: Three-Dimensional Printing	139
Polyjet Objet™ Printer	140
DLP: Envisiontec® Perfactory™	141
Sintering and Direct Metal	142
RP Applications in Product Design	142
Computer Numerical Control	143
Full-Size VMC CNC Machines	146
Machinable Prototype Materials	146
Rapid Tooling and Molding	147
Which Technology Is Best?	148
File Preparation	148
Other File Formats	149
RP Cost-Saving Tips	150
Secondary Processes to RP Parts	150
Painting	150
Electroplating	150
Machining	151
Threaded Inserts	151
Installing the Inserts	151

UV Cure Sealing of Foam Parts 151
RP Casting Patterns 151
Reverse Engineering 152
Innovative Applications of RP 152
   RP and Surgical Planning 152
   RP and Training Models 153
      Molecular Modeling 153
   RP-Produced Medical Products 153
      Investment Cast Orthopedic Implants 153
   RP and RE Combined into a Product and Service 155
      Crowns in One Visit 155
   RP and Tissue Engineering 157
      Envisiontec Bioplotter 158
   RP and Pharmaceuticals 160
   RP and Analysis 160
      Programmable RP Molding 161
      Printed Food and Inkjet Proteins 161
      Direct Manufacturing Freedom of Creation 162
      Direct Manufacturing: The Center for Bits and Atoms 162
Conclusion 163
Resources 163
   References: Print and Online 163
   References: Websites 163
   References: Professional Societies 164
   References: Universities and Organizations 164
Acknowledgments 165
Endnote 165

OVERVIEW

The past decade has seen an explosion of rapid prototyping (RP), rapid tooling, and reverse engineering (reverse modeling) technologies. All of these technologies have become more readily available, less expensive, and more flexible and capable each year. RP has been widely available for less than 20 years. These technologies put exciting and unprecedented capabilities into the hands of the designer to develop, iterate, and manufacture products. In parallel with the growth of RP, computing power has grown by orders of magnitude and plummeted in price. Computer-aided design (CAD) applications that not so long ago required a $50,000 workstation running a proprietary operating system can now be run on a computer worth less than $5,000 and an inexpensive operating system (OS) with high-end graphics. Desktop replacement laptops are making this computing power portable. Affordable CAD solid modelers and high-speed Internet connections allow designers and engineers to work from any location and transmit files to in-house RP resources, or remote service bureaus, and to receive parts quickly via courier service.

   Key advantages of RP include being able to model directly from your three-dimensional data and the ability to quickly have a real part in your hands. Rapid tooling methods allow you to make preproduction, and sometimes even production, parts for testing and timely evaluation before moving to hard tooling.

Before RP, to get a part required a detailed drawing that was then interpreted by a machinist or model maker to fabricate the part. Parts were designed to fit the limitations of machine tools, further limited to what could be communicated in a dimensioned drawing. Free form and complex surface parts can now be fabricated easily. Before RP, models took days or weeks and were expensive. RP can make parts that are nearly impossible to build from a drawing, with no drawings required. Nested assemblies are also possible, in which case objects may be built inside of other objects. Direct manufacturing is even emerging as a category in which parts are built from data files, on demand, without tooling.

Rapid tooling is a growing technology that is an RP process, as applied to producing tooling used in high-volume manufacturing processes, such as injection molding. The use of RP to produce patterns used in another process to produce tooling is sometimes referred to an indirect RP process.

Reverse engineering (RE) is a broad term for a process that may include starting with a physical object and using scanning and digitizing technology to produce a three-dimensional computer model of the object for reproduction. There are many important applications for RE, such as digitizing hand-sculpted models, the production of patient-specific prosthetics, scanning and reproduction of rare or fragile medical specimens, and the generation of CAD data from parts for which CAD data are not available. Makers of digitizing equipment prefer to call this process reverse modeling rather than RE.

Together, computer numeric-controlled (CNC) machining, RP, RE, rapid tooling, and direct manufacturing are a family of highly capable and flexible tools that can get a needed part in your hands for evaluation and in some cases can even generate the final product.

As good as three-dimensional CAD has become, there is still no substitute for seeing a real part in your hands and seeing how it really looks, feels, behaves, and fits with other parts. RP has become an essential tool in product development as well as scientific visualization. RP technology is also being adapted to numerous new medical applications, such as custom prosthetics, implants, and tissue engineering.

RAPID PROTOTYPE TECHNOLOGY

There are two basic types of RP available, additive and subtractive. Additive modeling is like building a sculpture from clay, adding material until the final shape is produced. Subtractive modeling starts with a block of material, and a cutting tool removes material until the final shape is produced. This is a form of CNC machining. Roland DGA uses the term SRP™ (subtractive rapid prototyping) to describe its CNC machines and computer-aided manufacturing (CAM) systems that are optimized for prototyping, as opposed to industrial CNC for production machining.

Another term for rapid prototyping is the broader term *automated fabrication*. According to Marshall Burns, "Automated fabrication is a modern family of technologies that generate three-dimensional, solid objects under computer control."* As you can tell from this definition, RP is a subset of the larger category, that of digitally controlled fabrication technologies. Automated fabrication, especially digitally controlled additive fabrication, is still relatively new. There exists a further category of direct manufacturing and manufacture-on-demand opportunities that has only begun to be explored. This other category of RP is referred to as automated forming, in which a material is shaped and formed under computer control, without fixed tooling. Automated fabrication may include new technologies for building engineered tissue scaffolds with RP and inkjet technology. Some of these applications are described at the end of this chapter.

Another category of RP technology is the use of reverse modeling in conjunction with RP. Case examples of this are included in the chapter.

Additive object modelers work in similar ways. They assemble slices or layers of material to develop a three-dimensional object. Think of it as taking a cutting out of a series of flat paper dolls and then stacking them up to make a solid paper doll. Additive layered manufacturing methods use a variety of materials, from photoreactive polymer, to plastic melted through a nozzle, to paper cut with a laser, to powders that are hardened layer by layer, and inkjet-style modelers to produce a free-form solid object. The resolution and surface finish of the model are controlled by how each layer is laid down and by the size of line or dot used to progressively harden the build material. Each RP method has its own advantages and limitations in prototyping and development of medical devices. RP additive modelers fall into two general categories: Industrial-grade RP machines can produce high-accuracy parts, have large price tags ($75,000 to $250,000 and up), and require a special shop environment. Office-based three-dimensional printers are designed to be easy to use, can operate in an office, and are in a price range less than $40,000.

Subtractive rapid prototyping (SRP™) is a term developed by Roland DGA, a maker of third- and fourth-axis CNC milling machines, to identify it in the RP market. These machines are designed to be easy to operate by users not extensively trained as machinists. Many operations and functions, such as material setup, tool speed, and feed rates, are preprogrammed, and a tool path generation program is bundled with the machine to allow the user to perform a relatively simple setup and to allow the machine to run unattended as it produces a final CNC machined part.

In medical device product development, the RP technology used is not an end in itself. The designer needs to become familiar with the range of technologies available to make a rational decision based on the criteria important to the project. Some of these considerations and questions to ask when deciding which RP technology is appropriate are as follows:

- Do we need RP models occasionally, or do we require a large number of iterations and models?
- Do we want to have an RP machine in-house, shared between a group of designers, or will we use a service bureau?
- If we bring it in-house, what are the costs of ownership?

---

* Marshall Burns, *Automated Fabrication* (Englewood Cliffs, NJ: Prentice Hall, 1993).

Rapid Prototyping for Medical Devices 131

- Will the vendor company be able to provide good support after the sale?
- What functions do the parts need to perform?
- Do we require parts that have the mechanical properties of the final material?
- Does the model need to be of medical-grade materials?
- Are we making parts that are especially large or small?
- How much detail do we need?
- What is the smallest feature size we are trying to build?
- What surface finish do we need to have?
- Does the model require built-in colors?
- What is our manufacturing workflow?
- How does the RP technology we choose best fit into that workflow?

Keep in mind that not every RP technology one can find in the literature is commercially available. There are actually relatively few major companies in the market. Some machines that were once marketed are no longer sold, and other technologies exist as research prototypes in various stages of development. When choosing a system that meets your needs for product development, it helps to filter out the various approaches that are not readily available, and focus on the ones that are. Then, narrow that list to a short list of technologies that meet your practical needs.

If your goal is to use RP technology in an innovative way, investigating the numerous methods that are either in development or have fallen by the wayside may provide the building blocks you need to deploy RP methods in entirely new areas. New RP technologies developed in universities may be available for license. Also, as some of the earlier technologies go off-patent, they can provide platforms for innovative new medical applications. This chapter includes several examples of innovative applications of RP technology that go beyond using RP to make prototype parts.

Following are some of the representative applications of RP technology in medical device R&D:

- A painted visual model for trade shows, investor presentations, internal review, or photo shoots
- A pattern for making copies in soft tooling, for example, casting in room-temperature vulcanate (RTV) molds
- Multiple copies of a visual model
- Models for fit and clearance checks
- Models for human factors and ergonomic studies
- A model used for bench tests in which mechanical function is most important
- A prototype model that is to be used as part of an investigational device
- A model that is a master for a downstream manufacturing process such as investment casting
- A model that is large and bulky, such as an engine block or a museum model of an animal
- A model requiring very fine, jewelry-like detail, such as a small medical device
- A model that is optically clear and acts like a light pipe
- A model that is complex and would be difficult or impossible to machine

- A model that is in color and represents areas such as fluid flow patterns in a part or charged areas of a macromolecule
- Direct production of low-volume or bridge tooling
- Direct manufacturing of a difficult-to-manufacture or low-volume part
- Packaging of RP and RE technology into an innovative combination to provide a product or service
- Some types of tissue engineering

All of these applications are possible with the appropriate use of RP technology.

RP cuts steps and time out of the product development process. Iteration, the development of a product in evolutionary steps, is absolutely required for design and innovation. The more efficiently these iterations are produced, the more quickly decisions can be made to get to the next step in the process and identify the time to stop iterating and start producing. Every company, especially start-ups, has a "burn rate" and consumes money just standing still. It is imperative to pack the highest number of iterations into the shortest amount of time, with the least overhead expense. Consider also that if you are working on an important problem, you can be sure other smart people are looking at the same problem, too. RP, properly used, is a tool to stay ahead of competition, quickly reduce your concepts to practice, and boil these concepts down into marketable products fast and first. Choosing the best RP technology for your needs moves the product development process forward the fastest, at the lowest cost, and with the results that you want. RP technology is a means to an end. Starting with clear goals in mind and having a basic understanding of the capabilities of competing RP technologies can help to efficiently sort through the array of approaches and marketing claims by RP manufacturers and vendors and help you to choose the approach that best fits your business, engineering, and design needs. The RP field is evolving quickly, with new technologies and materials being introduced constantly.

This chapter gives an overview of materials and methods, as well as links to company websites. Links to websites covering the RP field in general and discussion groups are also included. These discussion groups can be important sources of information, ranging from actual users of RP machines and their capabilities and limitations in real-world use to a place to find answers to specific questions. Numerous case study examples are included, both of RP in use and innovative applications of RP.

IN-HOUSE RP VERSUS SERVICE BUREAUS

Unless a company produces a large volume of parts, has a need for on-demand prototyping, needs to keep prototyping in-house for confidentiality reasons, has specialized needs, or uses RP as part of a manufacturing process, an outside service bureau may be an appropriate option.

RP Service Bureaus

Service bureaus vary widely in their range of services and whether they offer secondary operations, finishing, and additional services. Service bureaus range from solo operators with one RP machine to full-service model shops. Some of the larger service bureaus offer several RP technologies (e.g., SLA®, FDM™, SLS™, CNC) and three-dimensional printing, all under one roof, so it becomes easier to choose the right approach for a given job.

The value of service bureaus is that they make available to you the use of machinery that would be prohibitively expensive to own as well as the assistance of skilled operators. The other value service bureaus can offer is a package of services. They can make an RP part and offer secondary operations, such as milling and drilling, light assembly, painting, RTV casting of less expensive copies in urethane, and painting. Many medical device companies do not want to bring these types of activities in-house; therefore, sending this work outside can be the most appropriate option. When looking for a service bureau, find a company that offers the right combination of services offered, price, quality, speed of delivery, and reliability.

OFFICE-BASED RP MACHINES

Some of the newer office-based RP machines are from 3D Systems (InVision™ multijet modeling [MJM]), Stratasys® (Prodigy Plus™), and Z Corporation (Z Printer 310). Some of these solutions bring in-office prototyping into a range less than $40,000. Solidscape sells its T66 model for less than $50,000, which is intended for production of smaller lost-wax investment casting masters. 3D Systems markets a similar system capable of producing wax masters, the InVision HR 3-D Printer. Roland sells its line of easy-to-use three-axis CNC milling machines from less than $4,000 to more than $25,000. These solutions make bringing RP in-house a more viable option. Your needs in terms of turnaround, part functionality, detail, surface finish, and volume of prototypes, and whether you need to do any secondary finishing operations in-house, will help determine whether an office-based three-dimensional printing solution is right for your application. Do not forget to factor in the cost of consumables, maintenance, and the cost of a sufficiently skilled person to operate the machine. When looking for an in-house RP solution, consider whether the finished part from the RP machine is as close to the finished product you want as possible. Analyze whether you save money over the long run. How soon does the machine pay for itself in your situation? Do you need to protect confidential information? Can you split the cost by pooling this resource among several design and engineering groups? Do you have an existing manufacturing workflow where an RP machine can fit? These are some of the considerations and strategies for bringing RP in-house.

TYPES OF AVAILABLE RP TECHNOLOGIES

3D SYSTEMS: SLA®

SLA is a process invented by Charles Hull and developed by 3D Systems of Valencia, CA. The acronym SLA (stereolithography apparatus) comes from the name of the company's first machine, the SLA-1, introduced in 1988 and a registered trademark of 3D Systems (http://www.3Dsystems.com). As of 2012, SLA was the most common RP system in use. Numerous service bureaus offer SLA part production, competing on price, speed of delivery, and ease of ordering. Other companies now offer similar UV laser- and photopolymer-based RP, including Sony in their Solid Creation System (SCS®) line of RP machines.

In stereolithography, a UV laser is used to trace the surface of a photoreactive polymer that hardens to produce a solid object based on a three-dimensional computer file, usually in .STL (stereolithography) format. The stereolithography process builds the object in layers, as if you were building an object of stacked pieces of paper. A base on an elevator starts at the top of a tank of plastic and drops a small amount every time a new layer is laid down, and this "grows" the part. Support structures are required to support cantilevered areas of the part. These vertical supports are removed during finishing. When completed, the part is ready to remove from the tank. The part is then placed in a postcuring oven, where it is cured under a UV lamp to harden any uncured polymer. The part will have a characteristic stair-step finish equal to the per-slice resolution of the stereolithography machine. This stair-step finish is usually removed by sandblasting the parts, giving the parts a translucent frosted finish. Stereolithography machines require a controlled and vented shop environment.

Stereolithography machines are limited in the size of parts produced by the width and depth of the liquid material vat. Larger parts may be produced by making a large part (such as large instrument housings) in smaller sections, bonding the sections together with stereolithography resin.

Stereolithography machines are expensive pieces of capital equipment and require special setup and venting, as well as trained operators. Some larger corporations with specialized or high-volume prototype requirements have chosen to bring stereolithography in-house. Most start-ups, small companies, and consulting offices find using a service bureau vendor to get stereolithography parts to be quite convenient and cost-effective.

STEREOLITHOGRAPHY MATERIALS

Common materials for stereolithography rapid prototypes include the 3D Systems Accura® resins and the DSM Somos® line of resins (http://www.dsmsomos.com). DSM offers resins with expanded materials properties, such as flexibility or clarity. Newer composite SLA materials are being developed that are loaded with ceramic fillers for added strength. Huntsman Advanced Materials (http://www.renshape.com) offers a line of specialized SLA materials, including medical-grade resins, acrylonitrile–butadiene–styrene (ABS)-like materials, and selectively colorable resins. 3D Systems recently announced its Accura Bluestone™ line of composite materials for high-heat applications.

SLA parts made from commodity prototyping resins are quite strong; however, they may fracture if overstressed, drilled, or milled. These parts can be milled and drilled with care. An advantage to the harder resins is that they are less prone to warping or sagging in thin unsupported sections, and take paint finishes very well. If snap fits are required, specify one of the flexible stereolithography resins, for example, DSM Somos. Check with your service bureau on the availability and properties of these resins.

The flexible grades are similar in properties to polypropylene; however, the parts may still break if flexed too much. Optically clear grades of stereolithography materials are also available, allowing the prototyping of light pipes and clear parts for evaluation of internal components and fluid flow tests.

SLA parts can be sensitive to heat and humidity. Thin or unsupported sections can warp and sag under heat and pressure, or from some paint solvents. Therefore, appropriate care must be taken in shipping and storing stereolithography parts.

Stereolithography parts range from clear amber in color to milky white or clear, depending on the material. The transparency of stereolithography parts can be an advantage when evaluating parts together in assemblies. Because it is a wet-build method, SLA gives one of the better surface finishes of the RP methods, with tolerances close to that of CNC machining. Feature sizes as small as 0.01 inch are achievable. The ultimate resolution depends on the beam size of the SLA machine and the step increment in the z-axis. The trade-off for more detail is slower build times, and therefore a more expensive part. Check with your vendor to find out the smallest feature its machine will produce.

Colored areas may also be built into stereolithography parts. This is often done with stereolithography models produced for surgical planning. With a colored area, the location of an area of special interest, such as nerves or tumors, may be highlighted to assist the surgeon planning an operation. To produce parts of a stereolithography model that are selectively colored, a special stereolithography material (available from Huntsman Advanced Materials) is used that contains a dye that activates at a higher energy level than that to cure the clear polymer. Two .STL files are produced, one with the normal anatomy and one with the areas of interest. The models are overlaid and run together, and the stereolithography machine is programmed to apply a higher power setting to the laser that is curing the areas of surgical interest in that file. This results in a model in which the normal anatomy is clear and the areas of interest are highlighted in pink or red.

Rapid prototyping stereolithography resins and machines are being constantly developed and improved. Visit industry websites regularly to learn of new developments in stereolithography technology. Be sure to look at the examples and applications sections to see examples of RP applied to medical device design and anatomical visualization.

At this time most stereolithography materials are not U.S. Pharmacopeia USP Class VI or medical grade. Stereolithography parts may be used for in vitro (benchtop) or preclinical testing; however, only parts fabricated from medical-grade materials are appropriate for clinical use. Huntsman Advanced Materials advertises USP Class VI resins for use in stereolithography machines (http://www.huntsman.com, http://www.renshape.com).

Another application of stereolithography technology is QuickCast™, developed by 3D Systems. In this application an SLA model is produced that is hollow inside, with a thin supporting lattice. This produces a model with as little material volume as possible, which in turn is used to produce an investment casting pattern. The SLA material burns into a small volume of ash when the ceramic shell of the investment casting mold is fired.

Sony: SCS™

SCS is a stereolithography system made by Sony Precision Technology. It is similar to 3D Systems SLA in that it uses a UV laser to draw layers. Sony uses two laser beams and makes machines to build larger-size stereolithography parts.

3D Systems: SLS™

SLS stands for selective laser sintering, a process patented by Carl Deckard in 1989 and a trademark of 3D Systems, which acquired the DTM Corporation of Austin, TX, and the SLS process in 2001. In this process a laser traces a beam onto the surface of a container of fusible powder. The laser heats the particles of powder and sinters them together into a solid section. An elevator drops by a small increment and another layer is sintered to the preceding layer. The process builds in layers, similar to stereolithography, except using dry powder instead of liquid polymer as a medium. The SLS process does not require the use of support structures as in stereolithography and fused deposition modeling (FDM), as the part is supported by the uncured powder material as it is lowered into the powder chamber.

One advantage to the SLS process is its versatility. Almost any material that can be powdered and sintered may be used to produce a part. Parts made from sintered nylon, for example, are quite tough and flexible. SLS process build materials include glass-filled rigid plastics, elastomers, and metals. Because the SLS process allows the fabrication of sintered elastomers, making prototypes of rubber parts, such as shoe soles and custom-shaped orthopedic brace padding, is possible.

Another use of the SLS process is the production of injection mold tooling and tooling inserts. The SLS process allows the production of injection mold tools with built-in conformal cooling channels.

Another example for the SLS process in medical device design is fabrication of sintered metal parts such as laparoscopic grasper jaws that model the characteristics of powdered metal injection-molded (MIM) parts. As-built SLS metal parts are green and require postcuring in a special oven to achieve full strength and density. SLS powdered metal parts may be infiltrated with bronze to increase strength and density and eliminate porosity.

SLS is an RP technology requiring specialized capital equipment and skilled operators. It is best to utilize this technology through a service bureau. The 3D Systems website provides links to a number of qualified service bureaus offering SLS part-building services.

Stratasys: FDM

FDM is a process invented by Scott Crump and developed and marketed by Stratasys corporation (http://www.stratasys.com) of Eden Prairie, MN. In this process, a thin cord of plastic material is extruded through a nozzle, and strands of molten material are deposited layer by layer to produce a final part. The process is similar to building a model with a very small hot-glue gun. Because the part is being formed in air, cantilevered sections require a supporting structure to prevent sagging. This support structure is deposited during the build process, and broken away from the part when it is completed. Another method is to make the supports using water-soluble material, which then allows the construction of complex details that are not damaged when the support material is removed. The FDM process is limited to those thermoplastic materials that may be formed into beads or cords, heated, and deposited. FDM materials are supplied by the manufacturer on preloaded spools.

Rapid Prototyping for Medical Devices

FDM material is typically lower in cost, relative to volume, than the SLA or SLS processes. FDM machines are also capable of producing parts from medical-grade materials. These materials are available in spools from the manufacturer. The most common build material is ABS plastic.

The cost of FDM machines has dropped significantly. At this time, office-based FDM RP three-dimensional printers are available in a range less than $25,000, making them affordable to have in-house at a facility that produces enough volume of models to justify the purchase price, maintenance, and consumables costs. The lower cost machines are limited in some of the features they offer, like water-soluble support deposition and the materials they can run.

RESOLUTION AND SURFACE FINISH

On the higher end machines, resolution may be one of four settings. Maximum resolution is 0.005 inch. Accuracy is ±0.005 inch on models up to 5 inches. Accuracy is ±0.0015 per inch on models greater than 5 inches. On the lower end office-based machines, maximum resolution is 0.010 inch.[*]

Surface finish is not as smooth as the wet processes like SLA or PolyJet. As-built FDM models are somewhat porous. Because FDM parts can be made of plastics like ABS, however, they may be readily sanded, primed, and painted. FDM can also produce large parts up to 23 × 23 × 19 inches in the larger machines.

FDM models can be quite robust, and made from a number of engineering plastics, including ABS, polycarbonate, and nylon. In the following example, FDM parts were used to make a surgical tool based on surgeon input. Often, a surgeon will visit with the engineer, design a product in CAD based on the surgeon's input, and have a working model ready for evaluation the next day (see Figure 7.1).

> Sofamor Danek engineers designed a ratcheting counter-torque surgical instrument using both prototyping technologies. The instrument is used to fasten set-screws to a corrective implant on a patient's vertebrae and to break off the screw heads at a preset torque level. The existing method required surgeons to use two separate tools, working them in opposing directions, using both hands. Engineers chose the FDM Titan™ for the ratcheting portion and the Eden PolyJet™ system for its extension assembly. The extension comprises two concentric tubes or *cannulae,* one that slides inside the other. The Eden was used for this assembly because engineers wanted excellent detail on the inner and outer diameter and the smoothest possible surface finish. The FDM Titan produced a working, durable polycarbonate ratchet that withstood testing on steel set screws and required only one hand to control.[†]

FDM models may be used as masters for investment casting of orthopedic implants. In a case study from *Modern Casting Magazine,*[‡] Biomet, Inc. (Warsaw, IN),

---

[*] Specifications supplied by Stratasys, Inc., http://www.stratasys.com, http://www.dimensionprinting.com/3d-printers/3d-printing-comparison_chart.aspx (accessed 8/7/2012).

[†] Stratasys Corporation case study, http://www.stratasys.com/Resources/Case-Studies/Medical-FDM-Technology-Case-Studies/Medtronic.aspx (acccessed 8/7/2012).

[‡] *Modern Casting Magazine* (November 2001). Rapid prototyping provides speed and cost-effective castings. American Foundry Society.

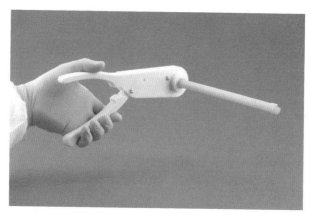

FIGURE 7.1 Figure shows a combination of polycarbonate FDM and Polyjet parts in a functioning surgical ratchet. (Courtesy of Stratasys, Eden Prairie, MN, and Medtronic Sofamor Danek, Minneapolis, MN.)

engineers designed an orthopedic implant in CAD and then reviewed the design with the foundry to determine gate and vent locations. The model was saved as an .STL file and built in pattern wax using FDM. The model was smoothed and then mounted on a casting tree and dipped in ceramic slurry. The tree was processed at 1900°F to fire the ceramic and melt out the wax pattern. The fired investment shell was then ready for casting with steel. Using these RP processes, an implant in CoCr or stainless steel can go from design to casting in as little as two weeks. Once the design was tested and verified, the design was moved into quantity production with hard tooling.[*]

SOLIDSCAPE

Solidscape, Inc. (Merrimack, NH; http://www.solid-scape.com), manufactures the T66 Benchtop and T612 Benchtop systems. These systems are not RP machines per se, as they are not intended to produce a functional part. Their purpose is to produce highly accurate master patterns for lost-wax (investment) casting or RTV molding. Because Solidscape's systems are able to build using extremely thin layers, models produced exhibit excellent surface finish and tight tolerances (see Figure 7.8 later in this chapter).

The maximum build platforms are somewhat smaller than most RP machines (6 × 6 × 6 inches on the T66 Benchtop and 6 × 6 × 12 inches on the T612) and dictate the markets and applications that Solidscape targets. Although patterns for toys, small medical devices, aerospace components, and consumer goods are commonly produced by Solidscape users, Solidscape systems are especially popular in the jewelry industry. This is because most jewelry consists of intricate designs that are traditionally cast using the lost-wax process.

The Solidscape system works by melting and depositing the build material (a wax-like thermoplastic) and a dissolvable wax support structure (to fill cavities and brace undercuts and cantilevered sections) in very small droplets through a piezo inkjet.

---

[*] Stratasys no longer supports the use of wax material in its machines. Wax masters may be produced with the Solidscape ModelMaker system, or the 3D Systems InVision system.

Rapid Prototyping for Medical Devices   139

The support material is dissolved using a heated solvent after the part is complete. After each layer build there is a milling step where the droplets are milled flat before the next layer is deposited. This contributes to the high accuracy of the process.

As discussed, the Solidscape systems produce master patterns for lost-wax casting. One company that uses Solidscape systems in medical device manufacturing is Interpore Cross. Interpore Cross, a division of Biomet (Warsaw, IN), manufactures and markets spinal implant and orthobiologic devices. The Solidscape systems are used to produce the GEO™ Structure Vertebral Body Replacement implants. This spinal implant device is a latticed structure that comes in a variety of shapes and sizes. Interpore Cross features one of the largest installations of Solidscape systems, with more than 30 machines in operation.

LOM™

LOM stands for laminated object modeling, a process originally developed by the Helisys Corporation. LOM uses a web of paper or other flexible sheet material and cuts this sheet material with a computer-controlled laser cutter. These sections are then laminated together with an adhesive to produce a final part. Excess material is sliced into blocks during the process and broken away from the part when finished. LOM was intended as a way to build large models from inexpensive materials. LOM has been used in pattern making for large castings and to produce large free-form models with thick wall sections. LOM has also been popular for producing architectural models. The technology had some early teething troubles, such as the laser causing the paper material to sometimes catch fire. Helisys ceased operations in 2000 and was succeeded by Cubic Technologies. The LOM process is currently marketed by the Stereoniks Corporation of Carson, CA.

Variations of the LOM process are seen in modelers from Solidimension (Israel), makers of the SD300 desktop three-dimensional printer. This modeler uses a LOM-type process laminating thin sheets of a polyvinylchloride (PVC) plastic material to produce models, with future plans to offer ABS and polycarbonate materials. Another variation of the LOM process is the Kira paper laminating process (PLT), which uses a knife to cut layers of material. The LOM process has a number of intriguing possibilities, as any material that can be supplied in sheet form (e.g., sheet metal, plastics, and composites that may be cut and laminated) is a candidate for LOM and related processes. Javelin 3D (Draper, UT) uses LOM-type technology in its MedLAM™ and CerLAM™ process to construct alumina–ceramic composite constructions in the shape of bones from computed tomography (CT) scan information, and other alumina ceramic objects.

Z Corp.: Three-Dimensional Printing

Z Corp. makes a line of machines referred to as three-dimensional printers.[*] Z Corp. three-dimensional printers use a powder-binder technology invented at and patented

---

[*] Three-dimensional printers are a general category of easy-to-use, office-based machines for RP applications.

by the Massachusetts Institute of Technology (MIT). First, the three-dimensional printer spreads a thin layer of powder. Second, an inkjet print head prints a binder in the cross section of the part being created. Next, the build piston drops down, making room for the next layer, and the process is repeated. Once the part is finished, it is surrounded and supported by loose powder, which is then shaken loose from the finished part.[*] The low-end office-based machines sell for less than $26,000 and use inexpensive consumables. The build material may be either starch based or plaster based (see Figure 7.2). The Z Corp. three-dimensional printers use Hewlett-Packard inkjet heads to deposit binders and food coloring–based dyes in layers on the build material. The surface finish of the models is grainy, and the models are porous and somewhat fragile. The strength of the models may be increased by the use of infiltrants supplied by Z Corp. These are wax, rubber, cyanoacrylate, and epoxy materials, and the model is painted or dipped in these materials.

Because of the lower cost of materials, the Z Corp. three-dimensional printer is particularly suitable for the production of large, bulky models on their larger machines. The resolution of the process is less than that of other processes. The process has difficulty with small radii (>0.5 mm) and small feature sizes.

A recent development from Z Corp. is the Z-cast process. This is the process of producing a plaster-casting mold directly, without the need for a lost-wax or sandbox casting pattern. The mold is printed using a plaster ceramic material. The material currently allows for the casting of low-melt-temperature metals, such as aluminum, zinc, and magnesium. Tolerances and finish of the part are similar to sand casting.

A unique feature of the Z Corp. three-dimensional printing technology is the ability to print models in color. This is accomplished by adding a color print head to the system, and printing food color–based dyes on to the build material. This feature has become popular in the production of visual communication models, such as models of fluid flow patterns, mold flow analysis, temperature maps, and stress pattern analysis. Figure 7.3 gives an example of the modeling of macromolecules with the Z Corp. Z810 three-dimensional printer. (ZCorp was acquired by 3D Systems, Rock Hill, SC, in January of 2012.)

Polyjet Objet™ Printer

Polyjet is a technology developed by the Objet company (Rehovot, Israel; http://www.2objet.com). Objet makes the line of Eden™ RP machines, distributed in North America by Stratasys Corporation. PolyJet can be thought of as three-dimensional printing with stereolithography-like photopolymers. The Objet deposits a very thin layer of photopolymer with an inkjet-type print head that is cured with a UV lamp. A water-soluble gel support structure is built at the same time to support cantilevered areas of the model. This support is washed away when the model is complete.

The PolyJet is suitable for use in an office environment. The PolyJet is capable of very fine detail, with X, Y jet resolution of 600 × 300 dots per inch (dpi) and a z-axis layer of 16 microns (0.0006 inch). This has made the PolyJet popular with users making small objects requiring very fine detail and smooth surface finish. Material

---

[*] See http://www.zcorp.com/en/home.aspx (accessed August 7, 2012).

Rapid Prototyping for Medical Devices

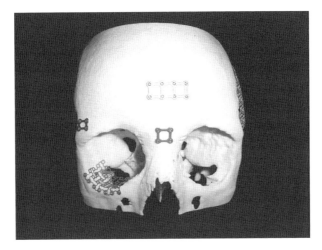

FIGURE 7.2 Three-dimensional printed model used for surgical planning. (Courtesy of Z Corp., Rock Hill, SC.)

properties are similar to those of stereolithography parts. Objet was acquired by Stratasys (Eden Prairie, MN) in 2012.

DLP: ENVISIONTEC® PERFACTORY™

Digital light processing (DLP) is a photopolymer method to build parts. Envisiontec GmbH (Marl, Germany; http://www.envisiontec.de) markets this technology in its Perfactory system. In this process, an entire image is projected onto the surface of a vat of photopolymer. The Perfactory lens system from Envisiontec is based on Texas

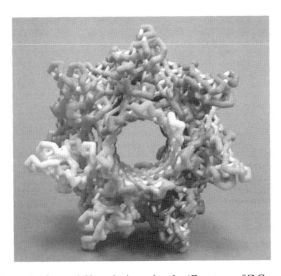

FIGURE 7.3 (**See color insert.**) Hemolysin molecule. (Courtesy of Z Corp., Rock Hill, SC.)

Instruments DLP technology. In this method, a microelectromechanical systems (MEMS) chip reflects an image off millions of mirrors through an optical engine into the surface of the resin to be cured. In this system, a layer of material is exposed at one time, rather than traced with a single or dual laser. The system uses a visible light projector bulb to cure the resin, and therefore no UV laser or jetting technologies are involved. The Perfactory is one of a new generation of RP machines meant for in-house prototyping and the direct manufacturing market, suitable for nonshop environments.

SINTERING AND DIRECT METAL

A rapidly developing area using RP-layered manufacturing technology is the direct metal process. This process has matured from expensive and somewhat limited machines of a few years back to systems capable of direct manufacture of fully dense metals with properties and constructions difficult or impossible to achieve with conventional casting and machining methods.

Among the vendors for these direct metal systems is Arcam AB (Moldnal, Sweden; http://www.arcam.com), with its EBM (Electron Beam Melting) machine. EOS (Munich, Germany; http://www.eos.info) produces the EOSINT line of machines used in laser sintering of plastics, foundry sand, and direct metal applications.

Another recent development has been the commercial release of the Solidica (http://www.solidica.com) system, a unique method of ultrasonically welding thin sheets of metal (e.g., aluminum) into a form, with an intermediate milling step between layer construction. The result is a metal matrix construction with finished milled features. This system is capable of laminating different metals into this metal matrix, as well as embedding functional elements, such as embedded sensors, ceramics, and fiber optics. Solidica was founded by Dawn White, PhD. This construction method allows, for example, the production of aluminum injection mold tooling with conformal cooling channels for optimized cycle times. Also in this space is the Ex-One Corporation ProMetal™ process for layered manufacture of tooling (http://www.extrudehone.com). Artist Bathsheba Grossman (see the section "Molecular Modeling") uses the ProMetal method to produce her sculptures.

RP APPLICATIONS IN PRODUCT DESIGN

Following are two examples of RP used to streamline and accelerate the product development process. In the first example, Equilasers, a manufacturer of laser systems based in San Jose, CA, needed a design for the housing of a new Nd:YAG cosmetic laser system, the Equilase 30™. The industrial and mechanical design was done, and the panels were fabricated from SLA parts. The size limitation on SLA parts was overcome by the parts being grown as smaller sections and then bonded together with SLA resin and painted. The project went from a clean-sheet concept design stage to a finished unit, ready to crate and ship to an overseas trade show in four weeks (see Figure 7.4). The parts were designed as detachable panels with production in mind, and they included all of the mounting hardware, wall thickness,

Rapid Prototyping for Medical Devices

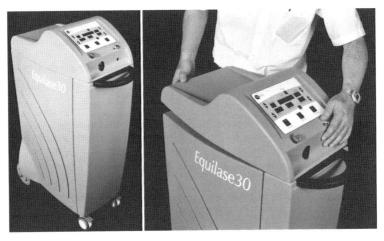

FIGURE 7.4 Large painted functional stereolithography RP panels. (Kucklick Design for Equilasers, Inc.)

and draft required when the parts were to be pressure formed. The parts were robust enough for functional testing and shipping.

In the second example, Sleep Solutions, Inc. used RP to iterate the product development and clinical testing process of the NovaSom QSG™ system. The original product was a test unit enclosed in a sheet metal project box, which needed to be redesigned for quantity production, as well as to have the look of a friendly, easy-to-use medical instrument for home use. The unit also had to be radio frequency interference (RFI) shielded and very durable for multiple shipping and reuse. Also, because the unit was to be compact, design for assembly issues needed to be resolved before committing to hard tooling. An iteration of the design was produced in RP to test and debug the design. A final SLA master was produced, and several cast urethane duplicates were produced with RTV silicone tooling (see Figure 7.5). The units were assembled using threaded inserts, just as the final plastic parts would be. These units were used for mechanical and assembly testing and electronics package development, and also in final clinical validation while the injection mold tooling was in process. Once the tooling was done, injection-molded parts were produced in a durable engineering plastic, with confidence in the fit and function of the final parts that had been verified with RP before the hard tooling was cut. RP was a useful tool to move this project forward quickly, and it allowed several design and validation activities to proceed in parallel, with high levels of confidence in the final results.

COMPUTER NUMERICAL CONTROL

CNC machining was originally developed by John Parsons with the assistance of MIT, Wright-Patterson Air Force Base, and the U.S. Air Force around 1947. The original purpose was to machine accurate curved objects that required complex jigs. Parsons originally conceived of the basis of the idea while working as a machine

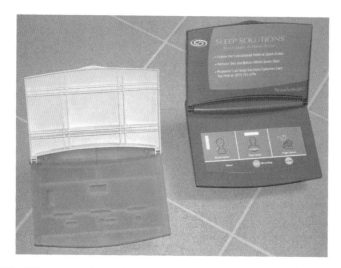

FIGURE 7.5 RP prototype (stereolithography and cast urethane) parts and injection-molded final design of the NovaSom QSG™. (Kucklick Design for Sleep Solutions, Inc.)

shop apprentice in 1929, and later while producing complex helicopter rotor blades at his own company for the military. The first CNC machine was built in 1949. In 1952 the first commercially available CNC machines were produced, and they were accepted into industrial use by 1957. One of the reasons CNC took so long to be accepted was that some of the companies involved (IBM and General Dynamics) saw "no application for it at all." In fact, a paper submitted by one of Parson's associates, Frank Stulen, to the American Helicopter Association on the use of CNC to produce helicopter rotor blades was rejected as "pure nonsense." CNC was also rejected at the time by the auto industry. It was finally the dogged persistence of John Parsons and his associates like Frank Stulen, and the intervention of the Air Force, by its purchasing a number of the first CNC machines and distributing them into the aircraft industry to help produce the new generation of advanced jet aircraft (the B-47), that finally led to the acceptance of CNC technology. CNC is now considered one of the cornerstones of the "Second Industrial Revolution."* CNC is but one of a number of revolutionary technologies (e.g., the personal computer, magnetic resonance imaging [MRI]) for which many experts originally saw no market or useful purpose.

Numerous small CNC machines available are driven by inexpensive personal computers. These range from light training models to smaller versions of industrial-grade machining centers. DesktopNC.com is a comprehensive resource of nearly every active (and inactive) manufacturer of small CNC milling machines (http://www.desktopcnc.com/index.htm).

Given the reasonable cost of smaller CNC mills, as well as lower cost domestic and import full-size machines, available new and used, it can be tempting to bring

---

* See http://machinist.org/uncategorized/the-invention-of-cnc-machining/ (accessed August 7, 2012).

CNC machining in-house. When considering bringing CNC machining in-house, it helps to ask the following questions:

- Do we have a specific need to manufacture or prototype in-house?
- Are we willing to hire or train a skilled machinist to operate this machine?
- How much work could we get done outside for the cost of the machine, plus the cost of a skilled operator (or a skilled operator already on staff, taken away from his other responsibilities)?
- Does the small CNC machine we are considering have the power to machine all of the materials we need to work with (e.g., ferrous metals), or do our needs require a full-size machining center?
- Will the machine be used enough hours per day to justify the cost of the capital to purchase it, and the ongoing expenses of facility overhead, taxes, and maintenance?

Small start-up companies operating on investment capital can find that it is difficult to justify bringing CNC machining in-house, unless there is a specific reason for doing so. Some companies find that having a simple manual mill and lathe that can be operated by an engineer with sufficient skills can be adequate for proof-of-concept work, where it makes more sense to send out more complex or higher volume jobs to a dedicated outside machine shop. Manual Bridgeport-type knee mills can also be retrofitted with two- and three-axis CNC drives and controls, although this can make them more cumbersome to use as manual machines. The use of the CNC function also requires special training, which can be difficult to retain for the casual or occasional user.

There are more than 47 makers of desktop milling machines with nearly 100 models available, with prices ranging from less than $5,000 to more than $40,000. Machines listed as educational are meant to train machinists to operate larger machines. Rapid prototype and hobbyist machines are usually not suitable for cutting ferrous metals (iron, steel, and stainless steel) and are limited to machining jeweler's wax, modeling foam, chemical wood, and sometimes plastic. Some of the larger machines can handle machining brass and aluminum. When considering a desktop milling machine, carefully evaluate whether the machine will handle the types of materials you want to cut. Desktop machines also tend to use only one tool at a time, unlike the tool-changing capabilities found in full-size machining centers.

Roland (http://www.rolanddga.com) offers a line of easy-to-use desktop CNC machines marketed as subtractive rapid prototypers (SRP®). The smaller machines (MDX 15 and 20) are capable of machining wax, foam, and plastics at slow feed rates. The MDX 500 and MDX 650 machines are capable of milling nonferrous metals like brass and aluminum. A unique feature of the MDX 20 (about $5,000) is that it is a combination lightweight tabletop three-axis mill and a three-dimensional scanner. The MDX 650 offers an optional tool changer for up to eight tools and an optional fourth-axis rotary material holder. They are bundled together with simple-to-use software, which allows a user with little or no previous machine shop experience to make parts. The drawback to these higher-end machines is their being limited in the materials they can machine, and their somewhat high cost (about $20,000, not including optional accessories).

FULL-SIZE VMC CNC MACHINES

Haas Automation (Oxnard, CA), Fadal (Chatsworth, CA, a division of ThyssenKrupp, Germany), Mori Seiki (Japan), Mazak (Japan), Daewoo (Korea), and Chevalier (Taiwan) are manufacturers of CNC vertical machining centers (VMCs). Recently Haas and Fadal have both begun to offer tool room VMC CNC machines capable of both CNC and manual operation in the $20,000 range, and mini-VMC machines in the $30,000 range. These machines claim to be easy to use for operators not familiar with traditional CNC G-code programming. In contrast to the desktop machines, these VMCs require 230 volt (V) of single- or three-phase power. Industrial-grade CNC machines also require a separate computer program to generate tool paths, the series of cuts that the machine makes to produce a final shape from a block of material. Examples of these programs are Mastercam (http://www.mastercam.com), Surfcam (http://www.surfcam.com), and Gibbs CAM (http://www.Gibbscam.com). When looking for a CAM package, it is important to determine how it will be used and how well it works with the CAD program you are using. A good place to start would be your CAD vendor, to see whether it has a good CAM solution that works seamlessly inside of your current CAD program. Analyzing your requirements and streamlining your workflow are vitally important before you go through the time and expense of implementing an in-house CNC machining solution.

Full-size CNC VMCs have the advantage of being able to cut any machinable material. They also offer turrets that hold multiple tools. Using these industrial CNC machines and the programs to run them, however, requires an operator with a significant amount of machine shop knowledge and training. This is why many small start-up companies conserve their cash and send machine shop work out to skilled and reliable outside vendors.

MACHINABLE PROTOTYPE MATERIALS

For prototype models in inexpensive materials, a number of foam, chemical wood products, styling, and tooling board materials are available.

The most popular and inexpensive is urethane, or surfboard foam. This can be easily hand shaped and sanded and can be machined on any milling machine. The drawback of urethane foam is its porous surface and production of gritty foam dust residue when sanded. Another variation of this material is polystyrene surfboard foam. These materials are available at many hobby shops or surfboard supply shops.

Ren Shape® pattern-making materials are manufactured by Huntsman Advanced Materials. There are two basic types, styling boards and tooling boards. Styling boards are lower-density, lower-temperature materials designed for dimensional stability and ease of machining. Tooling boards are made for dimensional stability and heat resistance in the range from 232°F to 496°F, for such applications as the production of vacuum-forming molds and other high-temperature pattern-making applications.

Machinable wax is used to produce tooling masters for lost-wax casting or nonporous casting masters that release easily from RTV silicone rubber mold-making materials. Pattern-making wood includes medium-density fiberboard (MDF), plank pine, and chemical wood. Most of these materials are available from Freeman Manufacturing and Supply (Avon, OH; http://www.freemansupply.com). Prototyping plastics commonly used and readily available for machining are Delrin® acetal (easy to machine, chemical and solvent resistant), ABS plastic (good general purpose plastic, less expensive), polycarbonate (very tough and strong plastic, harder to machine with good surface finish), and acrylic (readily available at hobbyist plastic shops, hard, machines with good surface finish, can be polished). All of these materials except Delrin can be easily bonded with proper adhesives. These materials are available from any large plastics supply house. Two that I have used are Polymer Plastics Corporation (http://www.polymerplastics.com) and Port Plastics (http://www.portplastics.com). Ren Shape materials, machinable wax, and pattern-making wood products are available from Freeman Manufacturing and Supply. Freeman also makes available online more than two hours of excellent video tutorials on how to use various casting and prototyping materials, as well as sample kits of various molding, casting, and machinable materials. Prototype metals include easy-to-machine grades of brass and aluminum. Obomodulan® is a polyurethane prototyping board in several densities made by the Obo-Werke GmbH of Stadhagen, Germany (http://www.obo-werke.de).

For those who do not want to own a milling machine or even a CAD program, machined parts can be designed and purchased online (http://www.emachineshop.com). The eMachineShop® site has a built-in draw program and an online quotation function for those who have an occasional need for machined parts and sheet metal prototypes.

RAPID TOOLING AND MOLDING

Several technologies have been developed to directly manufacture steel tooling for plastic injection molding. One of the barriers to acceptance is that the majority of these methods rely on some form of laser sintering and require postprocessing to turn the sintered RP tool into a usable, fully dense part. One potential advantage to RP tooling is in the free-form modeling capabilities inherent in RP. 3D Systems advertises its Laserform® material. This system allows the production of steel inserts for low-volume injection molding (20,000 to 50,000 shots.) One unique feature of the system is the ability to build into the tooling insert conformal cooling channels for specialized applications. Newer materials such as 3D Systems Laserform A6 can produce production-grade tools with good heat transfer characteristics.

Mold inserts may also be made from RP part masters by an electroforming process. Here, an RP part is used as a master, and a thick layer of copper is deposited on to the master, removed, and backed with epoxy. This is repeated until an A and B side of the mold is produced. The prototype core and cavity are then mounted into a mold base for prototype injection or compression molding. This service is offered by the Repliform company (http://www.repliforminc.com).

Another vendor who has entered the rapid tooling market is Protomold. By offering a defined set of mold-making services that are readily achievable within its CNC machining capabilities (part size, minimum feature size, minimum corner radius, limits on side actions, etc.) and an Internet storefront with online quoting, getting prototypes of many types of injection molded parts is fast, easy, and surprisingly inexpensive (http://www.protomold.com). Protomold keeps a fairly complete inventory of most types of molding plastics and can mold parts from customer-supplied material as well. Several other companies are also offering these types of rapid-turnaround injection-molding services.

WHICH TECHNOLOGY IS BEST?

Every RP technology has it own strengths and limitations. There is no one RP approach that is best for every application. The best technology is the one that best meets the requirements for what you want to accomplish. Therefore, first determine which factors are most important: speed, size of parts, surface finish, minimum feature size, materials properties, in-house or outsourced, cost, and convenience. Is the model for visual evaluation? Will it be a master for other reproduction processes? Will it be used for mechanical testing? Will the RP part be used as a tool or mold? Does the part need to be made of a medical-grade material? Answering these questions will help you to make the best choice of the numerous RP technologies available to you. In practice, 3D Systems SLA and Stratasys FDM make up the majority of models made at service bureaus. Z Corp.'s three-dimensional printing system is a popular in-office system for those applications that can work with its surface finish and feature size limitations, and secondary operations requirements (wax, cyanoacrylate, and epoxy, and infiltration to strengthen the part). For parts that must be made of a specific material, and not just a representation of it in an RP material, CNC machining is the best approach, although this may be more costly than RP, and you are limited to geometry that can be made with mill and lathe machine tools.

FILE PREPARATION

To produce an RP part requires a three-dimensional digital file of your part geometry, typically from a three-dimensional CAD or three-dimensional modeling program (e.g., SolidWorks™, Pro/Engineer™, Autocad™, Alias™, Rhino™, etc.). You must have a program capable of producing either a solid model or a closed-surface model. Two-dimensional drafting files (e.g., Autocad.dwg) will not work for processes such as SLA or FDM. Check your three-dimensional CAD software to be sure that you can export your three-dimensional model as an .STL file.

Three-dimensional scanners can also produce meshes that can be turned into .STL solid models. This is discussed in Chapter 9. The .STL files may also be produced from MRI and CT data. Mimics™ software from Materialise NV (Belgium) translates CT or MRI data into three-dimensional CAD, finite element meshes, or RP data (http://www.materialise.com). Protomed, Inc., in Arvada, CO, specializes in producing stereolithography models for surgical planning from MRI and CT scan data (http://www.protomed.net). Two other programs for converting CT and MRI scans are VG Studio Max (Heidelberg, Germany; http://www.volumegraphics.com), a voxel-based modeler for animators; and Vitrea (Minnetonka, MN; http://www.vitalimages.com), a high-end solution for radiologists.

An .STL file is a polygon mesh surface file that is sliced up in the SLA machine's preprocessing software. This produces a series of outlines of part sections, or slices, that are then filled in by the SLA machine's UV laser. In a polygon mesh file, a surface is described by a series of tessellated (tiled) triangles. The size and number of these triangles determine the resolution of the model. The higher the number of triangles, the higher the resolution and the smoother the model; however, this results in larger file sizes. Use the preview setting of your CAD program's .STL output function to see the effects of higher and lower triangle resolution settings, and how they affect the smoothness of the final .STL output file. If the file becomes overly large, try reducing the output resolution or compressing the file with a program such as WinZip™ before sending it to your service bureau.

OTHER FILE FORMATS

The majority of RP information is communicated in the .STL format. Some of the other more common neutral file formats available are as follows:

PLY format, or the Stanford triangle format. This is a simplified vertex and face description of a three-dimensional object. It is a simplified file format for the communication of three-dimensional surface models, usually acquired from three-dimensional scanners.

VRML (virtual reality modeling format). Based on Silicon Graphics (Mountain View, CA) Open Inventor file format for use in Internet applications. Inventor is yet another file format that is a superset of the VRML networked graphics data format. VRML is useful with communication texture and color data along with three-dimensional object information. Other three-dimensional formats, such as STL and PLY, do not support this type of color and scene data.

IGES (Initial Graphics Exchange Specification). An American national standard that is a neutral data format for the digital exchange of information among CAD systems and other applications. The standard is developed and maintained by the Initial Graphic Exchange Specification/Product Data Exchange Specification (IGES/PDES) Organization. IGES supports the representation of surfaces with smooth higher-order splines or nonlinear uniform rational B-splines (NURBS).

DXF (drawing interchange file). A file format developed by Autodesk, Inc. (Sausilito, CA) as a neutral file format for the communication of two- and three-dimensional vector information. DXF represents three-dimensional objects as polyface meshes and not smooth surfaces or NURBS.

STEP (Standard for the Exchange of Product Mode Data). An International Organization of Standardization (ISO) standard neutral file format for the communication of engineering solid model data generated from CAD programs.

For more information on the (numerous) three-dimensional file formats in existence, visit the Center for Machine Perception of the Czech Technical University department of Cybernetics (http://cmp.felk.cvut.cz).

RP COST-SAVING TIPS

The cost of SLA and other rapid prototype parts increases with the volume of the part. Larger-volume parts require higher expenses in machine time and materials costs. If a larger prototype is required, and cost is an issue, an RP method with lower material costs may be considered. A way to save cost with SLA, if a number of smaller parts are to be produced, is to run them all at one time, and incur only one setup cost or lot charge.

Another way to save costs is to produce only the part of the model that needs to be evaluated. For example, you may have only a connector interface that needs to be checked for function and fit. Save the part to a new CAD file and cut away the rest of the model so you are left only with the part of the model you want to evaluate. Save this section to an .STL file and send this to your service bureau for modeling. This will save the time and expense of producing the entire model in SLA.

If you are a company that operates globally, a way to speed product development and save time and costs with RP is to produce the CAD file in one country (e.g., the United States) and then transmit the data file over the Internet to an RP service bureau in a distant country (e.g., Australia or Europe). Then, have the model delivered by the service bureau to the local person in that country who will use the model. This can avoid issues with customs and overseas courier services. You will want to establish a good working relationship with the overseas service bureau before trying this on a critical project. Some companies with international offices use this method, designing in one location, and transmitting CAD data to be fabricated by an in-house manufacturing operation in another country.

With RP machines capable of printing in color (Z Corp.), a model can be built as one part, with different components printed in a different color. The model can then be sectioned in CAD, or sawn apart to analyze how components fit together. This saves the time of building the model in separate parts and assembling them.

SECONDARY PROCESSES TO RP PARTS

PAINTING

The most obvious secondary finishing process to RP parts is painting. Stereolithography parts are the easiest to paint, requiring only finish sanding and primer. SLS parts can be painted, depending on the material. Stratasys FDM models can be painted, but they require more finish work than stereolithography models. Z Corp. three-dimensional printed models can be painted, but they require more finishing and sealing work.

ELECTROPLATING

Another secondary operation that can be performed on RP parts is electroplating or vacuum deposition. This gives RP parts the look of metal parts, or it can be used for

MACHINING

RP materials vary in their machinability. FDM models are readily milled and drilled; SLA parts can be machined with care, although they may break easily.

THREADED INSERTS

RP parts can be assembled with machine screws if bosses are designed into the part and threaded inserts are used. These are more accurate and reliable than attempting to drill and tap RP material, and they will duplicate the way the final molded parts are likely to be assembled. Threaded inserts are available from Penn Engineering Corporation, makers of PEM® inserts (http://www.pennfast.com). These inserts are normally driven into injection-molded plastic parts with an ultrasonic welder.

Installing the Inserts

Use these inserts in RP and cast urethane parts as follows: design the bosses in your part to the interference fit specifications given for the threaded insert when driven in with ultrasound. This information is available in the product literature for the insert. To install the inserts, use a soldering iron set to the melt temperature of the RP plastic from which your part is made. A pointed soldering iron tip that fits into the brass threaded insert works particularly well. Place the threaded insert into the boss until the insert's lead-in taper holds it in position. Place the hot soldering iron tip into the insert, and gently press the insert into the boss as the soldering iron melts the plastic. Remove the soldering iron tip from the insert. You now have a reliable and reusable assembly thread in your RP part.

UV CURE SEALING OF FOAM PARTS

When making urethane or styrene foam models either by hand or on a CNC mill, you will find that these models can be fragile in their thin sections, dusty, and unable to be painted. Sealing the model helps make it stronger as well as able to take paint. Although you can use spackle or artist's gesso to seal the foam, the drawback to this method is that the gesso and spackle are heavy and can take a very long time to dry. A better solution is to use UV-curable surfboard polyester resin. These are low viscosity and easy to use and brush on the part. Putting the parts out in the sun for about an hour cures the resin. The result is a stronger, cleaner part. UV cure polyester is available from surfboard materials shops, or from Fiberglass Supply (Bingen, WA; http://www.fiberglasssupply.com).

RP CASTING PATTERNS

RP models may be used as masters to produce cast duplicates. Any casting method may be used, depending on the material to be cast. RTV silicone rubber is the most common. Other casting materials, such as dental alginate, may be used to produce wax patterns for making the plaster of dental stone molds.

When making a master for casting, factor in the shrink of the casting material. Casting materials can shrink significantly as they harden. The percentage of shrink is different for each material. The data sheet from the supplier will provide this information. If the castings are being done at the same vendor as the RP master, the vendor will have this information on hand and can build the shrink factor into the master part for you. This means that dimensions are critical; a cast part made from a casting material with a 2 percent shrink factor will need to be scaled 2 percent larger than the master if the final part is to be the same size as the original CAD model.

Masters are usually done at a higher resolution than visual-check or fit-check parts. They are sanded and painted to ensure that they release readily from the RTV mold and produce a smooth surface finish.

A twist on the use of RP casting masters is to use an RP model as a casting tool. SLA would work well, because it is not porous. If you have rubber grips or some other elastomer part to cast, try making the mold in RP, especially if you do not have access to a CNC mill. An RP mold, treated with mold release, can quickly produce a tool to cast silicone or urethane parts.

REVERSE ENGINEERING

RE is a natural companion to RP. It uses three-dimensional scanning techniques to generate a CAD model to produce a copy of the object with RP techniques. Scanner vendors like to call this process reverse modeling. It is very similar to the older process of taking a clay impression or making a plaster "splash" mold to duplicate a part. There are a number of very useful and important applications for these methods. The subject of RE will be handled in more detail in Chapter 9.

INNOVATIVE APPLICATIONS OF RP

This last section is a digest of a number of innovative uses of RP. Some of these applications are commonly used, others are in development, and yet others are a view into the future. Perhaps in one or more of them is the inspiration for your own groundbreaking innovation.

RP AND SURGICAL PLANNING

RP has given surgeons powerful tools in planning high-risk complex surgeries. This is especially useful in cases presenting significant anatomical variations or damage, such as deformity or trauma. RP models are now used routinely to plan challenging surgeries.*

When producing a model for surgical planning, it is often necessary to highlight areas of surgical interest or concern. To produce a stereolithography model that is

---

* For an interesting use of rapid prototyping using 3D Systems SLA process in surgical planning, see "Conjoined Twins Separation a Model Surgery," *Designfax Magazine* (November 2002), http://www.designfax.net.

selectively colored, use a stereolithography material containing a dye that activates at a higher energy level than that to cure the clear polymer.

Two stereolithography models are produced, one with the normal anatomy and one with the areas of interest. The models are run together, and the stereolithography machine is programmed to apply a higher power setting to the laser curing the areas of surgical interest. This results in a model in which the normal anatomy is clear and the areas of interest are highlighted in pink.

RP AND TRAINING MODELS

RP has found numerous applications in medical modeling.* Selective laser sintering has been used to reproduce the temporal bone, and the malleus and incus of the middle ear. The model was cut and shaved using a surgical drill, burr, and suction irrigator in the same way as a real bone.

Molecular Modeling

This chapter highlighted an example of a hemolysin molecule modeled in color with the Z Corp. three-dimensional printer. Bathsheba Grossman is a mathematician and artist in Santa Cruz, CA, who produces sculptures based on mathematical models and molecular information. Bathsheba was kind enough to share some of the details of how she prepares the molecule data set for burning into a glass block with CNC lasers:

> I get most of the glass done at precisionlaserart.com. To build a protein point cloud, I start with the PDB file, and my first aim is to turn it into a three-dimensional CAD model. The CAD software I use has a strong scripting language, so I do this by lexically converting the PDB into a script file. If ribbons or cartoons are required I use Kinemage as an intermediate step, since it writes a tractable ASCII format for these structures. If an electrostatic surface is required, I use GRASS (Graphical Representation and Analysis of Structure Server) to create the surface, and other software tools to smooth and condition it. Once I have the structure as a CAD file, I distribute points onto it. And lastly, I use some of my own software to dither these points, adding thickness to curves, and regulating the translucency of surfaces. So at the end of all this, I have a simple ASCII list of points, scaled to size, and that's what I send to the laser facility (see Figures 7.6 and 7.7).†

RP-PRODUCED MEDICAL PRODUCTS

Investment Cast Orthopedic Implants

Solidscape, Inc., recently announced the installation of its 32nd ModelMaker™ RP system in the production facility of Interpore Cross International. Interpore Cross is a medical device company with a complementary combination of spinal implant and orthobiologic technologies. The ModelMaker™ systems are used to produce the GEO™ Structure Vertebral Body Replacement implants, for which Food and Drug Administration (FDA) clearance was recently received. This spinal implant device is a latticed structure that comes in a variety of shapes and sizes.

---

* See "Rapid Prototyping of Temporal Bone for Surgical Training and Medical Education," *Acta Oto-Laryngologica* 124 (May 2004): 400–402.
† For more information on Bathsheba Grossman's sculptures, see http://www.bathsheba.com.

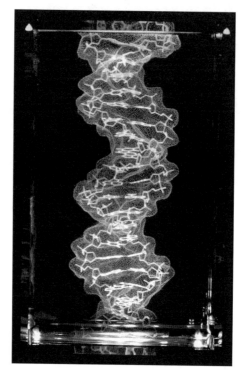

FIGURE 7.6 DNA model, laser engraved in glass. (Courtesy of Bathsheba Grossman, Santa Cruz, CA.)

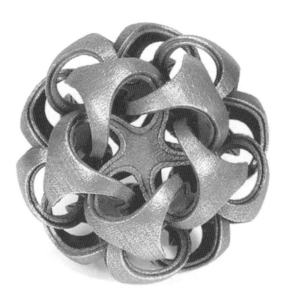

FIGURE 7.7 Quintron, metal print sculpture. Note the geometric complexity and nested shapes achievable with RP. (Courtesy of Bathsheba Grossman, Santa Cruz, CA.)

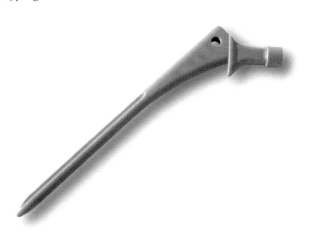

FIGURE 7.8 Hip implant stem-casting master in wax. (Courtesy of Solidscape, Merrimack, NH. Acquired by Stratasys, Eden Prairie, MN, in 2011.)

According to Solidscape,

"We evaluated a number of the RP systems available and determined the Solidscape technology to be the only system on the market capable of fabricating investment casting patterns that met the dimensional tolerances our products required," said R. Park Carmon, Vice President of Operations. "Application of advanced rapid prototype equipment to deliver production quantities is a good example of the innovative approach Interpore is taking to bring new products to the spinal market. The Solidscape system made that application possible"[*] (see Figure 7.8).

RP AND RE COMBINED INTO A PRODUCT AND SERVICE

Crowns in One Visit

Sirona Dental Systems (Germany) makes the CEREC® system for the chair-side production of dental crowns (see Figures 7.9 to 7.11). Rather than taking a physical impression, drilling out the box for the crown, and sending the patient home with a temporary crown to come back in a week or two while a dental lab produces a crown from the impression, the CEREC system gives the patient a permanent crown in one visit. This is done using a sophisticated three-dimensional scan of the tooth called a digital impression. The tooth is then drilled, and a second digital impression is taken of the box, or the cavity into which the crown will fit. The digital information from the scan of the intact tooth surface is combined with the box that the tooth implant will fit into. These data are then transmitted to a special milling machine that uses dental burrs to shape a blank of ceramic tooth crown material into the shape of the previous tooth surface and the box it is to fit into. The finished crown is then cemented in place, and the patient is sent home, with her permanent crown, precisely fitted, in one visit. This is an example of RE and RP applied to a medical product and service.

---

[*] Solidscape, Inc., press release, May 29, 2002.

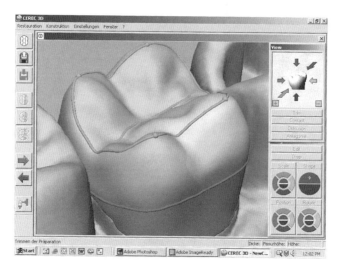

FIGURE 7.9 **(See color insert.)** The CEREC system. (Courtesy of Sirona Dental Systems, Germany.)

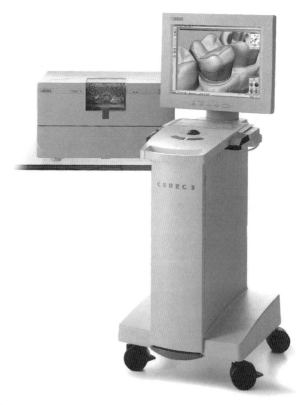

FIGURE 7.10 Milling the ceramic blank. (Courtesy of Sirona Dental Systems, Germany.)

Rapid Prototyping for Medical Devices

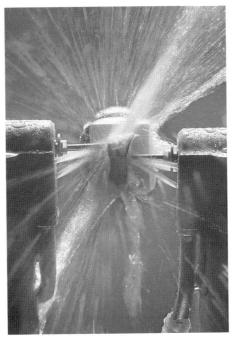

FIGURE 7.11 Three-dimensional data capture of a tooth. (Courtesy of Sirona Dental Systems, Germany.)

RP AND TISSUE ENGINEERING

Some of the greatest advances in technology have been the application of one technology redeployed into another area. One example is the combination of personal computers and Xerox® copier technology, which spawned the laser printer, and with it desktop publishing and graphics. Another is the adaptation of RP technology to the areas of tissue engineering (see Figure 7.12). RP is used to manufacture the framework onto which living cells attach and proliferate. A 1989 *Business Week* article gives a brief history and theory of tissue engineering:

> As early as 1979, Eugene Bell, professor emeritus of biology at MIT and the founder of Organogenesis, figured out how to grow skin in his lab. Since then, much of the field's progress stems from a 20-year collaboration of two fast friends—Joseph Vacanti, a pediatric surgeon at Children's Hospital, and Robert S. Langer, a chemical engineering professor at MIT. Their lab "seeded the entire country with people doing this work," says Dr. Pamela Bassett, president of medical consultants BioTrend in New York.
>
> The two, both 49, first met as researchers in the mid-1970s and started working on a way to grow tissue in the early 1980s. In 1986, they developed an elegantly simple concept that underlies most engineered tissue. Start with a scaffold, bent to any shape, made of an artificial, biodegradable polymer. Seed it with living cells, and bathe it in growth factors. The cells multiply, filling up the scaffold and growing into a three-dimensional tissue. Once implanted in the body, the cells are smart enough to recreate their proper tissue functions. Blood vessels attach themselves to the new

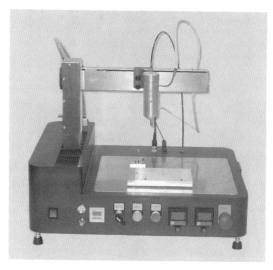

FIGURE 7.12 The Envisiontec Bioplotter. (Courtesy of Envisiontec GmbH, Marl, Germany.)

tissue, the scaffold melts away, and the lab-grown tissue is eventually indistinguishable from its surroundings.[*]

As you can see, the basic theory is to make a tissue scaffold with the desired shape and characteristics, and deposit cells and growth medium on the scaffold to grow tissue in a directed way. This is the famous "ear on a mouse," where a scaffold made of human chondrocytes (cartilage) in the approximate shape of a human ear was attached to the back of a mouse, and tissue grew around it to resemble the shape of a human ear. This feat earned a fair bit of notoriety for the experimenter, Linda Griffith of MIT, and a fair bit of misunderstanding of the concept in the popular press.

Alternatively, the scaffold is implanted, and the body supplies the tissue to grow onto the scaffold. When the scaffold has served its purpose, it is then broken down and absorbed into the body. The difficulty in using this approach to build larger tissues and organs is providing tissues within the engineered construction with oxygen and nutrients. One of the difficulties to overcome is the 2 mm rule from physiology. This rule states that no living tissue in the body can be more than 2 mm away from a blood supply. This is one of the major obstacles in building implantable solid organs using tissue engineering.

Envisiontec Bioplotter

Envisiontec GmbH (Germany; http://www.envisiontec.de) makes the Bioplotter® to build scaffolds for tissue engineering. The Bioplotter acts in a similar way to a rapid prototyping machine and uses cell cultures to build new structures layer by layer (see Figure 7.13).

---

[*] Catherine Arnst and John Carey, "Biotech Bodies," *Business Week* (July 27, 1998), http://www.businessweek.com/1998/30/b3588001.htm. See also The Human Body Shop, Doug Garr, *MIT Technology Review Magazine* pp. 72–79. (April 2001).

Rapid Prototyping for Medical Devices

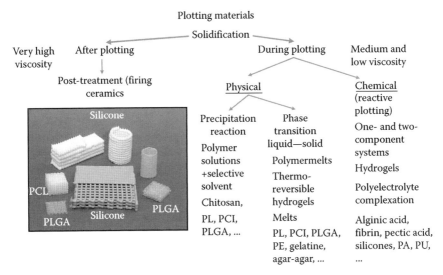

FIGURE 7.13 Tissue engineering plotting materials. (Courtesy of Envisiontec GmbH, Marl, Germany.)

The Bioplotter creates a digital data model of the structure to be built. It then dispenses cells, producing a three-dimensional arrangement of biological and biocompatible material.

Other work in this area is being conducted by Thomas Boland at Clemson University, SC, and Vladimir Mironov at the Medical University of South Carolina and the University of Missouri, Columbia:

> To print 3D structures, Boland and Mironov used a "thermo-reversible" gel recently developed by Anna Gutowska, research scientist at the Department of Energy Pacific Northwest National Laboratory. The non-toxic, biodegradable gel is liquid below 20°C and solidifies above 32°C. The team has done several experiments using easily available tissues such as hamster ovary cells. By printing alternate layers of the gel and clumps of cells onto glass slides, they have shown 3D structures such as tubes can be built up.[*]

The effect is evident when considering that similar to producing a colored document when a cartridge is filled with assorted ink colors, complex structures such as organs can be printed when a cartridge is replenished with different kinds of cells. That step, however, requires the discovery of a method to produce circulatory networks that would furnish nutrients and oxygen to the deeply embedded cells. To make that a reality, Boland and Mironov aspire to print a whole system of veins, capillaries, and arteries that would support whole organs.[†]

In a *Business Week* article, Neil Gross reported:

---

[*] "Ink-Jet Printing Creates Tubes of Living Tissue," *The New Scientist* (January 22, 2003), Charles Choi, http://www.newscientist.com/article/dn3292-inkjet-printing-creates-tubes-of-living-tissue.html (accessed August 7, 2012).

[†] "Desktop Printing of Living Tissue," *R&D Magazine* (March 2003, Vol. 45, Issue 3, p. 41).

Doctors may one day use a variety of rapid prototyping techniques to build replacements for bones destroyed by injury or disease. The Office of Naval Research (ONR) in Arlington, Va., pioneered such techniques for making plastic, metal, and ceramic parts from digital designs. Biomedical engineers picked up the trend, making plastic plugs to replace pieces of damaged bone. Three years ago, the ONR teamed up with Advanced Ceramics Research Inc. in Tucson for more advanced applications.[*]

Therics Corporation (Princeton, NJ; http://www.therics.com) applies RP methods to building bone graft material using RP technology.

For more information on the subject of tissue engineering and its current business and regulatory environment, see "Body by Science" by Aileen Constanz in the October 6, 2003, issue of *The Scientist*.

RP AND PHARMACEUTICALS

RP may have applications in the packaging of pharmaceuticals. According to Ed Grenda's RP report,

Medical dosages forms which would be difficult if not impossible to make any other way are in development. Using rapid prototyping it's possible to fabricate pills with precise and complex time release characteristics or that dissolve almost instantly. A recent patent describes the interesting possibility of combining one drug with a second compound that synchronously counteracts the first drug's side-effects within the same pill. Medications can be made more effective and safer in this way and drug companies may be able to realize stronger revenue streams from older drugs that go "off-patent" by providing them in novel and beneficial dosage forms.[†]

RP AND ANALYSIS

Another novel application of RP is using RP technology to facilitate an old analysis method: researchers at the University of Warwick have found a way to apply a test devised in the 1930s, once used to gauge the stress on the superchargers in Spitfire fighter planes, to model the stress that surgical procedures would put on an aortic aneurysm. As Rob Coppinger wrote in *The Engineer*,

Photoelasticity is a technique that has been used for decades in industry. It looks at the patterns of coloured light reflected from the surface of an object to gain a detailed understanding of the stresses on that object.

Initially surgeons had tried placing mechanical strain gauges on an aortic aneurysm as they manipulated it but found that the gauges themselves placed an unwelcome additional physical strain on the aortic aneurysm.

They turned to researchers at the University of Warwick led by Geoff Calvert who had an idea that would combine photoelastic stress analysis with the technology of rapid prototyping to solve the problem.

---

[*] Neil Gross, ed., "Developments to Watch," *Business Week Online* (June 23, 2003).
[†] *Printing the Future: The 3D Printing and Rapid Prototyping Source Book*, Ed Grenda, Castle Island Company, 2006.

The University of Warwick and UCL researchers took a three-dimensional scan of the patient's actual aortic aneurysm and used rapid prototyping technology to produce an exact latex duplicate of the aneurysm. They then covered the duplicate with a reflective coating and used photoelastic stress analysis to examine the stress on the model aneurysm as the surgeon manipulated it.[*]

Programmable RP Molding

Saul Griffith, while a graduate student at MIT, developed a programmable "printer" for eyeglass lenses. This is an RP device that curves a membrane to form a mold cavity. The idea was to solve the problem of stocking an inventory of costly or inappropriate eyeglass lenses to serve the vision care needs of millions in the developing world who cannot afford standard prescription ground eyeglasses. A company, Low Cost Eyeglasses, has been formed to make this solution available to those who need it (http://www.lowcosteyeglasses.net).

Griffith's advances in low-cost lenses sprung from his interests in rapid prototyping technologies and efficient manufacturing. Using a process dubbed programmable molding, he created a portable device similar to a desktop printer that can produce any prescription lens from a single-mold surface in five to 10 minutes.

The device casts the lenses by applying pressure and constraints to a programmable membrane, which becomes the mold surface when under pressure. The current device uses car window tinting film for the membrane and a reservoir of baby oil for applying the correct pressure. A large range of lens types, covering the majority of prescriptions, can be cast from two such mold surfaces.[†]

Printed Food and Inkjet Proteins

Shimadzu Biotech, in conjunction with Proteome Systems, makes the Chemical Inkjet Printer (ChIP) to deliver precise picoliter volumes of reagents for microscale on membrane protein digestion:

The novel ChIP technology offers researchers a revolutionary new approach to automatic protein processing, identification, and characterization. Developed jointly by Shimadzu Biotech and Proteome Systems with financial support from the Australian Government's START Program, the ChIP is a unique technology platform for executing micro-scale on-membrane chemistry that will have widespread applications in biomedical research and biomarker discovery.[‡]

Homaro Cantu is a chef at Moto restaurant in Chicago. He uses flavored inks printed onto edible paper.

[His] maki look a lot like the sushi rolls served at other upscale restaurants: pristine, coin-size disks stuffed with lumps of fresh crab and rice and wrapped in shiny nori.

---

[*] Rob Coppinger, "Making Bones about It" and "From Spitfire to Surgery," *The Engineer* (August 4, 2004), http://www.e4engineering.com.
[†] Lemelson MIT Program, press release, February 19, 2004.
[‡] "Shimadzu Biotech and Proteome Systems Win R&D 100 Award for Novel Chemical Inkjet Printer (ChIP) Technology," press release, July 23, 2004, http://www.shimadzu-biotech.net/pages/news/1/press_releases/2004_07_23_chip.php.

They also taste like sushi. But the sushi often contains no fish. It is prepared on a Canon i560 inkjet printer rather than a cutting board. He prints images of maki on pieces of edible paper made of soybeans and cornstarch, using organic, food-based inks of his own concoction. He then flavors the back of the paper, which is ordinarily used to put images onto birthday cakes, with powdered soy and seaweed seasonings.[*]

This is yet another example of technology being redeployed in innovative ways for uses for which it was not originally designed.

Direct Manufacturing Freedom of Creation

Freedom of Creation (FOC) is based in Amsterdam, The Netherlands. This is a collaboration of two design school classmates who produce direct manufactured furniture and lighting using RP techniques. FOC also has been doing interesting work in the area of three-dimensional printed textiles and is worth looking into for examples of innovative applications of RP (http://www.freedomofcreation.com). The work of the FOC team is available from Materialise, n.v., which sells a line of manufacture-on-demand lamps and home furnishings using RP technology (http://www.materialise.com/made/MGXcollection2004.pdf). FOC was acquired by 3D Systems in 2011.

Direct Manufacturing: The Center for Bits and Atoms

The Center for Bits and Atoms (CBA) is an initiative by the Massachusetts Institute of Technology coordinated by Neil Gershenfeld and Bakhtiar Mikhak. The CBA seeks to explore innovative ways to deploy digital technology, including ubiquitous computing, digital programming of living systems, RP, and automated fabrication.[1] One interesting exploration is the use of personal fabrication—that is, the use of digitally controlled RP technology to bring products and replacement parts to remote parts of the world without supply chain infrastructure. From the CBA mission statement:

> The Fab Lab program is part of the MIT's Center for Bits and Atoms (CBA), which broadly explores how the content of information relates to its physical representation.
>
> One of its grand-challenge research goals is to bring the programmability of the digital world to the physical world through the development of technologies to personalize fabrication rather than computation.[†]

The Fab Lab dream is to have technology that will allow a person to download a description of a product and send it to a general purpose fabrication machine, which will then produce a one-off example of the product, assembled, complete with functional parts and fabricated electronic circuitry.[‡]

---

[*] David Bernstein, "When the Sous-Chef Is an Inkjet," *New York Times* (February 3, 2005), http://www.nytimes.com/2005/02/03/technology/circuits/03chef.html (accessed August 7, 2012).
[†] See http://fab.cba.mit.edu/ (accessed August 7, 2012).
[‡] Katharine Dunn, "How to Make (Almost) Anything," *Boston Globe* (January 30, 2005), http://www.boston.com/news/globe/ideas/articles/2005/01/30/how_to_make_almost_anything/ (accessed August 7, 2012).

CONCLUSION

RP is a powerful way to accelerate product development when its capabilities and limitations are understood. Although RP build materials can often mimic but not exactly duplicate the properties of the final production material, they can provide a close enough representation to enable a design and engineering decision, which after all is the purpose of a prototype. It has been shown that RP is also an increasingly common aid in the planning and prepractice of complex surgeries. RP technology can also be used in the direct manufacture of some parts where it is appropriate.

Numerous technologies are available, and it is the task of the design manager and innovator to evaluate these options and choose the technology or combination of technologies that best gets the job done.

Variations of RP and RE technologies are also being deployed and recombined in new and innovative ways, such as for tissue engineering, and to accelerate product development and provide innovative new products and services to enhance human life.

RESOURCES

REFERENCES: PRINT AND ONLINE

Burns, Marshall. *Automated Fabrication*. Englewood Cliffs, NJ: Prentice Hall, 1993. This book gives some interesting history of RP and early innovative applications. The book is out of print, but it is readily available through Alibris.com.

Chelule, K. L., T. Coole, and D. G. Cheshire. "Fabrication of Medical Models from Scan Data via Rapid Prototyping Techniques." School of Engineering and Advanced Technology, Staffordshire University, http://www.deskartes.com/news/fabrication_of_medical_models_fr.htm.

Gebhardt, Andreas. *Rapid Prototyping*. Cincinnati, OH: Hanser-Gardener, 2003.

Grenda, Ed. Castle Island Company publishes the online Worldwide Guide to Rapid Prototyping: http://www.additive3d.com/eg1.htm.

Grimm, Todd A. *User's Guide to Rapid Prototyping*. Society for Manufacturing Engineers, Dearborn, MI, 2005, http://www.sme.org or http://www.tagrimm.com.

Prototype Magazine. http://www.edaltd.co.uk/magdownloads. *Prototype* is full of practical information and product specifications for RP and available for download in pdf format. It is part of the CAD server group of resources found at http://www.cadserver.co.uk.

Time Compression Technologies. http://www.timecompress.com. This publication is advertiser-supported publication covering the RP industry.

Wohlers, Terry. *Wohler's Report*. http://www.wohlersassociates.com. This yearly report provides in-depth market and technical information on RP.

REFERENCES: WEBSITES

CADCAM Net (http://www.cadcamnet.com) is an online subscription-based service that tracks news and developments throughout the CADCAM and RP space.

CAD/CAM Zone (http://www.mmsonline.com) is an online discussion forum for working machinists. It is a good place to go to see discussions on CNC machinery and software from people who make their living in the manufacturing industry.

DesktopNC.com (http://www.desktopcnc.com/index.htm) is a comprehensive resource of nearly every active or inactive manufacturer of small and desktop NC milling machines.

Fabbers.com (http://www.ennex.com/~fabbers/intro.asp) is a community of enthusiasts for direct manufacturing through RP technology. It is hosted by Marshall Burns (http://www.ennex.com).

Milwaukee School of Engineering (http://www.rpc.msoe.edu /medical.php) maintains a list of medical applications of RP.

Rapid Prototyping Mailing List (http://rapid.lpt.fi/.) is an ongoing conversation among more than 1500 people. Edited and categorized archives can be found at the RPML site of Helsinki University of Technology. The "Complete RPML Archives" are the entire contents of all messages posted since September 11, 1995. The list archives thousands of pages of information, which can be used as a source of advice, case studies, contact information, expert individuals, and market data.

The **Whole RP Family Tree** (http://ltk.hut.fi/~koukka/RP/rptree.html) is a compendium of RP that was, is, and is yet to be.

REFERENCES: PROFESSIONAL SOCIETIES

Computer Aided Radiology and Surgery (CARS) Society. http://cars-int.de/index.htm.
Index of CARS Resources. http://homepage2.nifty.com/cas/casref.htm.
International Society for Computer Aided Surgery. http://igs.slu.edu.
International Society for Computer Assisted Orthopaedic Surgery (CAOS). http://www.caos-international.org.
Society of Manufacturing Engineers (SME). http://www.sme.org/rapid. The SME organizes an annual event, the RAPID show, which is a tradeshow and symposium on all facets of the rapid prototyping and reverse engineering and modeling industry. It is a valuable event to attend if you have a special interest in this area. This is the largest event of its kind in North America.

REFERENCES: UNIVERSITIES AND ORGANIZATIONS

Many researchers refer to rapid prototyping by the name *solid freeform fabrication* and *functional freeform fabrication*. A number of projects are underway in tissue engineering, bioceramics, advanced ceramic aerospace materials, direct manufacturing technologies, and nanotechnology. This is a very quickly evolving field. Websites such as the DARPA (Defense Advanced Research Projects Agency) SFF site and the University of Texas, Austin SFF Laboratory are good places to look for links and breaking news. Here are a few of the universities and organizations working in this area:

Bone Tissue and Engineering Center of the University of Pittsburgh (BTEC).
Cornell University Functional Freeform Fabrication. http://www.mae.cornell.edu/ccsl/research/sff/and.
Defense Advanced Research Projects Agency (DARPA) Defense Science Office.
The Genetically Organized Lifelike Electro Mechanics (Golem) Project.
Laboratory for Freeform Fabrication and Advanced Ceramics, Rutgers University.
Laboratory for Freeform Fabrication, University of Texas, Austin.
Massachusetts Institute of Technology (MIT).
Milwaukee School of Engineering.
SFF Conference. The 16th annual meeting was held in 2005 in Austin Texas, and hosted the leading researchers in this field.

Stanford University.
University of Connecticut SFF Program.
University of Dayton.
University of Michigan SFF Laboratory.

ACKNOWLEDGMENTS

Thanks to Hendrik John (Envisiontec GmbH), Bathsheba Grossman, Joe Hiemenz (Stratasys), Jeroen Dille (Materialise n.v.), Bruce Lustig (Solidscape), Karen Kiffney (Z Corp.), Dr. Stefan Hehn (Sirona), Gary Sande (3D Systems), and Ed Grenda for their assistance and contributions to this chapter.

ENDNOTE

1. "Perhaps the most dramatic example at CBA of programming nature comes from my colleagues Joe Jacobson, Shuguang Zhang, and Kim Hamad Schifferli, who showed how to take a protein and stick a 50-atom gold nanocluster onto it. For proteins, their shape is their function. If you use the little antenna to send radio energy into it you change the shape. That means that you can, for example, take a repressor protein that shuts off expression of a gene, and under a radio signal you can release it and let the gene be expressed, and then reattach it. The reason that is so important is that cells run programs to make things. When a cell fabricates, say, a flagellar motor, it's running a complex program, and more importantly it's error-correcting; it's doing logic. The antennas provide handles for programming those pathways. Cells are terrible as general-purpose computers, but they function based on this amazing ability to compute for fabrication. ... The real breakthrough may, in fact, be biological machinery that is programmable for fabrication. This may be the next manufacturing technology." Edge Foundation, http://www.edge.org/3rd_culture/gershenfeld03/gershenfeld_index.html (accessed August 7, 2012). The foundation's website has many such thought-provoking interviews and biographies and is worth visiting.

8 Medical Applications of Rapid Technologies
Technology Update

Theodore R. Kucklick

CONTENTS

Rapid Technologies: It's Not Just for Prototyping Anymore	168
Digital Capture and VR Join the Family	168
Biomedical Reverse Engineering and Patient-Specific Data: A Critical Link	170
Osirix: A Powerful Open-Source Tool for Visualizing DICOM Data Sets	170
Surgical "GPS"	171
It's a Material Issue	174
Dancing a Jig	174
Rapid Technology Innovators	175
RTAM Custom-Made Veterinary Orthopedic Implants	178
Case Study 1	178
Case Study 2	179
Rapid Technologies and Tissue Engineering	180
Digital Scanning and 3D Geometry Reconstruction	180
Case Study 3	181
Resources	182
References: Website	182
Acknowledgments	182

Rapid technologies are a family of digital geometry capture, three-dimensional (3D) data processing, digital freeform fabrication, and virtual reality computer-aided design/computer-aided manufacturing (CAD/CAM) technologies that offer an expanded set of problem-solving tools for medical device research, development, design, and manufacturing.

Since *The Medical Device R&D Handbook, First Edition* was written in 2003–2004, there has been an explosion of applications of medical applications of rapid technologies. A few of these technologies were mentioned in the first edition. This chapter is an update on some of what has developed since that edition was published.

Collectively, these technologies have variously become known as "rapid technologies," including Rapid Technology and Additive Manufacturing (RTAM), Computer-Aided Radiology and Surgery (CARS), reverse engineering (or more properly 3D digital geometry reconstruction), and rapid prototyping (RP). At this time the nomenclature, like the field, is still evolving. If one is on the engineering side, the collective term is typically rapid technologies (or RTAM) or Medical Applications of Rapid Prototyping (MARP). Perhaps a collective engineering acronym could be MART (Medical Applications of Rapid Technologies), which would cover the spectrum of RP, rapid manufacturing, digital freeform fabrication, and 3D data capture and reconstruction.

There has been a significant interest in the application of these rapid technologies, and they offer intriguing possibilities for medical devices. My article "Rapid Technologies in Medicine: The Future is Now," which appeared in the Society for Manufacturing Engineering (SME) magazine *Manufacturing Engineering: Medical Manufacturing 2008 Yearbook*, traced the development of rapid technologies from their early days as a means of intermediate model-making to the 21st century, during which rapid technologies are now being deployed in direct manufacturing (i.e., medical devices) and for which the digitally fabricated object is no longer a prototype; instead, it is the finished product, skipping the intermediate steps of traditional fabrication and tooling.

RAPID TECHNOLOGIES: IT'S NOT JUST FOR PROTOTYPING ANYMORE

The best-known rapid technology is RP. In RP, a digital 3D model is used to drive a layered deposition freeform fabrication device (see Figure 8.1). Some of the most popular of these are the 3D Systems (Rock Hill, SC) stereolithography (SLA®), Stratasys (Eden Prairie, MN) fused deposition modeling (FDM™), EnvisionTec (Gladbeck, Germany) Perfactory® system, Z Corp. (Burlington, MA), 3D printers, and Objet (Rehovot, Israel) Polyjet™ (see Figure 8.2). Easy to use CNC-based tools are also becoming more capable and available as well. RP materials have evolved from being unsuitable for clinical use, to the point at which biocompatible RP materials are now used in Food and Drug Administration (FDA)-cleared commercial applications in dentistry and orthopedic surgery.

DIGITAL CAPTURE AND VR JOIN THE FAMILY

Allied to these systems are digital geometry scanning technologies, often referred to by the misnomer "reverse engineering. There are increasingly cheaper, sophisticated,

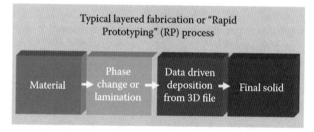

FIGURE 8.1 Typical RP or layered freeform fabrication process.

Medical Applications of Rapid Technologies

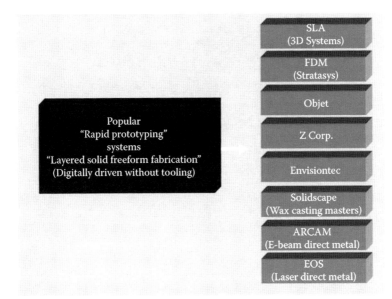

FIGURE 8.2 Popular rapid prototyping and direct manufacturing systems.

and capable systems for capturing 3D surface data for integration into CAD, by suppliers such as Roland DGA, Minolta, FARO, Z Corp. (Handyscan), and several others.

Tools to interactively sculpt 3D data sets in virtual reality with force feedback (haptics) are available from such companies as Immersion and SenseAble. These tools are becoming an important part of the rapid technology toolkit (see Figure 8.3).

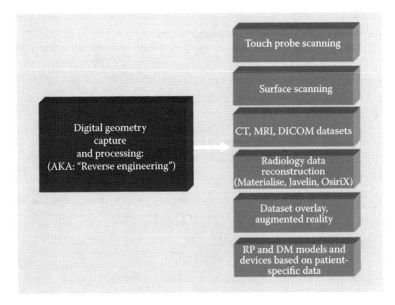

FIGURE 8.3 Digital capture modalities.

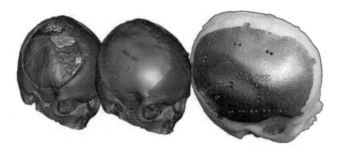

FIGURE 8.4 (See color insert.) Titanium skull plate made in direct metal from a 3D digital model derived from patient radiology data. (Courtesy of Materialise Leuven, Belgium, and Dr. Jules Poukens, Academic Hospital, Maastricht, Belgium.)

BIOMEDICAL REVERSE ENGINEERING AND PATIENT-SPECIFIC DATA: A CRITICAL LINK

Specific to medicine is the ability to generate 3D models from radiology data in the area of CARS. Computerized tomography (CT) scans and magnetic resonance imaging (MRI) and digital imaging and communications in medicine (DICOM) image sets can be turned into models using Materialise (Leuven, Belgium), Javelin, (Park City, UT), and OsiriX (The OsiriX Foundation; http://www.osirixfoundation.com) software. Together these rapid technologies offer a rich set of tools to solve clinical problems.

Figure 8.4 shows an example of a titanium skull plate generated with CT scan data, Materialise software, and direct-metal rapid manufacturing by Arcam (Mölndal, Sweden). The patient model was generated in Mimics™, the skull plate was designed in 3-matic™, and the plate was built in Ti6Al4V titanium with direct-metal rapid manufacturing.

One potential drawback of using radiology in generating images is that the patient is exposed to radiation (e.g., with CT scans) that they otherwise might not have been exposed to. When developing patient-specific solutions based on radiology, it is important that the clinical benefit outweighs the risk and cost of the additional imaging procedures.

Technology alone does not solve clinical problems. A clear understanding of the clinical need, the regulatory requirements, and the insurance reimbursement environment, and applying the appropriate technology are essential to developing and deploying an effective medical device innovation.

OSIRIX: A POWERFUL OPEN-SOURCE TOOL FOR VISUALIZING DICOM DATA SETS

Andrew Swift, MS, CMI (certified medical illustrator) is an expert user of Osirix. I asked him to share some information and images on the program. Osirix is an open-source DICOM viewer with powerful capabilities to manipulate datasets. Osirix is available on the Apple Macintosh platform only (OS 10.5 or higher) and is published by the Osirix Foundation and Pixmeo (Geneva, Switzerland).* Viewers are also available for the Apple iPhone and iPad. Swift described the process of using Osirix as follows:

> Osirix is an open source image processing software used in radiology. It is designed to aid in the visualization of diagnostic images specifically serial DICOM images. One functionality of the software allows the user to extract and render a three-dimensional virtual representation based on the tonal values captured during the scan. The Osirix software can assign transparency and color to select tonal values captured within each 16-bit gray-scale image. Thus colored each slice is stacked relative its position during the initial scan and it is these virtual stacks which are known as "3D Reconstructions." These 3D Reconstructions can be manipulated and then exported as still or moving images.

The software is used as an adjunct to understanding and teaching anatomical concepts. Specifically, Osirix is used to perform virtual dissection in a nondestructive and reversible fashion. Dissections can be made on data sets taken from living individuals.

With traditional dissection, superficial anatomy must be removed or distorted to visualize deep structures, creating an irreversible stepwise process from superficial to deep. With virtual dissection, select areas or entire pixel values may be removed or enhanced.

These virtual 3D reconstructions are tools to interactively perform virtual and nondestructive dissections on DICOM data sets imaged from living subjects. With this tool, the anatomist can perform virtual dissections and stage keyframes throughout the process. Once completed, the entire dissection is recorded from beginning to end by a virtual camera and saved as a movie file. Another application would be to scan a cadaver and use an imaging workstation in the cadaver lab as an adjunct to the dissection of that particular cadaver. This may also help reinforce anatomic relationships and facilitate the correlation of virtual versus actual anatomy (see Figures 8.5 to 8.8).

SURGICAL "GPS"

Allied with digital capture and scanning are digital guidance systems for more accurate surgery. One of the earlier companies in this space was Cybyon (Palo Alto CA, acquired by General Electric in 2004), which made a system that mapped an endoscope image with the patient's MRI and CT scan data, and accurately registered these 3D data sets to offer the surgeon an "augmented reality" view through the endoscope. This enabled the surgeon to avoid critical structures, such as arteries, when performing high-risk brain surgery.

Brainlab (Munich, Germany) makes several applications based on spatial navigation technology, in which a 3D scanner tracks fiducial markers in space. This allows

---

* "Advanced Open Source PACS Workstation DICOM Viewer," OsiriX, http://www.osirix-viewer.com/AboutOsiriX.html. (accessed August 7, 2012).

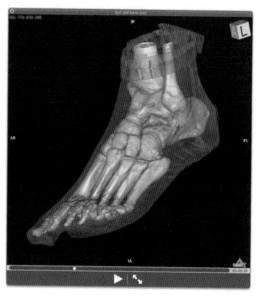

FIGURE 8.5 (**See color insert.**) Osirix reconstruction of foot and ankle. (Courtesy of Andrew Swift, CMI.)

the registration in space of surgical instruments to anatomical landmarks for faster and more accurate surgery. For videos and examples see http://www .brainlab.com.

Digital scanning and reconstruction are important tools in reconstructive surgery, dentistry, orthopedics, and anapalstology—the constructions of aesthetic prosthetics (see Figure 8.9).

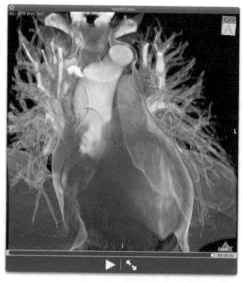

FIGURE 8.6 (**See color insert.**) Image of heart and pulomonary vessels. (Courtesy of Andrew Swift, CMI.)

Medical Applications of Rapid Technologies 173

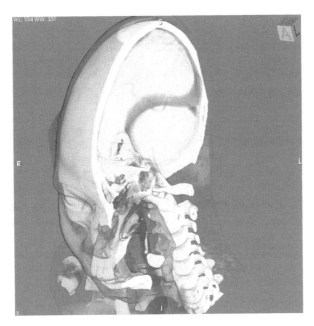

FIGURE 8.7 (**See color insert.**) Digital reconstruction of cranial anatomy from radiology data. (Courtesy Andrew Swift, CMI.)

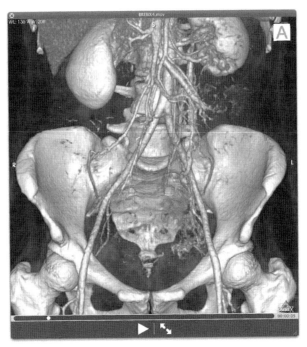

FIGURE 8.8 (**See color insert.**) Digital reconstruction of kidneys and abdominal vasculature from radiology data. (Courtesy Andrew Swift, CMI.)

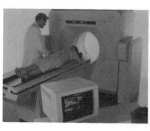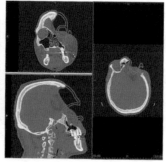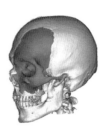

FIGURE 8.9 (**See color insert.**) Process of capturing radiology data for 3D reconstruction and implant production. (Courtesy of Materialise, Leuven, Belgium.)

IT'S A MATERIAL ISSUE

RP and prototype casting materials are usually not suitable for use in a production or human-use medical device. Some materials that are more suitable are the PC-ISO polycarbonate build material from Stratasys and the Hapco (Hanover, MA) line of FDA-approved casting materials. 3D Systems, in conjunction with Dreve (Germany), has developed the materials for the V-Flash™ rapid direct manufacturing system for hearing aid shells. Digital direct metal fabrication with laser and e-beam has proved to be an effective technology for producing implants directly from digital files, using titanium and cobalt-chrome alloys with high purity and good materials properties.

DANCING A JIG

Another effective way to deploy rapid technologies is building molds, jigs, and fixtures with rapid prototyping methods (see Figure 8.10). Jigs and fixtures are less

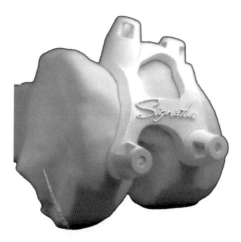

FIGURE 8.10 Biomet signature RP-generated drill guide based on patient's radiology data. (Courtesy of Biomet Inc., Warsaw, IN.)

sensitive to material choices than devices meant for body contact or implantation.[*] Several of these devices are now on the market for more accurately cutting bone during joint replacements and for putting the implant in place.[†] The first company in the space for total knee arthoplasty (TKA) jigs was OtisMed (Alameda, CA, acquired by Stryker in 2009), Signature™ from Biomet (based on modeling technology from Materialise, and using Stratasys part-building, released in 2008), and Visonaire™ from Smith and Nephew (S&N), released in 2011.[‡] S&N also announced a partnership with Brainlab (Munich, Germany) to utilize their guidance and positioning systems with their orthopedic implants.

RAPID TECHNOLOGY INNOVATORS

Following are just some of the innovators in rapid technology:

- MAKO Surgical (Ft. Lauderdale, FL). Produces the MAKOplasty robotic tactile feedback guidance system for precision resection of joint tissue for minimally invasive implant placement, based on patient radiology data.
- ConforMIS (Burlington, MA). Produces custom-made joint implants based on the patient's radiology data.
- Sirona Dental (Long Island City, NY). Makes the CEREC™ system that digitally scans dental anatomy and produces a ceramic replacement crown using CAD/CAM technology.
- Align Technology (Santa Clara, CA). Makes the Invisalign invisible orthodontic brace system and utilizes rapid technologies in their production process.
- Sensable (San Jose, CA). Dental Lab System offers an integrated suite that allows a dentist to digitally scan dental anatomy to design and build crowns and bridges. The technician then sculpts and designs the wax casting master in a digital environment, using the PHANTOM™ input stylus to provide virtual-reality force feedback.
- 3D Systems (Rock Hill, SC). Recently launched the V-Flash™, which enables direct digital manufacturing of custom hearing aid shells in an FDA-approved material.
- Biomet Corporation (Warsaw, IN). Has been using rapid technologies for several years to make customized implants for those patients who need customized implants, from data sets derived from CT scans. These have been used to treat patients with unusual anatomy, deformities, or tissue loss from cancer resection where no standard implant device exists

---

[*] "Ask the Experts: Patient-Specific TKR Instrumentation," ORTHOSuperSite, February 16, 2011, http://www.orthosupersite.com/view.aspx?rid=80597.
[†] Adolph V. Lombardi, Keith R. Berend, and Joanne B. Adams, "Patient-Specific Approach in Total Knee Arthroplasty," *Orthopedics* 31, no. 9 (September 2008): 927, http://www.orthosupersite.com/view.aspx?rid=31419.
[‡] "Smith & Nephew Launches VISIONAIRE Patient Matched Technology for Total Knee Replacement," Medical News Today, http://www.medicalnewstoday.com/articles/143015.php.

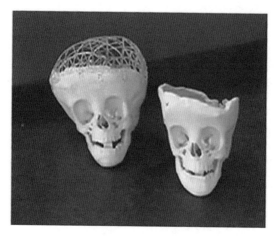

FIGURE 8.11 Bioabsobable cranial mesh used to treat conjoined twins. (Courtesy of Biomet PMI, Warsaw, IN; *Medical Applications of Rapid Prototyping* [DVD], 2007, SME.)

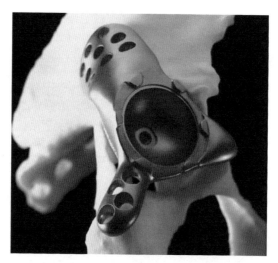

FIGURE 8.12 Patient-matched acetabulum implant. (Courtesy of Biomet PMI, Warsaw, IN.)

(see Figures 8.11 and 8.12). One example is a bioabsorbable cranial mesh to protect the brain of conjoined twins who were connected at the head (see Figure 8.11). The mesh was made from the patients' radiology data and was designed to dissolve over time as the child grew.*

At the *American Academy of Orthopaedic Surgeons* (AAOS) in 2008, Biomet launched their Signature™ positioning guides for knee replacement surgery. These

---

* For more information on this case example, see Ted Kucklick, *Medical Applications of Rapid Prototyping* (Dearborn, MI Society of Manufacturing Engineers, 2007).

Medical Applications of Rapid Technologies

single-use custom guides are built from the patient's radiology data and produced with Materialise software and Stratasys FDM to help ensure the accurate fit and function of the orthopedic implant.

EOS GmbH (Munich, Germany) and Arcam AB (Mölndal, Sweden) are pioneering the direct manufacturing of orthopedic implants suitable for human use from e-beam and laser energy-fused advanced engineering materials, such as cobalt-chrome and titanium.

Arcam uses a laser-based direct-metal system that uses an electron beam to melt and fuse metal layer by layer. An elevator drops the solidified part into a bed of powdered metal and thus "grows" the part. These direct-metal parts are used in custom-made implants and aerospace applications.

EOS GmbH recently began marketing implants for human use in Europe. Figure 8.13 shows examples, including an acetabular implant with complex features (see Figure 8.14). An advantage to rapid prototyping and manufacturing was stated by industry analyst Terry Wohlers, who noted that "complexity comes free." That is, it takes no longer to form a complex structure than a solid one. This can be an advantage when building scaffolds for tissue in-growth.

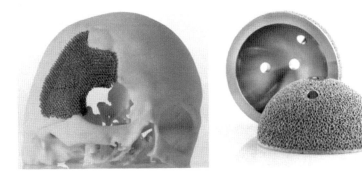

FIGURE 8.13 (See color insert.) Complex direct-metal mesh skull plate and acetabular cup implant. (Courtesy of Arcam AB, Mölndal, Sweden.)

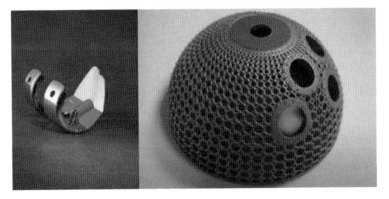

FIGURE 8.14 Laser-sintered direct metal knee and acetabular implants. (Courtesy of EOS GmbH Munich, Germany.)

RTAM CUSTOM-MADE VETERINARY ORTHOPEDIC IMPLANTS

Ola Harrysson, PhD, is director of the North Carolina State Edward P. Fitts Department of Industrial and Systems Engineering Rapid Prototyping and Additive Manufacturing Program. Most of his research involves RP, specifically the medical applications of RP. Dr. Harryson had graciously supplied the following two case studies of veterinary orthopedic examples of RTAM.

CASE STUDY 1

Aspen, a Labrador Retriever was diagnosed with a chondrosarcoma of the proximal portion of the tibia. A limb-sparing surgery was planned. A titanium alloy free-form implant was designed and fabricated via electron beam melting (EBM; see Figure 8.15). The implant has a solid proximal portion made to receive the cemented tibial component of a total knee prosthesis. Distally, the implant has a porous portion for bone ingrowth and an interlocking nail for initial fixation to the distal portion of the tibia on the mediolateral and craniocaudal radiographs of the limb made immediately after surgery. It has been paired with a commercial cementless femoral TKA component. Five custom-made titanium alloy bolts secure the implant to the distal portion of the tibia (see Figure 8.16).

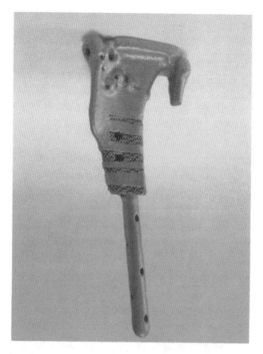

FIGURE 8.15 Implant fabricated on the EBM machine using Ti6Al4V.

Medical Applications of Rapid Technologies

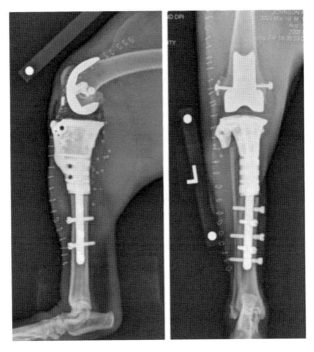

FIGURE 8.16 Radiograph of custom-made veterinary implant for Aspen.

CASE STUDY 2

Cassidy, a mixed-breed dog, had sustained a partial amputation of the distal portion of his pelvic limb distal to the stifle (knee) joint. A socket prosthesis was prepared but failed because of the high skin mobility and the dog's reluctance to wear it. A transdermal osseointegrated implant was designed and implanted. A prosthetic foot was secured to the osseointegrated implant after several months. The dog learned to walk on his prosthetic leg over a period of a few weeks (see Figure 8.17). Over time,

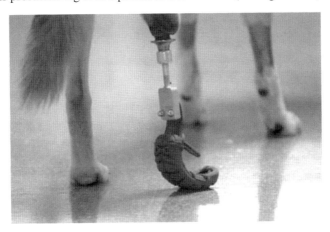

FIGURE 8.17 (See color insert.) Cassidy walking on his osseointegrated prosthetic.

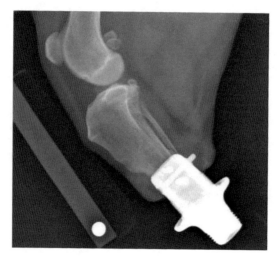

FIGURE 8.18 Radiograph of Cassidy's implant.

the bone-implant interface was stable and showed no sign of infection or loosening (see Figure 8.18).

RAPID TECHNOLOGIES AND TISSUE ENGINEERING

Tissue engineering methods using rapid technologies are being developed at the Medical University of South Carolina (Charleston, SC) under the direction of Dr. Vladimir Mironov. Here, inkjet printing technology is used to build constructs of hydrogels and living tissue with the goal of one day growing replacement tissues and organs (see Figure 8.19).[*] Other work in this area is being done at Wake Forest University by surgeon Anthony Atala, director of the Wake Forest Institute for Regenerative Medicine, focusing on the science of growing and regenerating tissues and organs.[†] Organovo (San Diego, CA) has recently announced the first commercially available bioprinter, the NovaGen MMX, which claims the ability to generate semisolid structures with three-dimensional structure and high cell viability.[‡]

DIGITAL SCANNING AND 3D GEOMETRY RECONSTRUCTION

Rapid technologies are used in medicine to scan facial features and rebuild them with anaplastology. The Johns Hopkins Hospital (Baltimore, MD) and its School of Arts as Applied to Medicine regularly use rapid technologies to scan, capture, visualize, and model medical data.

---

[*] For more information on this case example, see Ted Kucklick, *Medical Applications of Rapid Prototyping* (Society of Manufacturing Engineers, Dearborn, MI, 2007).

[†] For more information, see "TED Conference Video of Dr. Atala," http://www.ted.com/talks/anthony_atala_growing_organs_engineering_tissue.html (accessed August 7, 2012).

[‡] "About Us," Organovo, http://www.organovo.com/about, (accessed 8/7/2012).

Medical Applications of Rapid Technologies

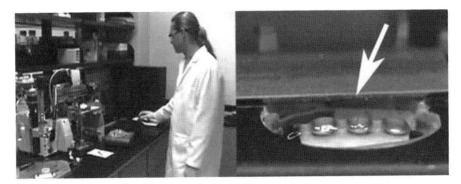

FIGURE 8.19 (**See color insert.**) Printed hydrogel biologic constructs incorporating living cells. (Courtesy of Vladimir Mironov PhD, MUSC, from the *Medical Applications of Rapid Prototyping* [DVD], 2007, SME.)

Direct Dimensions (Baltimore, MD) is a contract 3D scanning service. The following is a case study of a particularly challenging scanning project in conjunction with Johns Hopkins University:

Case Study 3

Pterosaurs are known more commonly as pterodactyls. Because their bones were hollow, the skeletons preserved very poorly, as they often were crushed by the weight of sediment.

Julia Molnar, a graduate student at Johns Hopkins University department of Art as Applied to Medicine, brought to Direct Dimensions a set of bone castings from a well-preserved pterosaur skeleton. For her master's thesis project, Ms. Molnar was studying the way in which pterosaurs would have taken flight.

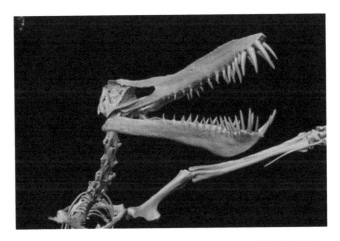

FIGURE 8.20 3D scanned pterosaur skeleton. (Courtesy of Julia Molnar and Direct Dimensions, Inc., Baltimore, MD.)

The castings of the 8-foot pterosaur skeleton were taken with a FARO Arm (Faro, Lake Mary, FL) equipped with the FARO noncontact laser line scanner.

Ms. Molnar described the process: "The scanning was challenging because there were many undercuts, particularly around the ribcage, and the casting is very fragile."

With these completed digital 3D models (see Figure 8.20), Ms. Molnar then created a 3D animation to show the launch movement in 3D Studio Max (Autodesk, Inc., Sausalito, CA) rendering and animation program.[*]

RESOURCES

REFERENCES: WEBSITE

Society for Manufacturing Engineers (Dearborn, MI). http://www.sme.org. One way to stay up-to-date with developments in Rapid technologies is through the Society for Manufacturing Engineers RAPID Show, which recently included a day-long special interest session on medical technology applications.

ACKNOWLEDGMENTS

The author would like to thank Materialise, Direct Dimensions, Biomet, Dr. Ola Harryson, Julia Molnar, and Andrew Swift for supplying case studies and images for this chapter.

---

[*] The author would like to thank Michael Raphael of Direct Dimensions (Baltimore, MD) for supplying this case study. For more case studies, see Ted Kucklick, *Medical Applications of Rapid Prototyping* (Society of Manufacturing Engineering, Dearborn, MI, 2007).

9 Reverse Engineering in Medical Device Design

Theodore R. Kucklick

CONTENTS

Value of Reverse Engineering in Patient Care 187
Reverse Engineering Methods 189
    Digitizing.. 189
        Case Study: Using a Low-Cost Scanner to Digitize a Vertebra 189
    Using a Flatbed Scanner for Three-Dimensional Reconstruction..................... 192
    Cannibalizing an Existing Device 193
        Why Reinvent the Handle?.. 194
    Case Study: Building on an Existing Product for Higher Performance............ 194
        Case Study: Making Your Own Stent 196
Where to Find Used Medical Devices and Equipment 196
Three-Dimensional Reconstruction 198
    Common Three-Dimensional Capture File Formats and Terminology............. 198
Continuity 200
    Automated Touch Probe... 201
    Light Beam Scanners 201
    Arm Probe Scanners...202
    Arm Probe Noncontact Scanners 202
    Three-Dimensional Image Reconstruction 203
Reverse Engineering and Inspection..203
Destructive Reverse Engineering 204
Reverse Modeling, Radiology, and Surgical Planning..204
Resources 204
    References: Print 204
    References: Professional Societies...205
    References: Three-Dimensional Information Websites 205
    Vendors: Bones and Bone Models 205
    Vendors: MRI and CT Reconstruction and RP Modeling.................................206
    Vendors: Reconditioned and Used Medical Equipment 206
    Vendors: Three-Dimensional Capture Equipment 207
    Vendors: Three-Dimensional Scanning and Manufacturing Inspection 207
    Vendors: Three-Dimensional Service Bureaus 207
    Vendors: Three-Dimensional Software 208
Endnotes...208

Reverse engineering (RE) is the process of taking something apart to see how it works and making a product that functions, in whole or part, like the original product, or as an intermediate step to an improvement on the original product. It is an attempt to recover as much of the "top-level specification"[*] of a product as possible, and to understand how and why a product works. Other related concepts to RE are reverse modeling and image reconstruction. This chapter will discuss the general subject of RE, review case examples, and provide a list of resources.

RE to some is a negative word. It is, but only if it is being used to take the technology and intellectual property of others, claiming them as your own, and avoiding the work of making your own original contribution. RE is a way to study what is already being done to make improvements, advancements, or new applications of existing technology. It is also a way to study existing products to develop compatible products or products that conform to standard clinical usage. Did you ever take things apart when you were growing up to see how they worked? (Most of the great inventors have.) Then you have engaged in RE. RE, properly used, is an important tool, a textbook, for advancing the state of the art in clinical technology.

> Reverse engineering has long been held a legitimate form of discovery in both legislation and court opinions. The Supreme Court has confronted the issue of reverse engineering in mechanical technologies several times, upholding it under the principles that it is an important method of the dissemination of ideas and that it encourages innovation in the marketplace. In *Kewanee Oil v. Bicron*, [the court called reverse engineering] "a fair and honest means of starting with the known product and working backwards to divine the process which aided in its development or manufacture."[†1]

Companies that make scanning devices prefer the term *reverse modeling*, as they find the term *reverse engineering* to be negative, implying that their equipment enables the improper taking of the design work of others. Reverse modeling, or more properly digital geometry capture, is actually a subset activity of RE. It is a digital version of the "plaster splash" method of copying geometry, which was once common in the automotive aftermarket design business.

RE serves an important function in the development of new medical device technology. Observing and studying accepted and proven technology is important when developing new products.

RE for the purposes of learning and making your own original contribution is appropriate. However, plagiarizing, pirating, and purloining another's product design and intellectual property is not. The German industrial designer Rido Busse developed the Plagiarius Award in 1977, in response to his designs being pirated by unscrupulous manufacturers.[‡] The motto of Aktion-Plagiarius is "Innovation vs. Imitation." The German Industrial Designers Association now awards the prize, a black garden gnome with a gold nose, to the most egregious

---

[*] David C. Musker, "Reverse Engineering," http://www.jenkins.eu/articles-general/reverse-engineering.asp#a3 (accessed August 11, 2012).
[†] Chilling Effects, "Frequently Asked Questions (and Answers) About Reverse Engineering," http://www.chillingeffects.org/reverse/faq.cgi (accessed August 11, 2012).
[‡] See Action Plagiarius (accessed August 11, 2012), http://www.plagiarius.com/e_index.html.

examples of design theft. "Winners" of this dubious distinction may be found at http://www.plagiarius.com/e_index.html. RE properly done is an educational exercise that leads to innovation. You look at what is being done and find where it does and does not work, identify areas where it does not meet customer needs, and build on this information to do better. We learn what is being done so that we can rise above the state of the art with our own original contribution.

The imitator dooms himself to hopeless mediocrity.

—**Ralph Waldo Emerson**[*]

An even more serious abuse of RE is the production of counterfeit products with faked approval stamps. Such counterfeit products have shown up in aircraft parts and pharmaceuticals. Fake products can result in unfounded liability claims against the legitimate manufacturer and damage to its branding and reputation. The industry needs to be vigilant against this dangerous criminal activity. This is not just pirating intellectual property; it is dangerous to public health and safety. MDDI Devicelink reports that "both finished goods and device parts have been successfully faked. For example, intra-aortic pumps worth $7 million were recalled after malfunctioning components were found to be counterfeit."[†] Recent news stories documented a medical device distributor prosecuted for selling fake hernia repair mesh, supposedly made by the Ethicon division of Johnson & Johnson.[‡] Patients found to have received this fake product had to undergo revision surgery to remove the counterfeit product. Some of the larger medical device manufacturers have taken stringent measures to curb gray market trade in their products to prevent fakes from entering their distribution chain. The International Anti-Counterfeiting Coalition (http://www.iacc.org) and CSA International (http://www.csa-international.org) monitor activity in the trafficking of counterfeit products.

If you discover a technology by RE that is patented, you cannot use it anyway, unless it helps lead you to your own original invention, or you compensate the originator by way of an agreed-to license and royalty, or work around the patent. If it is a trade secret, and you are able to arrive at the know-how to make the product independently, you can use this information. If the information disclosed in the product is neither patented nor a trade secret, it is available in the public domain and free for you to use, learn from, or build on. RE is also a way to discover what is already being done, and what is patent protected, so that you can avoid unintentional infringement. It is the responsibility of the designer and engineer to research prior art in the area in which they are working. With the placement of the U.S. patent library online, this has become a much easier task than in the past. The searchable library of issued patents and published applications can be found at http://www.uspto.gov.

---

[*] Ralph Waldo Emerson, "Address to Divinity Students," *Harvard Classics*, vol. 5 (1937): 39.
[†] "FDA Issues Alert on Counterfeit Polypropylene Mesh Used in Hernia Repair," http://www.infectioncontroltoday.com/news/2003/12/fda-issues-alert-on-counterfeit-polypropylene-mes.aspx (accessed August 11, 2012).
[‡] Rick Dana Barlow, "Facts on Fakes," *Healthcare Purchasing News* (March 2004).

Another use of RE is the legitimate practice of studying a technology or method that is being applied in one area and redeploying and repurposing it for a different use. This is how many important clinical advances have occurred. One prolific inventor for a major medical device company often starts his invention process with a trip to the hardware store. It was his observation of how lead weights were clamped to a fishing line that inspired an idea for replacing intercorporeal suture knots with a polymer bead clamped and melted to the suture. As many clinical innovations have probably come from the toy store and the tackle box as from the research lab. In another example, IDEO, an engineering and design consultancy based in Palo Alto, CA, keeps a library of interesting and clever mechanical devices from which its designers can study and draw inspiration.* Modifying and "hacking" existing technology have become popular pastimes. Two books on the subject of hardware hacking are *Hardware Hacking Projects for Geeks* by Scott Fullam (O'Reilly, Sebastopol, CA, 2003) and *Hardware Hacking: How to Have Fun While Voiding Your Warranty* by Joe Grand (Syngress, Rockland, MA, 2004).

The term *MacGyvering* (verb) has entered the popular slang lexicon to signify the act of recombining and repurposing objects and technology at hand.† Another term for this is *bricolage* (noun), an assemblage made or put together using whatever materials happen to be available. A *bricoleur* is one who invents his own tools and works with what is at hand. For example, the winning participants on the television series *Junkyard Wars* are the bricoleurs most adept at MacGyvering bricolage and show up the competition as mere bricklayers.

On the subject of RE, Pamela Samuelson wrote the following:

> Reverse engineering is fundamentally directed to discovery and learning. Engineers learn the state of the art not just by reading printed publications, going to technical conferences, and working on projects for their firms, but also by reverse engineering others' products. Learning what has been done before often leads to new products and advances in know-how. Reverse engineering may be a slower and more expensive way for information to percolate through a technical community than patenting or publication, but it is nonetheless an effective source of information. Of necessity, reverse engineering is a form of dependent creation, but this does not taint it, for in truth, all innovators stand on the shoulders of both giants and midgets. Progress in science and the useful arts is advanced by dissemination of know-how, whether by publication, patenting or reverse engineering.‡

Computer programs, software and firmware, as well as some circuitry are in a different category than physical parts when it comes to copying and RE. The software, electronics, and entertainment industries have erected a number of barriers against RE by use of copyright and licensing laws. Computer programs are copyrighted, and therefore copying any part of the program is prohibited. Also, computer programs are not sold to the end user; they are licensed. The end user does not take title to the program as property. As a condition of the license that is an agreement between

---

* Jeremy Myerson, *IDEO: Masters of Innovation* (New York: TeNeues, 2001).
† *MacGyver* was a popular television show in the 1980s about "the adventures of a secret agent armed with almost infinite scientific resourcefulness." The author has even seen *MacGyvering* listed in a German technology lexicon.
‡ Pamela Samuelson and Suzanne Scotchmer, "The Law & Economics of Reverse Engineering," *Yale Law Journal* (April 2002), http://ist-socrates.berkeley.edu/~scotch/re.pdf.

the seller and buyer, the right to use the program is controlled by contract, and the licensee submits to a number of terms and restrictions, including an agreement not to reverse engineer or decompile the software. The Digital Millennium Copyright Act (DMCA) goes even further by criminalizing the act of defeating anticopying locks and disseminating any copyrighted information thus obtained. To detect this, some software makers insert nonfunctional code and byte obfuscators into programs as markers to detect unauthorized copying. Software publishers have made it especially onerous for you to look under the hood and see how their software ticks.

Physical objects that are sold become the property of the purchaser. The owner is free to take apart the product to see how it works, unless the buyer and seller agree otherwise. Physical objects may be covered by copyrights and design patents. Boat hulls are subject to a special protection, from what is called the plug molding rule, or using a boat hull as a mold plug to make a duplicate of the hull.

RE can involve taking an existing part, and without the original drawings or computer-aided design (CAD) model, producing a duplicate. This has an important application in situations in which drawings or a CAD model to your own part no longer exist, if they ever did. Three-dimensional scanning technologies and rapid prototyping (RP) have greatly simplified the process of RE these types of parts.

RE tools also make possible the production of patient-matched and patient-specific prosthetics. With the availability of RE and RP and manufacturing, this is more feasible all the time. In Chapter 8, a case study is given for the Sirona Dental GmbH Cerec® system, which uses digital tools to capture tooth information and build a final dental crown while the patient waits. The use of RP-produced anatomical models made from patient magnetic resonance imaging (MRI) and computer tomography (CT) scans to plan complex surgeries has become commonplace. Stanford University is taking this a step further, by building patient-specific computer analysis models that allow, for example, for accurate modeling of blood flow in arteries, including fluid shear forces and vessel elasticity, which can help predict the results of vascular surgeries.[*]

RE tools may also be used to verify the accuracy of your own manufactured parts. For example, a molded part is scanned in three dimensions and then overlaid with the three-dimensional CAD model to check for deviations between the manufactured part and the base CAD model data. A number of service bureaus offer this capability.[†]

VALUE OF REVERSE ENGINEERING IN PATIENT CARE

When designing surgical devices, product acceptance is sometimes based on how closely the device works like the devices the surgeon is familiar with already. Surgeons, especially those who do a large volume of procedures, are sensitive to anything that disrupts their workflow, even if it is a better-performing product. Many times surgeons will accept or reject a product based on how it feels in their hands. If the feel of your product is not what they have come to expect from a product of the type you are designing, they may reject the product.

---

[*] See http://www.cicas.org/bits/home.php?pg=partlab.
[†] For example, see http://www.laserdesign.com and http://www.scansite.com; also see http://www.sculptors.org for information on art-based and sculpture-based services.

In this process it is vitally important to actually observe what surgeons do, rather than rely only on what they tell you, or worse, relying only on descriptions in textbook literature. To rely only on textbook or verbal descriptions of a surgical procedure can lead to embarrassing and expensive design mistakes. Direct observation gives you a more complete and accurate picture of how a product is actually used, and why existing products work the way they do.

Physician preference is often based on their particular training. This will affect how surgical procedures evolve over time, and sometimes surgeons use procedures that seem counterintuitive to one who is not a practitioner. There is also not one way of doing things. Different surgeons that study under different mentors at different schools will do procedures in their own idiomatic way. There will be regional and national preferences. For example, electrosurgical pencils in the United States are sold with push buttons. Surgeons in Europe prefer hand pieces with rocker switches. This has to do with the differences in the way the instrument is held in the hand and how the surgeon stands relative to the patient. Therefore, it is important to observe not only the handful of surgeons who are your close associates, but also a larger sample outside of your immediate board of advisors.

If you are a medical device designer, it is your responsibility to learn and know as much as possible about the way your product is used, and the beneficial outcomes it is supposed to produce for the patient, as well as to be aware of any problems your device might cause. You need to talk to end-users and have a deep understanding of their needs gained by direct observation. If you design surgical devices, this means observing surgeries. You also need to observe the patients your device will be used on. If you are a manager, this means sending your designers and engineers regularly into the operating room. The smart managers know this and do this.

Managers who keep their designers and engineers and product managers penned up in their cubicles are doing a disservice to their workers, their company, and the doctors and patients the company serves. The designers are not being given the tools they need to make knowledgeable contributions. (If you work for this kind of company, you may want to look for a better-managed place to work, with better training and growth opportunities.)

The practitioner and his support staff are motivated by patient care. This usually means providing the best care to the most patients at the most affordable cost. Look for ways that this has been achieved in existing products, and apply those lessons in your products.

Examining existing products, finding out how and why they developed, and carefully observing how they are used can help lead to innovative new products and procedures that will be accepted into the current surgical workflow.

RE in medical device design can fall into the following categories:

- Digitizing a part to make a duplicate, if allowable
- Taking things apart to see how they work
- Using a mechanism from one product to use in a new way in another product prototype
- Competitive product analysis
- Prevention of unintentional infringement

Reverse Engineering in Medical Device Design

- Detection of copying or infringement in a competitor's product
- Production of a replica or aftermarket part no longer supplied by a manufacturer
- Using an existing product as the basis of a new similar or compatible product
- Anatomical reconstruction for visualization
- Anatomical reconstruction to produce a fitted prosthesis
- Anatomical reconstruction to produce a replacement prosthesis

REVERSE ENGINEERING METHODS

DIGITIZING

Case Study: Using a Low-Cost Scanner to Digitize a Vertebra

The Roland MDX-20 is an inexpensive three-axis mill and three-dimensional scanner combination. While working on the design of an orthopedic implant, the RE capabilities of the MDX-20 made the design of a properly fitting implant possible.

One of the important features of an orthopedic implant is that it needs to fit closely to the bone where it is being placed for the bone to grow into the implant and anchor it in place. The product needs to fit closely to the lamina of the vertebral body for proper fixation. The lamina of the spine, however, is a complex surface for which it is difficult to make a model that fits to it properly.

Several attempts were made to look at spine vertebra models, measure landmarks with calipers, and build a model in CAD of an implant. Getting a rapid prototype implant to fit over the complex surfaces of the spine proved difficult and frustrating, resulting in several unsuccessful rapid prototype iterations.

When building an implant model from automotive styling clay onto a spine model, it became apparent that a digital "buck" or armature was needed to properly model the implant in CAD.

A spine model was obtained from Pacific Research Laboratories (Sawbones). This model was placed into the Roland MDX-20 and scanned (see Figure 9.1).

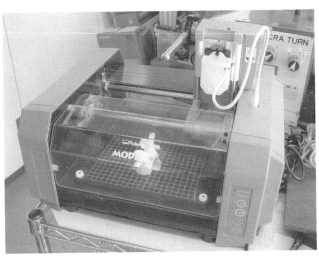

FIGURE 9.1 Setting up the spine model for scanning.

The MDX-20 has both a milling and scanning head. The cutting spindle head was removed, and the scanning sensor unit was mounted into the machine. The vertebra model was then mounted to the work area with adhesive clay. The surface of the model was scanned using the Roland's piezo needle touch probe scanning head. The MDX-20 is capable of scanning any firm object, such as metal, plastic, or clay. Parts that are made of rubber or do not have a firm surface cannot be scanned with the touch probe.

The Roland comes bundled with a simple-to-use program, Dr. Picza (see Figure 9.2). This program saves the scan data in a proprietary format (.PIX), which may then be exported as .DXF, .SAT, VRML, 3DMF, ACIS, or IGES.

In this example, the scan was exported as .IGES and opened in Rhino® (Robert McNeel Associates, Seattle, WA; http://www.Rhino3D.com) (see Figure 9.3). Rhino was used to trim and clean up and cap the open side of the mesh. Rhino is a relatively inexpensive ($895), easy-to-use program for producing and editing high-quality meshes. Another strength of the program is its ability to act as a three-dimensional hub, which means it can open a wide range of three-dimensional formats and export the edited mesh to yet another variety of formats. Rhino supports third-party plug-ins, including a plug-in to import Roland .PIX files directly into Rhino. This is useful for handling large, complex .PIX scan files from Roland DG scanners.

The inexpensive touch probe scanner shown in Figure 9.2 is useful for scanning one side of a surface at a time. You could scan two or more sides at a time

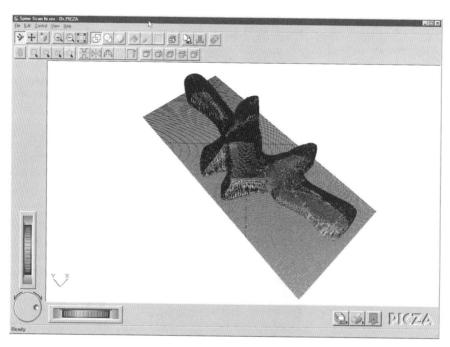

FIGURE 9.2 Scanned mesh in Dr. Picza capture program.

Reverse Engineering in Medical Device Design

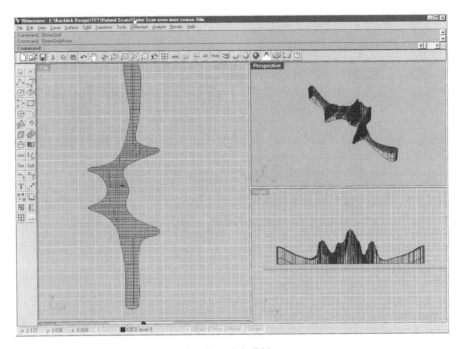

FIGURE 9.3 Editing three-dimensional mesh in Rhino.

and assemble the meshes in a three-dimensional editing program; however, this would be a lot of work (see Figure 9.3). Roland makes a line of noncontact rotary laser scanners if you need to digitize a part "in the round." Another option for capturing geometry is digitizing probe arms from Faro and Immersion Corporation.

Producing a high-quality watertight mesh is important when importing into a CAD solid modeling program. This means that the mesh is free of gaps or discontinuities. This is important for the mesh to turn into a complete solid when imported, instead of a collection of fragmented surfaces. Using this method, it may take a number of attempts to find the combination of file formats (.DXF, .IGES, .STEP, .SAT) that produces a solid model in your CAD program (see Figure 9.4).

This is a fairly simple demonstration of reverse modeling an anatomical specimen using inexpensive equipment and a mainstream engineering CAD program. This process of reverse modeling has been highly developed in the toy industry, where very complex models are sculpted, digitized, edited in a three-dimensional surfacing program, and output for prototyping and tooling.

Vendors can be an important resource for more sophisticated model production work. Programs such as Innovmetric's (Sainte-Foy, QC, Canada) PolyWorks™ offer sophisticated tools for handling and managing scanned point cloud data.

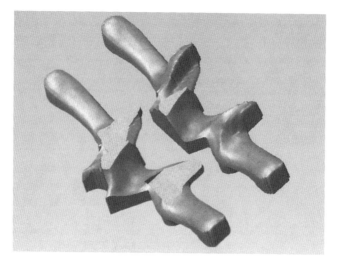

FIGURE 9.4 Solid CAD model of spine in SolidWorks. Features like the spinous process may be resected in CAD realistically. The lamina was sectioned with planes to extract curves for lofting a matching surface. (Example series T. Kucklick, Kucklick Design, Los Gatos, CA.)

USING A FLATBED SCANNER FOR THREE-DIMENSIONAL RECONSTRUCTION

With so many tools at our disposal, we can combine them to quickly and easily solve problems. The tools may not be shrink-wrapped together into one package, but with a little imagination they can be used in innovative combinations.

I once had a need to determine the volume of tissue heated by a radio frequency (RF) ablation device I was working on. The purpose of the device was to produce RF ablations in solid organs to treat cancerous tumors. Because the ablations were being made with multiple electrodes and produced an irregular shape, calculating the volume of the ablations might have been a challenge.

To solve this problem, chicken breast was packed into a metal cup. The cup acted as the ground electrode. The ablation needle device was inserted into the solid mass of chicken meat, and the device delivered energy according to a time- and temperature protocol.

The chicken was then frozen and sliced up to 3 mm sections with a commercial meat slicer. The slices were then put on letter-size overhead transparency plastic sheets. These were then placed on a flatbed scanner and, in order of the sections, scanned. The scans were saved as bitmap files and adjusted for brightness and contrast in Adobe Photoshop®. The scans were then imported into Corel Draw®, and the blanched, ablated area of the chicken was traced in the draw program. These outlines were exported as .DXF outlines and saved. These outlines were then imported into a CAD program (in this case Autocad®). The outlines were extruded into solid objects in the CAD program to a depth of 3 mm. Once the objects were generated in the CAD program, using the program's tools to calculate the volume of the ablation became a simple matter. To visualize the ablations, the sections were rendered in a

Reverse Engineering in Medical Device Design

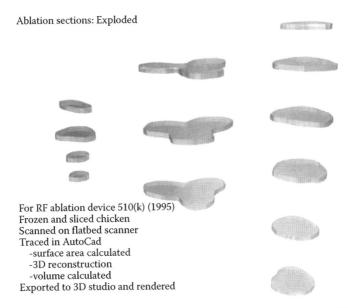

FIGURE 9.5 Three-dimensional tissue reconstruction using simple tools. (T. Kucklick for RITA Medical.)

three-dimensional program, 3D Studio® (see Figure 9.5). This allowed for the use of the data for interpretation and presentations. This was done with a combination of simple-to-use and readily available tools.

CANNIBALIZING AN EXISTING DEVICE

One of the ways to develop new medical devices is to cannibalize a device that is already in use.

When working on a project for a client, I needed a robust flexible catheter with a steerable end for a proof-of-concept prototype. I could have built this from scratch; however, I would have had to locate materials, get them in-house, and build up this assembly. The cost in billable hours to build from scratch would be higher than locating and buying a used device and cannibalizing the part I needed. I suspected that what I wanted was readily available off the shelf, in some form. At first I tried to find replacement parts for small endoscopes, but I found that these were limited in availability and quite expensive. I called one of my used equipment sources and found it had a pediatric bronchoscope from a German manufacturer with broken optics that was the right diameter and length for the device I wanted to prototype. The cost of this unit was about $600, which might sound like a lot, but a similar scope in good working order sells for more than $2,000. It was also less expensive than building the flexible component myself and charging the client for my time.

Getting the bronchoscope apart proved to be a little bit of a challenge. This unit was constructed to be watertight and quite resistant to disassembly. I had to resort to using a milling machine to carefully cut open the housing. Once I had the case open,

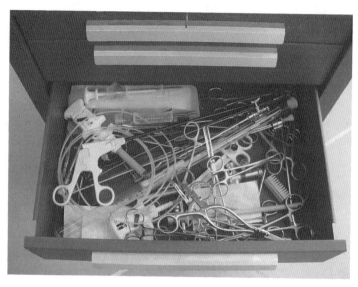

FIGURE 9.6 Assortment of medical devices for R&D.

I separated the flexible end of the bronchoscope from its case. Being able to cut open a piece of equipment like this was an education in itself, seeing how the device was constructed, how the fiber-optic bundles were laid out, how the steering actuation worked, and how it was engineered for reliability.

Once I had the flexible end of the device separated, I was able to concentrate on the more important part of the project, which was the connection mechanism between the flexible catheter and the actuation handle of the device that I was designing. This approach saved me time, gave me a reliable, high-quality steerable catheter quickly, got the device to proof-of-concept quickly, and saved the client money.

Why Reinvent the Handle?

Just cut off the part you do not want. When developing products, there are a number of common handles and actuators that may be readily adapted to a device on which you are working (see Figure 9.6).

One example of a common actuator is the handle of a disposable wire grasper. The three loops of the actuator are for the thumb and middle and index fingers, and they produce a pushing and retracting action. I have used this actuator for a number of projects. They are simple and inexpensive and are a convenient way to quickly and inexpensively build up a number of devices that require this type of actuator.

CASE STUDY: BUILDING ON AN EXISTING PRODUCT FOR HIGHER PERFORMANCE

When making an incremental improvement to a product, there is often a part that is not proprietary and that had been in clinical use for decades. Many times, surgical devices were originally borrowed from one type of surgical procedure and pressed into service in another specialty, thus becoming embedded into surgical practice by

Reverse Engineering in Medical Device Design

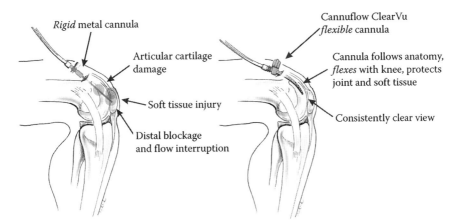

FIGURE 9.7 Example of using an existing product (a rigid metal cannula) as a platform for an improved version. (Illustration by T. Kucklick. Courtesy of Cannuflow, Inc., San Jose, CA.)

use and convention. This offers opportunity for improvement and innovation. A new feature can be added to this system that is higher performance, is less invasive or less traumatic to the patient, and uses an existing instrument, familiar to the surgeon as a platform for a new technology. An example of this is the ClearVu™ flexible arthroscopic cannula (see Figure 9.7).

The ClearVu device was designed to overcome the problems with rigid inflow–outflow cannulae commonly used in three-portal knee arthroscopy. Rigid metal cannulae were borrowed from the Veress needle, originally used in general surgery. Bob Bruce, an orthopedic physicians assistant in San Jose, CA, saw a need for a better cannula while observing the shortcomings of the rigid metal cannula in surgical practice. In arthroscopy, the joint space is distended with water, and the viewing scope and instruments are inserted into the joint through small incisions, or portals. Surgical efficiency depends on the surgeon having a constant flow of clear water through the joint, or the surgical field quickly becomes murky and obscured with blood and surgical debris.

The knee also needs to be bent during surgery, and the metal cannula does not bend. This caused the distal end of the cannula to become clogged with soft tissue and the inflexible cannula shaft to make dents in the sensitive articular cartilage of the inside joint surfaces of the knee. The main disadvantage to the surgeon was that when the rigid cannula dug into soft tissue at the distal end, the flow of fluid through the knee stopped and the surgical field quickly became murky and obscured by blood, and the sharp end of the cannula often skived and damaged articular cartilage.

In the process of designing the flexible section of the cannula, Bob discovered a number of innovative solutions to keep the cannula from collapsing and kinking during a procedure. Being a former U.S. Army Special Forces medic and an avid outdoorsman, he noticed that fishing rods were tapered to keep them from breaking when flexed. Bob adapted this observation to develop a patented progressively flexible tapered cannula, purpose built and optimized for consistent fluid flow during arthroscopic procedures.

Bob, being sensitive to surgeons' resistance to the unfamiliar, used an existing metal cannula, cut off the front of the cannula, and replaced it with a flexible plastic cannula shaft of his improved design and the familiar stopcock proximal end. Once this prototype was accepted by surgeons, he produced a molded version of the product. The Cannuflow® ClearVu™ is now being marketed worldwide and is a less traumatic, high-performance replacement for metal cannulae in three-portal arthroscopy. From the patient's point of view, there is less trauma and pain during and after surgery, and the arthroscopic surgeon can see what he is doing, without the surgical field being clouded with blood and debris.

Case Study: Making Your Own Stent

There are times when using an off-the-shelf item may not be the best way to go, and making a home-brewed version is the better solution.

On a cardiac device project I worked on, a stent-like device was needed. The only way we knew of to get stents was to buy a stent-and-delivery catheter at retail. This gave us a stent that was not quite what we wanted and was very expensive (about $2,000 each at that time). To save money, we took these precious devices and (carefully) cut them in half. Now they were only $1,000 each. There had to be a better and more cost-effective solution.

The stent we needed did not have to be anything special. We were pushing it into a lumen in an open procedure in bench and preclinical tests; they did not need the flexibility and trackability of a commercially available stent.

We searched and found some companies that make stents and stent prototypes. We contacted one of these companies and found out the process of making a stent is really not that exotic. Stents are made by laser-cutting tubing, and there are vendors that specialize in this work. It was a relatively simple matter of deciding what open diameter we wanted and finding a thin-wall hypodermic tube of that diameter, which was an off-the-shelf item at a hypotube supplier. The vendor had a pattern for a generic stent and cut a number of stents for us for a nominal lot charge. These stents were then collapsed down to their deployment size and used successfully in preclinical studies. The total cost per home-brewed stent was about $40 each.

WHERE TO FIND USED MEDICAL DEVICES AND EQUIPMENT

A lot of commonly used medical equipment is available for sale if you know where to find it. Buying used or refurbished equipment can be a cost-effective way to get equipment with which to work. This equipment comes on the market by way of liquidation auctions and sale of equipment from facilities that are upgrading their hardware.

Purchasing directly from a manufacturer is sometimes difficult, especially if you do not have a doctor or medical facility purchasing for you. The other issue with buying from manufacturers is their understandable reluctance to sell their equipment into the industry or to a potential competitor. Some equipment companies tightly control their distribution, will not send you a catalog, or even let you browse their online catalog without you having to fill out a qualifying lead form.

If you have to have a particular piece of equipment that is not available on the used equipment market, it helps to have connections with a doctor or facility within that specialty to get it for you. Companies regularly purchase competitor's equipment through friendly surrogates.

Most used equipment dealers are good sources of capital and durable equipment such as RF generators, endoscopy units, arthroscopy units, and common surgical hardware like forceps and retractors. Surgical disposables such as catheters, laparoscopic staplers, introducers, and so on, can be harder to find, however. The reason for this is that these items are packaged sterile and have a finite shelf life. Once the packaging expires, the device has little resale value to the reseller. This can be an advantage when looking for devices for parts. You may be able to buy expired disposables for a reasonable cost given that you want to dissect them anyway. The disadvantage is that you are limited to whatever stock is on hand, when and if they have it.

The way resellers sometimes get their equipment is by purchasing a liquidation lot from a hospital that is closing or upgrading equipment. The reseller will buy a palet load or container load at auction, and some of these disposables can be part of the lot. Ask your reseller if it ever gets disposables like this bundled in a liquidation lot. Since the reseller may have a limited market for these, you may be able to get a good deal on them. An advantage to going through a reseller is that most devices are resold without many regulatory controls. You also do not need to deal with the sales and marketing departments of the manufacturer, who will want to know all about who you are before selling to you.

If you need a specific piece of equipment, especially a newer item, be prepared to use your network to get it and pay list price for it.

Another way to get equipment is from a doctor who has excess equipment or is upgrading. This is why it helps to have a physician on your board of advisors who is practicing in the specialty in which you are designing equipment. At least one member of your advisory board should be adept at getting for you whatever devices you need to study to develop your products.

Another way to get some types of new and used equipment is to see whether the same or similar product is available for the veterinary market. Using these channels, you may find a device at lower cost, and with fewer restrictions when purchasing. For example, some manufacturers of endoscopes sell the same devices to the vet market as they do to hospitals.

Caution: When you purchase used equipment, purchase from an auction or from a practitioner; you do not know where the equipment has been. *Any device that has been used in contact with bodily fluids or mucous membranes is suspect and must be considered contaminated.* Most resellers are very good about providing clean and sanitary equipment, but some are not. I have seen examples of both. If you have access to a sterilizer (steam, autoclave, Steris, etc.) and the device can be sterilized this way, *wear protective gloves, disassemble, clean, and sterilize used devices before using or handling them.* Do *not* assume they are clean and sterile unless the vendor has certified them as sanitary or sterile or you can verify that they have been cleaned and sterilized.

Another way to sanitize devices is to cold soak the device in Cidex®-brand glutaraldehyde sterilant. Nooks, crannies, and valves in devices are places for organic gunk to hide. Endoscopes are especially prone to getting contaminated with biofilm and crud. Wear gloves, disassemble used equipment (as much as possible), always clean and sterilize before handling or using, and scrub yourself after handling by using the surgical scrub procedure. An exception to this is devices that are still in their factory packaging, where the packaging is intact and unopened.

Devices should be carefully cleaned and sanitized or sterilized after bench tests with tissue or preclinical animal studies. To avoid the possibility of serious illness, always use careful sterile and sanitary techniques when working with medical devices. Remember, if you can smell it, it is alive (with germs) and needs to be decontaminated. If you can see blood, assume that it is contaminated with bloodborne pathogens (e.g., AIDS or hepatitis) and take appropriate precautions.

THREE-DIMENSIONAL RECONSTRUCTION

Some of the subject of three-dimensional reconstruction has been covered in Chapter 8. The process of three-dimensional reconstruction involves taking data from one three-dimensional object and bringing that information into a three-dimensional computer program, where the data may be used or manipulated and a three-dimensional object produced, based on the captured three-dimensional data set. This sounds simple in concept; however, as with most things, the challenge is found in the details. One important thing to remember is that all of these data-capture methods yield some type of point cloud. This means a group of data points that are then interpolated by software to form a plane or surface. Once the surfaces are built, these can be closed to form a CAD solid. Once the points are captured and surfaces or solids are generated, they become "dumb" objects, as they were not built parametrically.

The other general concept to keep in mind is scan resolution. The higher the scan rate and the tighter the mesh, or number of triangles (polygons), the larger the file size. There is a trade-off between capturing enough data to produce a usable model and capturing too much and ending up with a large and cumbersome file size.

In each capture method, there is an art to getting a clean and usable data set. Sometimes it is simpler to just have a CAD draftsman use a set of calipers, take some measurements, and build a parametric solid model, instead of using automated data capture tools, especially if the desired end result is a feature-based CAD model.

COMMON THREE-DIMENSIONAL CAPTURE FILE FORMATS AND TERMINOLOGY

The majority of rapid prototype information is communicated in the .STL (stereolithography) format. Some of the other more common neutral file formats available are as follows:

PLY format, or the Stanford triangle format. This is a simplified vertex and face description of a three-dimensional object. It is a simplified file format for the communication of three-dimensional surface models, usually acquired from three-dimensional scanners.
VRML (virtual reality modeling format). Based on Silicon Graphics (Mountain View, CA) Open Inventor file format for use in Internet applications. Inventor is yet another file format that is a superset of the VRML networked

graphics data format. VRML is useful with communication texture and color data along with three-dimensional object information. Other three-dimensional formats, such as STL and PLY, do not support this type of color and scene data.

IGES (Initial Graphics Exchange Specification). An American national standard that is a neutral data format for the digital exchange of information among computer-aided design (CAD) systems and other applications. The standard is developed and maintained by the IGES/Product Data Exchange Specification (PDES) Organization. IGES supports the representation of surfaces with smooth higher order splines or nonlinear uniform rational B-splines (NURBS).

DXF (drawing interchange file). A file format developed by Autodesk, Inc. (Sausalito, CA) as a neutral file format for the communication of two- and three-dimensional vector information. DXF represents three-dimensional objects as polyface meshes and not smooth surfaces or NURBS.

STEP (Standard for the Exchange of Product Mode Data). An ISO standard neutral file format for the communication of engineering solid model data generated from CAD programs.

The basic difference between formats is this: DXF, STL, and PLY produce a polygon or *polyface mesh*. This means that a surface is made up of flat triangles that approximate the surface. A polygon mesh is a mathematically simpler way to describe a surface. DXF is a popular three-dimensional animation format, because a model is built using the smallest number of triangles to keep the three-dimensional file size small, and then the model is smoothed out visually when it is rendered in the animation software's shader. This works very well for animations that need to operate with limited hardware resources, like video game controllers. The results look smooth, but the underlying model may be roughly tessellated (faceted). Most three-dimensional programs can generate a .DXF file. NURBS produce a smooth surface and are more mathematically complex than a DXF polygon mesh. High-end surfacing programs can produce NURBS (e.g., Rhino and Alias®). *Parametric models* are feature-based solid models in which the model is described by geometric features (extrusions, revolved profiles, fillets, etc.), and each of these features may be edited according to precise values. Parametric models are generated by engineering CAD programs, for example, Pro/Engineer, SolidWorks, and AutoCAD.*

Digital Imaging and Communications in Medicine (DICOM) is not really a single-file format, but rather it is a way to organize radiology scan information under a common format. It contains information such as the CT or MRI image scans, their order, and slice thickness. A DICOM file is needed to then process through a software product like Materialise (Leuven, Belgium), Mimics®, or SimPlant® to produce an .STL file for the generation of a final three-dimensional physical model using rapid prototyping equipment.

---

* See Reverse Engineering, CT to CAD, http://www.nasatech.com/NEWS/rtb.brf.im3_0125.html (accessed August 11, 2012).

CONTINUITY

The mathematical smoothness of a surface is described by its continuity (see Figure 9.8). C0 continuity occurs when two lines or surfaces meet, but they are not curved or tangent. This is continuity by position only. C1 continuity occurs when a line or surface join and are curved, but they are not tangent (smooth). C2 continuity occurs when lines or surfaces meet and are both curved and smoothly tangent. Continuity becomes important when patching and cleaning up a captured mesh. Often, a captured mesh will have gaps where it lacks continuity and needs to be patched in a three-dimensional surfacing program (see Figure 9.9). Sometimes the mesh will have kinks where there is a C0 or C1 continuity and a C2 smoothness is desired. This can be accomplished in a three-dimensional surfacing program;

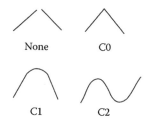

FIGURE 9.8 Types of continuity.

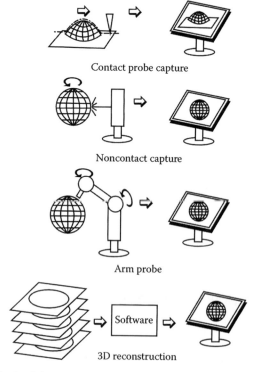

FIGURE 9.9 Methods of three-dimensional capture.

however, the time and expense in cleanup of the mesh should be allowed for in the project schedule and budget. Curve analysis tools in surfacing and CAD programs can help reveal creases and lack of desired continuity.

One difficulty in producing a rapid prototype model from captured point cloud data is ensuring a watertight mesh. This means that the surfaces may not have any gaps or lack of continuity. These gaps will result is an .STL file with holes and an unbuildable part. Sometimes mesh editing is required to patch up a model before it can be built successfully.

The four basic ways to achieve three-dimensional reconstruction are as follows:

- Automated touch probe scanning
- Light beam scanning
- Arm probe capture
- Data set reconstruction

AUTOMATED TOUCH PROBE

Automated touch probe scanners are a simple and convenient way to capture three-dimensional information. Inexpensive three-dimensional scanners like the MDX-20 described earlier in this chapter are available from Roland Corporation (Irvine, CA) and are bundled with capture software. Automated touch probe scanners of this type are limited to scanning one surface of an object at a time (see Figure 9.9).

LIGHT BEAM SCANNERS

Light beam scanners are noncontact probes that capture point cloud data. One type of scanner operates with a stationary beam, and the object is rotated to capture the point cloud. In the other, the object is stationary and the scanner moves to capture the image. One of the considerations in optical three-dimensional scanning is that the scanner requires a surface of uniform color and reflectivity to produce a clean scan. This may require that reflective parts be coated with powder. This can be a limitation, depending on the object to be scanned. If the object is, for example, a rare bone specimen or archeological object, the curator may object to having the object coated with nonreflective media. Also, for surfaces that require high-precision scanning (e.g., polished engine cylinder head surfaces), spray-on powders may actually produce a false picture of the geometry.[*]

Noncontact light beam scanners range from simpler models like the Roland LPX-250 to highly sophisticated (and expensive) models from Konica Minolta, Cyberware, and 3dMD. Noncontact light beam scanners work in similar ways, by projecting a beam of light to a surface and capturing z-axis height information with very accurate range finding, and then building this information with software into a surface that accurately represents the scanned object.

---

[*] Albert Shih, "Three Dimensional Precision Optical Measurements" (paper presented to SME, University of Michigan Engineering Research Center for Reconfigurable Manufacturing Systems, May 9, 2005).

Medical applications of three-dimensional scanning include a medically oriented hardware and software combination from 3dMD (http://www.3dmd.com) and a digital ear impression product for fitting hearing aids by Cyberware (Monterey, CA; http://www.cyberware.com). Cyberware is a pioneer in the high-end noncontact scanning industry, and its website provides numerous application examples. Cyberware noncontact scanners are an essential tool in movie digital special effects production. Other uses for noncontact digital scanning are in prosthetics, for which a digital model is made of a residual limb for fitting, whole-body scanning for the video game industry, anthropometric studies, and the apparel industry. Polhemus (Colchester, VT; http://www.polhemus.com) specializes in digital motion capture and is an important technology in human factors gait analysis and realistic animation of video game characters. Polhemus also makes a device, the VisionTrak, for analysis of eye movements. This is used in human factors studies of vision, as well as in the advertising industry, where eye movements are tracked to study the effectiveness of advertisements and whether the viewer is reading the ad or just looking at the pictures.

An application for digitizing and RE is the production of burn masks. These are custom-fitted dressings that prevent the formation of disfiguring facial scars on burn victims. Total Contact Incorporated (Germantown, OH; http://www.totalcontact.com) specializes in the production of these masks.[2]

ARM PROBE SCANNERS

Contact probe scanners are available from Faro (Lake Mary, FL; http://www.faro.com), Immersion (Microscribe; San Jose, CA; http://www.microscribe.com), and Romer/CimCore (Farmington Hills, MI; http://www.cimcore.com).

Arm probe scanners are a way to digitize objects with a higher degree of user control than automated scanning methods. Arm probe scanners are popular in manufacturing environments such as automotive and aerospace. Arm probe scanners can plug directly into three-dimensional surfacing programs such as Rhino, where a user can trace an object and see the surfaces built in the computer. Arm probe scanners are also important as inspection equipment.

Arm probe scanners have found applications in medicine. Orthopedic surgeons often need accurate spatial information to place implants. Several three-dimensional systems have been developed and marketed to help the surgeon place joint prostheses (e.g., the BrainLab System, Munich, Germany). Some of these systems use noncontact three-dimensional positioning methods. Microscribe arms have been combined with Phillips CT scanners to provide more accurate biopsy needle track placement in a stereotactic application.*

ARM PROBE NONCONTACT SCANNERS

These devices are a hybrid of a coordinate measuring machine (CMM) arm or articulated arm and a noncontact laser scanner head. One of the advantages of this type of

---

* See "Philips Medical Systems Customizes Immersion's Microscribe Technology," http://www.emicroscribe.com/Pdf%20files/Phillips_Case_Study_final.pdf (accessed 8/11/2012).

device is that the arm probe orients the data capture scanning head in space and helps to organize the point cloud data, especially when in comes to knitting together captured surface patches. Scanners mounted on an articulating arm allow the user to "paint" the surface with the scanner and watch the surface develop on a computer screen. These devices are made by companies such as Metris, Perceptron, Laser Design, and Kreon.

THREE-DIMENSIONAL IMAGE RECONSTRUCTION

Another method of producing a three-dimensional data set is by taking a serialized two-dimensional data set, for example, CT scans, and building this into a three-dimensional data set. Several companies offer this service and can provide a rapid prototype model for surgical planning and training. Using RE tools is also an important way to produce organ phantoms (training models) for surgical training.

One of the more ambitious three-dimensional image reconstruction projects is the Visible Human Project® of the National Library of Medicine. In 1993 researchers at Colorado State University took the cadaver of a Texas death row inmate, froze it, and sliced it into 1 mm sections. Each section was digitally photographed, and the resulting images were processed into a highly detailed three-dimensional database. Several more donated cadavers have since been processed and added to the database.[*]

Image reconstruction software to turn two-dimensional CT and MRI scans into three-dimensional data sets is available from Materialise, n.v. (Leuven, Belgium). Materialise sells its Mimics software to generate .STL files from CT scans. Materialise also offers a suite of applications for surgical planning and for editing and manipulating files in .STL format. These include Simplant, SAFE®, and SurgiGuide® products. Materialise also has published numerous case surgical studies on its website (http://www.materialise.com).

Javelin3D (Salt Lake City, UT; http://www.javelin3D.com) offers its Velocity® software for MRI and CT scan three-dimensional reconstruction.

REVERSE ENGINEERING AND INSPECTION

One important use of RE and reverse modeling and data capture is applied in part validation and inspection. Traditionally, inspections are performed with gauges or coordinate measuring machines (CMMs). The limitation of these methods is the relatively small number of data points that may be inspected. Also, these types of inspections measure discrete points or line traces. Reverse modeling is a powerful method of part inspection. In this method, a finished part is scanned with high-accuracy three-dimensional digital capture tools, and then the scanned model is overlaid on the CAD file, which is theoretically accurate. The use of fiducial markers helps to align and register the scanned data set to the CAD data set. Inspection analysis software such as PolyWorks (http://www.innovmetric.com) is used to analyze the deviations between the CAD model and the manufactured part. The power of this method is the ability to apply geometric tolerancing analysis tools in software,

---

[*] Thomas McCracken, *New Atlas of Human Anatomy* (Metro Books, New York, 1999), "The Visible Human Project," http://www.nlm.nih.gov/research/visible/visible_human.html (accessed August 11, 2012).

as well as the ability to color map dimensional variances. This gives the ability to visualize not only discrete inspection points, but also, for example, the flatness of a surface, with its high and low areas revealed.

DESTRUCTIVE REVERSE ENGINEERING

CGI Corporation (Capture Geometry Internally) makes a system for progressively milling and scanning an object, referred to as cross-sectional scanning. The part is obviously sacrificed in the process. This, however, is one way to obtain the internal geometry of a part or product assembly (http://www.reverse-eng.com).

REVERSE MODELING, RADIOLOGY, AND SURGICAL PLANNING

Interesting work in the area of three-dimensional reconstruction and surgical planning is being done at Stanford University (Stanford, CA), where vascular procedures are preplanned for improved outcomes with the Advanced Surgical Planning Interactive Research Environment (ASPIRE) system. For example, a vascular graft procedure is planned by scanning the patient's anatomy and building a dynamic flow model that represents both the pulsatile flow of blood and the elasticity of the vessel wall. This allows the modeling of a vascular system and the ability to test different grafting approaches. This also allows the ability to choose the procedure that will produce the best flow with the least turbulence in the blood flow, to prevent thrombosis and improve outcomes.

On the electronics side of RE, there is a company near Colorado Springs, CO, Taeus International, founded by Arthur Nutter. Taeus is short for Tear Apart Everything under the Sun. Taeus is expert at dissecting electronics and microchips, looking for evidence of purloined technology in high-stakes patent litigation cases for clients such as Intel, HP, and Texas Instruments.[3]

RE and reverse modeling are essential components in the toolbox of the medical device designer. Used properly, it helps to accelerate innovation, conserve capital, and produce devices that are compatible with standard surgical use and convention. It is an essential tool for competitive analysis. It is a way to learn accepted and successful design and assembly techniques. It helps to cross-pollinate technology from one field into a new area of application. It can be the seed and inspiration for your own original contribution.

RE and reverse modeling tools are becoming more powerful and less expensive all the time. Check with industry publications, informational websites, and industry conferences to keep up to date with the latest developments.

RESOURCES

REFERENCES: PRINT

Brown, Sam. *Forensic Engineering: An Introduction to the Investigation, Analysis, Reconstruction, Causality, Risk, Consequence, and Legal Aspects of the Failure of Engineered Products.* Humble, TX: ISI Publications, 1993.

Reverse Engineering in Medical Device Design

REFERENCES: PROFESSIONAL SOCIETIES

ACM Siggraph (http://www.siggraph.org) is the computer graphics special interest group of the Association for Computing Machinery (ACM). Siggraph puts on an annual conference and trade show that is one of the more important events for anyone working in the computer graphics and three-dimensional modeling field. Any piece of equipment or vendor you can think of exhibits at this huge event. (The 2004 attendance was over 27,000.)

Society for Manufacturing Engineers (http://www.sme.org) organizes an annual event, the RAPID show (http://www.sme.org/rapid), which is a trade show and symposium on all facets of the rapid prototyping and reverse engineering and modeling industry. It is a valuable event to attend if you have a special interest in this area. This is the largest event of its kind in North America.

REFERENCES: THREE-DIMENSIONAL INFORMATION WEBSITES

3DLinks.com. A very useful compendium of information on three-dimensional capture devices and three-dimensional products.
Computer Aided Radiology and Surgery (CARS) Society: http://cars-int.de/index.htm.
Index of CARS Resources. http://homepage2.nifty.com/cas/casref.htm.
International Society for Computer Aided Surgery. http://igs.slu.edu.
International Society for Computer Assisted Orthopaedic Surgery (CAOS). http://www.caos-international.org.

VENDORS: BONES AND BONE MODELS

Aptic Superbones
Phone: 866-265-BONE (2663)
http://www.discountbones.com
Synthetic bone models mimicking cortical and cancellous bone structure.

The Bone Room
1569 Solano Avenue
Berkeley, CA 94707
Phone: 510-526-5252
http://www.boneroom.com
Natural bones and skeleton specimens of all kinds, animal and human.

Pacific Research Laboratories (Sawbones)
10221 SW 188th Street
P.O. Box 409
Vashon, WA 98070
Phone: 206-463-5551
Fax: 206-463-2526
http://www.sawbones.com

Vendors: MRI and CT Reconstruction and RP Modeling

Biomedical Modeling, Inc.
http://www.biomodel.com

Protomed
http://www.protomed.com

Vendors: Reconditioned and Used Medical Equipment

Arthroscopy and Medical Equipment International
7440 SW 50th Terrace, #108
Miami, FL 33155
Phone: 305-662-2855
Fax: 305-662-1170
http://www.artroscopia.net
Source for new and used arthroscopes and orthopedic RF generators.

eBay
http://www.ebay.com
Medical equipment is also available on eBay, although the selection for a particular use may be limited.

Medical Resources
550 Schrock Road
Columbus, OH 43229
Phone: 800-860-4716
Fax: 614-433-7387
Broad range of supplies; good for some hard-to-find items.

Paragon Medical
P.O. Box 770187
Coral Springs, FL 33077
Phone: 800-780-5266 or 954-345-3990
Fax: 954-340-2457

United Endoscopy
10405 San Sevaine Way, Suite B
Mira Loma, CA 91752-1150
Phone: 951-360-0077 or 800-899-4847
Fax: 951-360-0066
Good prices on used endoscopy equipment; may have some disposables such as laparoscopic staplers, in stock.

Whittemore Enterprises, Inc.
1114 Arrow Route

Rancho Cucamonga, CA 91730
Phone: 800-999-2452 or 909-980-2452
Fax: 909-989-9976
Email: sales@wemed1.com
http://www.wemed1.com
Whittemore has a fully stocked showroom with a huge variety of surgical hardware and equipment; it is worth the visit to browse for an afternoon.

Vendors: Three-Dimensional Capture Equipment

Cyberware, Inc.
2110 Del Monte Avenue
Monterey, CA 93940
Phone: 831-657-1450
http://www.cyberware.com

Faro
125 Technology Park
Lake Mary, FL 32746
Phone: 800-736-0234 or 407-333-9911
http://www.faro.com

Immersion Corporation
801 Fox Lane
San Jose, CA 95131
Phone: 408-467-1900
Fax: 408-467-1901
http://www.microscribe.com

Roland DGA
15363 Barranca Parkway
Irvine, CA 92618-2216
http://www.rolanddga.com

Vendors: Three-Dimensional Scanning and Manufacturing Inspection

CavLab
http://www.cavlab.com
One of the largest service bureaus offering three-dimensional modeling and inspection.

Vendors: Three-Dimensional Service Bureaus

Javelin 3D
http://www.javelin3D.com

Vendors: Three-Dimensional Software

3dMD
http://www.3dMD.com

Alias
http://www.alias.com
Makers of Alias and Maya® high-end surfacing and animation programs.

Materialise
Technologielaan 15
3001 Leuven, Belgium
Phone: +32 16 39 66 11
Fax: +32 16 39 66 00
http://www.materialise.com
Mimics®, Simplant® SAFE®, and SurgiGuide® software.

Robert McNeel & Associates
3670 Woodland Park Avenue North
Seattle, WA 98103
Phone: 206-545-7000
http://www.Rhino 3D.com

VG Studio Max
Volume Graphics GmbH
Weiblinger Weg 92a
69123 Heidelberg
Germany

Vital Images, Inc.
5850 Opus Parkway, Suite 300
Minnetonka, MN 55343-4414
Phone: 952-487-9500
http://www.vitalimages.com

ENDNOTES

1. The website Chilling Effects is a joint project of the Electronic Frontier Foundation and Harvard, Stanford, Berkeley, University of San Francisco, University of Maine, George Washington School of Law, and Santa Clara University School of Law clinics. The site includes a detailed list of frequently asked questions on the subject of reverse engineering.
2. For more information on the use of fitted masks to prevent hypertrophic scarring, see Walsh, Nicolas E. et. al. "Computerized Manufacturing of Transparent Face Masks for the Treatment of Facial Scarring," *Journal of Burn Care & Rehabilitation* 24 (2003): 91–96; Leonardo Ciocca, DDS, PhD, and Roberto Scotti, MD, DDS, "Integration of

Laser Surface Digitizing with CAD/CAM Techniques for Developing Facial Prostheses, Part 1: Design and Fabrication of Prosthesis Replicas," *International Journal of Prosthodontics* 16 (2003): 435–441.
3. Based on his experience in the patent litigation area, Mr. Nutter has an interesting rule of thumb on patent claims: "Most large technology companies sit on thousands of patents, but only a few claims are solid enough to hold up in court. Nutter can tell the good ones by using what he calls the "three-fingers" rule. 'If you cover up a claim with just three fingers, it's probably a pretty good claim,' he says. 'Claims that go on paragraph after paragraph are too vague and almost impossible to make stick.'" Tomas Kellner, "Silicon Strip Search," *Forbes Magazine* (March 28, 2005).

10 Prototype or Produce? How to Decide

Theodore R. Kucklick

CONTENTS

Traditional Model-Making Tools 211
See What Has Already Been Solved 212
Rapid Prototype Options 213
    Short-Run Manufacturing Options 213
    Short-Run Injection Molding 213
Production Tooling 214
A Simple Decision Tool 214
Conclusion 215
Resources 215
    References: Print 215
    Vendors 215

When you are using seemingly more expensive mass production methods how do you decide whether to go: prototype or low production? The answers might surprise you. Here is some advice and a handy tool to help.

You need to make a few devices. These are going to be for a preclinical study or a pilot clinical study, or possibly a beta launch to test the market. You do not want to spend more than needed, but you also do not want to paint yourself into a corner if you have to make more units that you anticipated.

When developing a product, a good practice is to use real production processes, real production methods, and real production materials wherever possible, and to design for manufacturing as early as possible. Planning is especially critical when developing Food and Drug Administration (FDA) Class III devices. Once the PMA (Pre-Market Approval) dossier is set, reopening with material and design changes can be difficult and expensive.

"Hardware store" materials are good for conceptualizing a product and learning what you need to know during initial proof-of-concept bench testing. These materials can help iterate an idea quickly and inexpensively. When progressing beyond this, however, think strategically, like a pool player. Take your shot, but set up your next shot in the process. This way you won't wind up "behind the eight ball."

TRADITIONAL MODEL-MAKING TOOLS

Given all of the emphasis on the high-technology (and sometimes high-cost) tools available, it is possible to overlook some of the affordable and readily available

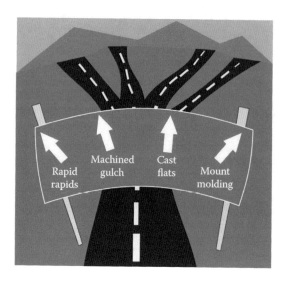

modeling tools that have served designers for decades. Some of these are styling and plasticene (Sculpey) clay, foamcore (great for making mockups of instrument housings and cases), surfboard foam, and room-temperature vulcanate (RTV) molding with urethane. Another readily available prototyping material is acrylic plastic, which is available at plastics hobby shops such as TAP Plastics. These readily available materials require no special tools much beyond an X-acto® knife, woodworking tools, and sandpaper. Other readily available materials include piano wire and brass and aluminum tubing from the hobby shop. PVC tubing is readily available from lab supply houses, and medical device fittings are available from companies like Qosina (http://www.qosina.com) that carry nearly any kind of luer fitting and stopcock you might need and that have a generous sampling policy. RTV casting and urethane molding have been a staple of designers and professional model-makers for years. Materials and step-by-step how-to videos on RTV silicone molding and casting are available from Freeman Supply (Avon, OH; http://www.freemansupply.com).

Simple model-making materials, used resourcefully, can help you iterate ideas quickly and affordably, in the concept and preclinical stage, before spending capital money on more expensive models and tooling.

SEE WHAT HAS ALREADY BEEN SOLVED

Many seemingly sophisticated medical devices had humble origins. Dr. Julio Palmaz got the idea for the coronary stent from chicken wire. If orthopedic repair implants look like refined versions of items from the hardware store, it is because not too long ago, as can be seen at the history display at the Academy of Orthopaedic Surgeons (AAOS, Rosemont, IL), that is where surgeons got their orthopedic repair hardware before they were specially manufactured. The solutions to many problems are already out there.

RAPID PROTOTYPE OPTIONS

Rapid prototype (RP) technology is getting better all the time, with improved speed, accuracy, and material choices. Getting the right combination of material, surface finish, and feature resolution remains challenging. Methods that can produce small feature sizes (Polyjet) can be useful for prototyping close-tolerance fit check parts and even some larger catheter tubes and are also capable of rapid prototyping rubber parts. Some medical-grade polymer material options are now available (3D Systems, Stratasys). Direct-metal e-beam and laser-sintering now make titanium and cobalt-chrome implants, without expensive investment casting, possible (EOS, Arcam). RP methods are capable of production medical parts, such as orthopedic implants and hearing-aid shells.

It is possible to use RP to make shapes and structures that are difficult or impossible to duplicate with conventional machining and molding. This is good if you need this capability, but it is not good if you get carried away and prototype something with unmoldable features, such as undercuts and lack of draft angles, that require you to redesign the prototype for molding later.

SHORT-RUN MANUFACTURING OPTIONS

The trade-off when working with short-run manufacturing options is usually between lower setup and tooling costs and higher per-part costs. Remember, it is the total costs that count and the ability to create a final usable part in the fewest number of steps. At the lower end, options include vacuum forming, casting in RTV silicone molds, machining, pressure forming, foam molding, and reaction injection molding. Typically, these methods are most useful for enclosures. For devices, machining may be a good option for metal parts and smaller quantities of items, like plastic handles. If you are going to make larger quantities later, check that your material is appropriate and available for production. You do not want to validate a part in a machined material that is not available or inappropriate in an injection-molding process. You may also avoid the cost and having to repeat expensive biocompatibility testing. For medical devices, extrusion can be a useful option, as the tooling costs are usually fairly low compared with injection molding. Design for manufacturing early, and plan your shots.

SHORT-RUN INJECTION MOLDING

Injection molding in aluminum tooling has become more readily available, less expensive, and easier to use. An advantage of short-run injection molding is the ability to mold parts in the final material that you want to use in production as well as the ability to use materials not available in stock shapes for machining. Typically, parts for medical devices are small and therefore the shot sizes are small. Many resin manufacturers are willing to send a sample of resin (about 20 lbs) for evaluation. This may be enough resin to run hundreds of smaller parts. Following this method, you will have parts that are in their production form, rather than a facsimile version for bioburden, package validation, and biocompatibility testing. Short-run soft tooling can also serve as bridge tooling to produce parts for clinical trials and marketing samples while production tools are being made. One company that specializes in aluminum soft tooling is Protomold (http://www.protomold.com). Use their website to upload computer-aided design (CAD) models and checked for their moldability (e.g., wall thickness, draft angles, and undercuts) and to generate a quote for tooling and piece parts. Protomold has many in-stock resins, or they can mold in customer-supplied material.

PRODUCTION TOOLING

When you reach production tooling, the last thing you want to make is an expensive, finely machined class-A polished "boat anchor" (useless mold). Take the necessary steps to ensure that what you can make lots of are (1) what you really want, (2) really work, and (3) really sell. One way to save money at this stage is to use Master Unit Die (MUD) Base tooling. This is a modular mold frame system that may be less expensive than a fully custom mold. Use less-expensive tooling, to start, and take the money you make on the product to pay for better tooling if the product is a winner. If it is not a winner, you have avoided buying an expensive boat anchor.

Another powerful tool for controlling overall costs is to design out labor costs whenever possible and make the mold do the work. Labor costs and secondary operations can be difficult to remove once they are "baked into the cake."

A SIMPLE DECISION TOOL

Remember, it is the total costs of your development program that count. The goal is to get where you need to go, in the fewest number of steps, spending the least amount of money. You can run the graph shown here in Excel or MathCad. Put your setup costs on the y-axis and plot the cumulative costs (setup + part costs) slope on the x-axis. You may be surprised to find that, in the quantities you need to make, a

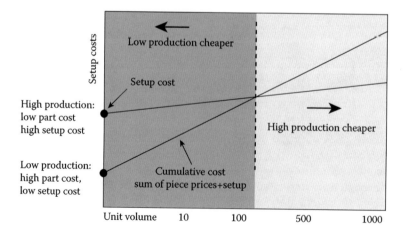

higher production method with higher tooling and setup costs is less expensive overall than a lower production method with high per-part costs, high labor content, and no economies of scale. Reducing the data to a chart not only can help you decide which option to use but also can help you sell the program to management.

CONCLUSION

Knowing the range of options to make the best design decisions will help you get to your end result in the fewest number of steps spending the least amount of money. Great places to see the range of vendors that serve the medical device industry include the Society for Manufacturing Engineering (SME) RAPID show, the Medical Device and Manufacturing Show (MD+M Show; http://www.canontradeshows.com), Orthopedic Manufacturing and Technology Show (OMTEC; http://www.orthoworld.com), and the Orthopedic Design + Technology shows (ODT; http://www.odtexpo.com).

The method with the lower upfront costs may not be the cheapest in the long run when cumulative costs and trade-offs like biocompatibility of materials unit cost and labor content are taken into account.

RESOURCES

REFERENCES: PRINT

Harvey, James A. *Machine Shop Trade Secrets: A Guide to Manufacturing Machine Shop Practices*. New York: Industrial Press, 2005.

Lefteri, Chris. *Making It: Manufacturing Techniques for Product Design*. London: Laurence King Publishing, 2007.

Meyers, Arthur R., and Thomas Slattery. *Basic Machining Reference Handbook*. New York: Industrial Press, 2001.

Thompson, Rob. *Manufacturing Processes for Design Professionals*. The Manufacturing Guides Series. London: Thames and Hudson, 2007.

———. *Product and Furniture Design*. The Manufacturing Guides Series. London: Thames and Hudson, 2011.

———. *Prototyping and Low-Volume Production*. The Manufacturing Guides Series. London: Thames and Hudson, 2011.

Trudeau, Norman. *Professional Modelmaking*. London: Phaidon Press, 1995.

VENDORS

Freeman Supply
1101 Moore Road
Avon, OH 44011
Phone: 440-934-1902
http://www.freemansupply.com
Source for RTV commercial prototype and casting materials, foundry supplies, and machinable media from REN Shape,™ foams, and pattern-making supplies, to casting wax. An extensive library of how-to videos is also available.

Douglas and Sturgess
730 Bryant Street
San Francisco, CA 94107-1015
Phone: 415-896-6283
http://www.artstuf.com
Source for sculpting clay and craft mold-making supplies. How-to information is also available on their website.

Instructables
http://www.instructables.com
More do-it-yourself information brought to you by Squid Labs (formerly of MIT Media Lab).

MAKE Magazine
http://makezine.com
Treasury of do-it-yourself technology projects.

11 Elements of Injection Molding Style for Medical Device R&D

Theodore R. Kucklick

CONTENTS

First Rule: Consistent Wall Thickness 219
    Consistent Wall Thickness: Ribs and Bosses 220
    Consistent Wall Thickness: Core Out Thick Sections 221
Second Rule: Designing in Adequate Draft 222
Third Rule: Radius Your Corners 222
    Two Ways Molds Are Made 223
Fourth Rule: Specify the Friendliest-to-Mold and Least Expensive Material 223
    Plastic Materials, Filled Plastics 224
        Glass 224
        Barium 224
        Plastics Additives to Watch for 224
Fifth Rule: Use Straight Parting Lines 224
Sixth Rule: is "Do It in the Mold" 226
    Product Design Principle 226
    Money-Saving Trick: Two Housing Shells from One Molded Housing Shell 226
    Side Hole without a Side Pull 226
    Molded-In Hinges 228
Surface Finishes 228
    Notes on Surface Finishes 229
    Finish and Draft Angle 229
    Surface Finish and Elastomers 229
    Preengineered Molds 229
New Capabilities: Mold Flow and FEA (Finite Element Analysis) 229
    Gating 229
    Edge Gate or Tab Gate 230
    Post Gate 230
    Subgate or Tunnel Gate 230
    Hot Tip 230
Locating the Gate to the Part 230
Part Ejection 231
Gluing, Joining, Fastening 232

    Inserts 232
    Ultrasonic Welding 232
    Heat Staking 233
    Interference Press Fit Bosses 233
    Snap Fits 233
    Adhesives 233
Sterilization and Bioburden 234
Sterilization Effects on Plastics 235
    Choosing a Biocompatible Material 235
    Colorants 236
    Other Molding Methods 236
        Silicone Molding 236
        RIM Molding 236
        Foam Molding 237
        Styrofoam Molding 237
    Inspection and Acceptance Criteria 237
Glossary 237
Resources 239
    References: Print 239
    References: Online 239
Acknowledgments 240

Once upon a time, not that many years ago, injection molding was virtually off limits to research and development (R&D). There were limited options to make small parts on manual presses in aluminum tools; however, if you wanted a part, you usually machined it. In that case, only after you were really, really sure of what you wanted, after hand-drawn paper production drawings were generated, after these drawings were sent to the tool and die shop, and then after several weeks or months, an expensive hardened tool steel injection mold would be produced.

With a combination of advances—such as computer-aided design (CAD) solid modeling software becoming mainstream, advances in computer numeric-controlled (CNC) and computer-aided manufacturing (CAM) milling technology, and the ability to easily transmit CAD data—reliable, inexpensive aluminum prototype injection molding is now easily within the reach of the R&D designer, at a price point about one-fifth to one-tenth of the cost of a steel tool just a few years ago, and lead times one-eighth to one-twelfth that of conventional steel tooling. CAD has made steel tooling faster and more predictable as well. Readily available molding analysis tools can spot potential problems in the molded part, so that they can be corrected before the CAD file is ever sent to the tool shop. Parts can now be made with production materials in an R&D setting and can be tested and debugged before committing to hard tooling. This work can be completed before they are sped to market with soft "bridge" tooling, while the hard tooling is being produced, shaving weeks or months off of the launch schedule.

Now that injection molding is a viable tool to iterate with, it is time to learn some of the basics of good injection mold style. Following these simple guidelines will

Elements of Injection Molding Style for Medical Device R&D

help you generate the parts you want with the dimensions you want, and with the fewest undesirable mechanical and cosmetic issues. Additionally, there are a number of clever tips and techniques for producing complex geometry without resorting to potentially expensive side-action slides, as well as ways to produce some features in the mold, to eliminate secondary assembly operations.

This chapter will give you some of the basics of plastic part design. It is tailored to the needs of the R&D engineer producing short-run parts. High-production part design is a specialty all its own and is beyond the scope of this chapter. If, however, a part is initially designed according to good practice and style, then it is more likely that it will scale up into production with fewer headaches.

Before you begin: The best way to approach an R&D project is to think ahead to how something will be molded, assembled, and manufactured. If you are making a one-off prototype that is just for proof of concept, you need not worry too much about manufacturability. If, however, you are starting to make multiples for clinical builds, and the project is moving quickly, thinking ahead to manufacturing can save many headaches down the road. I have seen more than one product whose design is moved quickly through R&D, is frozen, and then is moved into scale-up without considering design for manufacturability. This has resulted in mass-produced prototypes with intractably high labor costs, lacking mating and aligning features, with difficult-to-mold features or wall sections, or requiring needlessly complex and expensive tooling to make the now-frozen design. All of this is avoidable with a little manufacturing design preplanning and foresight.

FIRST RULE: CONSISTENT WALL THICKNESS

The first rule of designing a good injection-molded part is to design the part with consistent wall thickness. Plastic is melted and shot into a mold hot under high pressure. It shrinks when it cools. The thicker the wall, the longer to cool, and the more the material shrinks. Thick and thin walls in the same part result in uneven shrinkage, warping, potential internal voids, and a potentially bad part.

Think about how a plastic part is molded. When hot melted plastic is squirted into a mold cavity under high pressure, the plastic is hottest in cases in which it is first squirted in and cools as the plastic flows away from the injection gate. From there, the plastic fills and "packs" the mold and starts to cool. You want to design a part that allows the plastic to flow, is the easiest to fill, and avoids the combination of thick and thin wall sections that tend to result in shrinking and warping.

Determining which nominal wall thickness to use depends on the plastic. Each plastic has its own optimal nominal wall thickness. A starting point nominal wall for smaller parts (the scale of handles, and small to midsize enclosures that are typical of medical device parts) is about 2 mm (0.08 inch). Smaller parts can be thinner, and larger parts may need to be thicker. Some plastics such as acrylic are more tolerant of thick sections, whereas others like polycarbonate (PC) and acrylonitrile–butadiene–styrene (ABS) are not. Table 11.1 shows minimum and maximum nominal wall thicknesses for common plastics.

The second part of the wall thickness rule is to avoid thick wall sections (see Figure 11.2 later in this chapter). Overly thick wall sections consume excessive

TABLE 11.1
Minimum and Maximum Nominal Wall Thickness Ranges for Common Plastic Resins

ABS	0.045–0.140
Acetal	0.030–0.120
Acrylic	0.025–0.500
Liquid crystal polymer	0.030–0.120
Long-fiber reinforced plastics	0.075–1.000
Nylon	0.030–0.115
Polycarbonate	0.040–0.150
Polyester	0.025–0.125
Polyethylene	0.030–0.200
Polyphenylene sulfide	0.020–0.180
Polypropylene	0.025–0.150
Polystyrene	0.035–0.150
Polyurethane	0.080–0.750

Source: Courtesy of Protomold, Maple Plain, MN, and http://www.manufacturingcenter.com.

amounts of material, shrink more, take longer to mold and cool, and are prone to molded-in stress and internal voids. Use the least thick wall section that will give you a structurally sound part (see Figures 11.1 and 11.2).

CONSISTENT WALL THICKNESS: RIBS AND BOSSES

Ribs and bosses are highly useful features for stiffening a part and for generating assembly features. The features, however, generate a wall thickness issue that may not

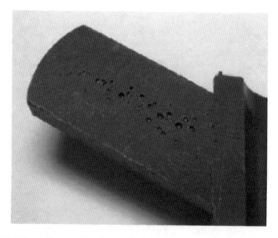

FIGURE 11.1 Thick section voids from shrinkage. (Courtesy of Protomold Inc., Maple Plain, MN.)

Elements of Injection Molding Style for Medical Device R&D

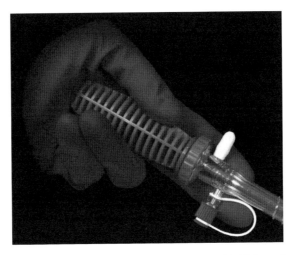

FIGURE 11.2 "Cored out" handle on medical device to avoid thick sections. (Courtesy of Cannuflow, Inc., San Jose, CA.)

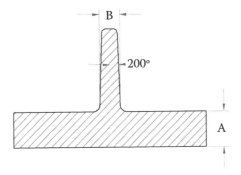

FIGURE 11.3 Rib example. Rule of thumb is that ribs thickness "B" is 60% of nominal wall thickness "A."

be immediately apparent. Where a rib joins a wall, there is an increase in the nominal wall at that intersection. This thick spot will take longer to cool and will shrink more than the material around it. This can result in molded-in stress and undesirable "sink marks" (see Figure 11.3).

Another use for ribs is for flow channels to direct the flow of plastic around a hole feature and to reduce knit lines.

CONSISTENT WALL THICKNESS: CORE OUT THICK SECTIONS

Thick cross sections of plastic are not desirable. However, when a space-filling feature like a handle is molded, the way to accomplish this is by "coring out" this feature rather than making it from a solid piece of molded plastic (see Figure 11.2).

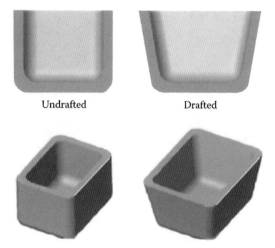

FIGURE 11.4 Drafted and undrafted part. (Courtesy of Protomold Inc., Maple Plain, MN.)

SECOND RULE: DESIGNING IN ADEQUATE DRAFT

Designing in draft, especially if you are used to dealing with machined or extruded parts, can take some getting used to. Draft is the taper given to a part to allow it to be removed from the mold.

Designing draft into a part takes a bit of strategy and understanding how the mold will fit together to form the part (see Figure 11.4). One important concept here is the "A" and "B" sides of the mold. The "A" side is the cavity side, the one that forms the outside of the part. The "B" side is the "core" or the part of the mold that forms the inside of the part. To understand how mold tools work begin by taking a molded plastic part and press modeling clay onto the part. This will produce a negative of the part and give you an idea of what the mold that made the part looked like. Look at how the part is drafted so that it could be removed from the mold.

If a surface is textured, it requires more draft. Textured surfaces typically require at least 1.5 degrees of draft per 0.001 inch of texture depth.

THIRD RULE: RADIUS YOUR CORNERS

When thinking of plastic parts think in terms of avoiding stress risers, notches, molded-in stress, and shrinkage. Sharp inside corners are harder to fill and make weak spots in a molded part. Note in Figure 11.5 how square corners form a local thick section and a place for shrinkage and molded-in stress to occur. In CAD it is very easy to design parts with sharp interior corners. Take the time to radius these corners wherever possible. Here is a simple rule of thumb for radii:

Inside wall thickness = one-half of nominal wall thickness
Outside radius = 1.5 × wall thickness

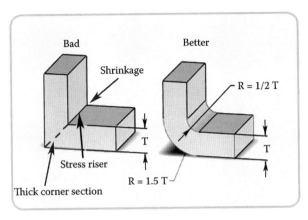

FIGURE 11.5 Radius corners for consistent nominal wall thickness.

Notice how a sharp corner will produce an increase in the nominal wall thickness in that area, greater shrinkage, and warping in the direction of the inside of the corner.

Two Ways Molds Are Made

Aluminum prototype molds typically are made by machining the mold cavity with an end mill, usually a "ball" end mill that is rounded on the cutting end. This will produce a cavity with a minimum corner radius equal to the diameter of the ball end mill. If designing a part intended to be made in an aluminum tool, it is important to not design critical features that cannot be formed by milling. One type of feature would be a deep narrow rib or hole feature, especially if there is little or no draft. In this case, the depth of the hole would be limited to the depth of the cutting tool.

The other method of forming a mold cavity is in ferrous tool steel (e.g., P-20) with an electrical discharge machining (EDM) electrode. With this method, a positive shape carbon "sinker" electrode in the form of the part is made, and this carbon electrode emitting a high-voltage spark erodes the mold cavity into the tool steel in the shape of the electrode. It is possible to form features in the positive shape of the carbon electrode that are not possible to machine into a negative cavity. The capabilities and limitations of these methods will affect the kinks of features you can design into a part. Discuss these with your tooling vendor as you develop you part.

FOURTH RULE: SPECIFY THE FRIENDLIEST-TO-MOLD AND LEAST EXPENSIVE MATERIAL

When designing medical parts it is tempting to use an exotic engineering plastic when an easier to process and more available commodity material would work just as well. High-performance engineering plastics tend to run at higher temperatures and can be several times the cost of a commodity plastic. For example, there is no need to mold the handle of a medical device out of a high-performance engineering resin like polysulfone unless it is meant to be steam sterilized, or has to withstand high temperatures. Often, ABS or a PC/ABS blend will work just as well, be easier to mold, have lower material costs, and have a better surface finish. Overspecifying the material does not make a better part. It can result in a part that is harder to produce, with a higher cost per part. The other risk of using an exotic material is availability. If the resin is discontinued by the supplier, this can be a real headache, especially if you are producing a device under a Food and Drug Administration Pre Market Approval (FDA PMA) and you are locked into using a specific material. Changing a material can mean reopening the PMA submission, triggering a Supplemental Application to obtain the change approved. It can take several months for the FDA to review the application and this can involve significant expense. Better to ensure that your material is readily available in the future. By all means, use an engineering resin if it is needed and meets a requirement that a commodity plastic cannot. For example, polyetheretherketone (PEEK) is a high-performance plastic often used for spinal implants, is highly biocompatible, and is specified in cases in which very high stiffness and heat resistance are needed. Just ensure that the decision to use a high-performance engineering resin adds value and is not just overengineering the part. More information on plastics for medical devices can be found in Chapter 1, "Introduction to Medical Plastics."

PLASTIC MATERIALS, FILLED PLASTICS

You may want to modify the properties of a stock resin to increase its stiffness, to make the material radiopaque, or to increase its surface lubricity. Plastics can be compounded with additives to achieve this. Here are some common fillers:

Glass

Glass is added typically to increase stiffness. PC is a common plastic to load with glass. The drawback to a glass- or mineral-filled resin is that it can be abrasive and cause wear to the mold tool.

Barium

Barium is added to give radiopaque properties to plastics and to catheter tubing to increase lubricity. Tungsten also may be added to make a plastic part radiopaque. Talk to your medical plastics compounder to discuss your options.

Plastics Additives to Watch for

There is greater sensitivity to what were once thought innocuous additives to common plastics (see Figure 11.6). Two of these are phthalates in polyvinylchloride (PVC; Bis(2-ethylhexyl)phthalate [DEHP]), which is a common plasticizer in flexible PVC; and Bisphenol A (BPA), which is commonly found in PC. Both substances are coming under increased scrutiny, so as your development program moves forward, check to see if your device materials contain these substances, if they are allowable in your device, or if a DEHP- or BPA-free alternative must be found. In the European Union, devices containing DEHP must disclose this on the label.

FIFTH RULE: USE STRAIGHT PARTING LINES

Sometimes a part is designed with what is called a "stepped" parting line. This occurs when the two halves of the mold are not flat to each other. Although some

Elements of Injection Molding Style for Medical Device R&D

	Some brand names	Mechanical properties		Moldability characteristics						Relative cost
		Strength	Impact	High temp-strength	Warp and dimensional accuracy, molded	Fills small features	Voids in thick	Sink in thick	Flash	High temp on mold & ejectors	
Acetal	Delrin, Celcon	Medium	Medium	Medium-low	Fair	Fair	Poor	Good	Good	Fair	Medium
Nylon 6/6	Zytel	Medium	High	Low	Fair	Excellent	Good	Fair	Poor	Fair	Medium
Nylon 6/6, glass filled	Zytel	High	Medium	High	Fair	Good		Good	Fair	Fair	Medium
Polypropylene	Maxxam, Profax	Low	High	Low	Fair	Excellent	Poor	Poor	Poor	Good	Low
High-density polyethylene (HDPE)	Dow HDPE, Chevron HDPE	Low	High	Low	Fair	Excellent		Poor	Poor	Good	Low
Polycarbonate	Lexan, Makrolon	Medium	High	Medium-high	Good	Fair	Fair to good	Fax	Good	Good	Medium-high
Acrylonitrile butadiene styrene (ABS)	Lustran, Cycolac	Medium-low	High	Low	Good	Fair	Good	Fair	Good	Good	Low
Polycarbonate/ABS Alloy	Cycoloy, Bayblend	Medium	High	Medium	Good-excellent	Fair	Good	Fair	Good	Good	Medium
Polybutylene terephthalate	Valox, Crastin	Medium	High	Low	Fair	Fair		Fair	Fair	Good	Medium-high
Polystyrene	Styron	Medium-low	Low	Low	Good	Good		Fair	Fair	Good	Low
Thermoplastic elastomer	Isoplast, Santoprene	Low	High	Low	Poor	Excellent		Good	Poor	Excellent	Low-medium
Acrylic	Plexiglass-Acrylite	Medium	Low	Low	Good	Fair		Good	Good	Good	Medium

FIGURE 11.6 Properties and moldability of common plastics. (Courtesy of Protomold Inc., Maple Plain, MN.)

features can be done only with a stepped parting line, a stepped parting line results in a more complex (and expensive) mold tool, and one that is more prone to wear. Angled mating surfaces can rub against each other in a way that two flat mating surfaces do not. This can result in galling in aluminum tools, shortening tool life, or causing unwanted "flash."

SIXTH RULE: IS "DO IT IN THE MOLD"

PRODUCT DESIGN PRINCIPLE

To avoid labor costs, design features "in the mold" even if the tool is more expensive (within reason). These can be snap fits, features to capture components, or combining features that would be assembled from several parts into one part. Labor costs never go away and unnecessary labor leads to process variability. Tooling costs can be amortized, and if a feature is "in the tool" it is less likely to suffer from variability. Calculate a quick financial model to see whether your expected consumption volumes and labor savings offset the cost of a more complex tool (for a simple modeling tool, see Chapter 10, "Prototype or Produce"). Anything saved past breakeven is "found money."

MONEY-SAVING TRICK: TWO HOUSING SHELLS FROM ONE MOLDED HOUSING SHELL

This money-saving trick relies on a concept known as "rotational symmetry" In this example, two identical molded shells fit together to make a complete case for a surgical power supply (see Figure 11.7). A number of complex features were incorporated to capture circuit boards and electrical connectors. Not all housings lend themselves to this process; however, when it works, it can cut your tooling costs in half.

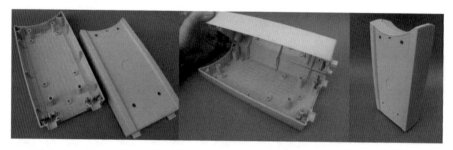

FIGURE 11.7 Two identical shells that form one housing. (Courtesy of T. Kucklick for Starion Instruments, Sunnyvale, CA.)

SIDE HOLE WITHOUT A SIDE PULL

One way to make a side hole perpendicular to the direction of pull of the mold is to use a side action core. This adds cost and complexity to the mold. Another way to get a side hole if the geometry allows it is to form the hold using a shut-off (see Figures 11.8 and 11.9).

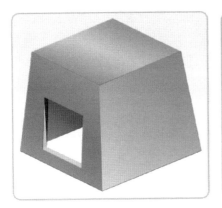
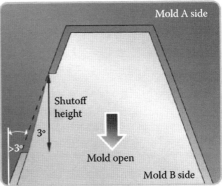

FIGURE 11.8 Forming a side-window feature with a shutoff. (Courtesy of Protomold Inc., Maple Plain, MN.)

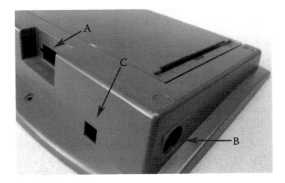

FIGURE 11.9 Features "A" and "B" were formed with side-action slides. "C" was formed with a shutoff. (Courtesy for T. Kucklick for Novasom, Glen Burnie, MD.)

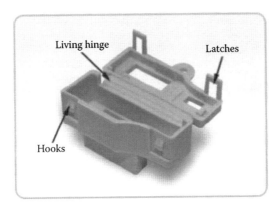

FIGURE 11.10 Prototype part with multiple molded-in features. (Courtesy of Protomold Inc., Maple Plain, MN.)

TABLE 11.2
Society of Plastics Industry Mold Polish Finishes

Mold Finishes

Current SPI		Equivalent (pre-1988)
Diamond-polished surfaces		
A-1	Grade #3, 6000 Grit Diamond Buff	#1
A-2	Grade #6, 3000 Grit Diamond Buff	#2
A-3	Grade #15, 1200 Grit Diamond Buff	#2
Paper Grit-polished surfaces		
B-1	600 Grit Paper	#3
B-2	400 Grit Paper	#3
B-3	320 Grit Paper	#3
C-1	600 Stone	#4
C-2	400 Stone	#4
C-3	320 Stone	#4
Sandblasted finishes		
D-1	600 Stone and Dry Blast Glass Bead #11	#5
D-2	400 Stone Prior and Dry Blast #24 Oxide	#5
D-3	320 Stone and Dry Blast #24 Oxide	#5
Unfinished: EDM surface or noncosmetic "as machined"		

Source: SPI Mold Finish Guide ref #AR-108 (SPI, Washington, DC).

Note: These mold finish specifications are available from the SPI at http://store.plasticsindustry.org. Included in the kit is a molded plaque with examples of these mold finishes (product order ref AR-106). Examples of surface finishes may also be available from your molding vendor. For specialized textures, see www.mold-tech.com , (Mold-Tech, a Standex Company, Salem, NH).

MOLDED-IN HINGES

There are several ways to form molded-in hinges (see Figure 11.10). One is a "living hinge," which is a thin area that acts as a hinge. The best materials for living hinges is polyethylene of polypropylene. Lining hinges work well for "clamshell" containers or other hinged features. One caveat for living hinges in medical devices is any embrittlement that may happen if the plastic is radiation sterilized.*

Another way to form a hinge is with a snap-fit type hinge. Examples of these hinges can be found in cosmetics boxes. Look for clever examples of injection molding and keep a collection of them to use for ideas when you have a design problem to solve.

SURFACE FINISHES

The surface finish of a molded part can vary from noncosmetic "as-machined" machines to a "Class A" diamond polish (see Table 11.2).

---

* For more on living hinge design, see "Living Hinge," http://www.efunda.com/designstandards/plastic_design/hinge.cfm, (accessed August 11, 2012).

Notes on Surface Finishes

Typically, the more highly polished the finish, the more expensive the tool. A class A-1 diamond polish can take up to two hours per square inch in labor to produce and can be rather expensive. Normally, aluminum tools for R&D use are given a low to medium cosmetic finish. Surface roughness of the finish is usually measured in microinches. Some molding vendors may have their own in-house standard finishes. Other specialty mold finishes are hard chrome plating or Teflon coating.

Finish and Draft Angle

When molding in a rigid plastic, if a surface is more polished, it typically releases more easily and may require less draft. If a surface is textured, it requires more draft. Textured surfaces typically require at least 1.5 degrees of draft per 0.001 inch of texture depth. The direction of polish can have an effect on removing a part from the mold. In draw polishing the tool is polished parallel to the direction of the pull of the tool. This makes the part easier to eject, but it may a more expensive polishing method.

Surface Finish and Elastomers

The rule of the "smoother the finish the easier the ejection" does not apply to elastomers, which tend to stick to smooth surfaces. For example, a polished mold core in which the thermoplastic elastomer (TPE) shrinks onto the core and sticks to a smooth surface can be a problem. Sandblasting the mold surfaces when molding in TPE helps it release from the mold surface and prevents sticking.

Preengineered Molds

In cases in which you want to make more parts than an aluminum tool, but do not need a full custom tool, you can save money by using a preengineered mold. These tools are built with standard features and dimensions to save money and to simplify setup and storage. One popular system is the Master Unit Die (MUD) base by Detroit Mold Engineering (DME; Madison Heights, MI). By having a preengineered frame and using the mold as an insert, you can save costs for certain tools. Ask your molding vendor about your options for using a preengineered mold system.

NEW CAPABILITIES: MOLD FLOW AND FEA (FINITE ELEMENT ANALYSIS)

Within the past few years, analysis packages have become mainstream, easier to use, and within the reach of most designers. These packages are now available as program plug-ins for many popular CAD packages.

Gating

There are a number of ways to form a path to inject plastic into a mold and each of these methods has relative advantages. There are two main considerations with gating, (1) the physical "vestige," "remain," or surface imperfection at the gate; and (2) the cosmetic appearance or "gate blush." The amount of allowable imperfection at the gate needs to be considered as well as the cost of different gating options.

EDGE GATE OR TAB GATE

An edge or tab gate is the simplest and cheapest type of gate. The injection nozzle is positioned at the parting line of the mold and a "runner" or "sprue" is cut into the mold as a conduit path for the plastic to enter the mold. If you have ever built plastic model kits, you will be familiar with these as the "tree" that holds the parts together. After the part is ejected, this sprue is manually cut off. Because the edge gate must contact the outer surface of the part, there will always be some noticeable gate remain. One disadvantage is the cooling of the plastic along the runner before it enters the mold. This sometimes requires a larger gate at the part, which results in a larger vestige or remain when it is trimmed. The amount of vestige or remain should be specified in the inspection and acceptance criteria for the part.

POST GATE

With a post gate, plastic is injected through one of the ejector pin bores, and the sprue is ejected when the ejector pin pushes the part out of the mold. The postshaped sprue is then manually cut off. The advantage of a post gate is that the gate vestige can be located on a noncosmetic area of the part.

SUBGATE OR TUNNEL GATE

In the subgate or tunnel gate design, the plastic is injected into the mold below the parting line in the B side of the mold. When the part is ejected, the gate sprue is automatically sheared off. This process leaves a vestige on the outer surface of the part, but it eliminates the manual operation of trimming the gate.

HOT TIP

In the hot tip method, the injection gate has a thermostatically controlled heater, and the plastic is shot in to the mold without losing heat along a runner. This method requires a dimple or depression in the part and leaves a small vestige or nub at the injection gate. The advantage is that there is no gate to trim, and the plastic flows better through the mold. Because it is heated, it requires a smaller gate than a runner gate, which is advantageous with larger parts. A disadvantage to the hot tip method is that once the location of the gate is set, it might not be able to be relocated without completely remaking that side of the mold.

LOCATING THE GATE TO THE PART

Selecting a gate location at one time was a matter of using one's best experience and judgment. Once a decision was made, the steel was cut, and if the decision was correct, good parts were made. With the availability CAD analysis programs like Moldflow® (Autodesk Inc., Sausalito, CA), several gating scenarios can be tried and

Elements of Injection Molding Style for Medical Device R&D

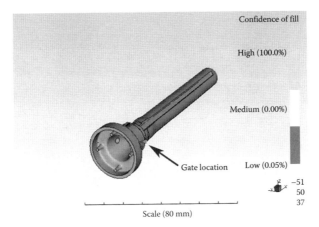

FIGURE 11.11 (**See color insert.**) Screenshot of Moldflow analysis of confidence of fill. (Courtesy of Cannuflow Inc., San Jose, CA.)

analyzed on the CAD model, and the gate location can be optimized (see Figure 11.11). Confidence in filling the mold, time to fill, and generation of knit lines can be predicted during analysis. With this data, potential problems with the part can be identified and corrected in the CAD model before the mold is produced. Ask your tooling vendor if they have this capability.

PART EJECTION

To remove a part from a mold requires ejector pins and a place for these pins to push against the part (see Figure 11.12). An important part of the design process is deciding

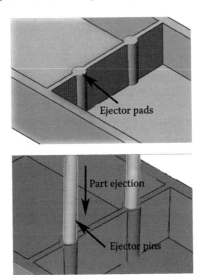

FIGURE 11.12 Ejection of parts with ejector pins. (Courtesy of Protomold Inc., Maple Plain, MN.)

where and how to locate the ejector pins and to ensure that the pins have a surface to push against to eject the part (see Figure 11.12). These pins will leave marks on the part, so normally the ejection is done against the noncosmetic side of the part.

GLUING, JOINING, FASTENING

The subject of adhesives is handled in more detail in Chapter 2, "Basics of Medical Device Adhesives." Here are some considerations when joining molded plastic parts.

INSERTS

Threaded inserts such as PEM® inserts made by the Penn Engineering Company (Danboro, PA)* are a great way to add reliable and durable brass threads to assemble plastic housing shells. There are versions for press-fitting, heat or ultrasound staking, and molded-in inserts (see Figure 11.13). These inserts are available from your local industrial fastener distributor. In an R&D environment, you may not have an ultrasonic staking machine to drive in staked inserts. An easy way to stake in these inserts is with an adjustable heat soldering iron and a pointed soldering iron tip. Adjust the soldering iron to the melt temperature of the plastic you are using, insert the tip of the soldering iron into the top hole of the insert, let it warm up a bit, and press it into the molded hollow boss. With a little practice you can get acceptable results with this simple and inexpensive method.

ULTRASONIC WELDING

Ultrasonic welding is a great way to assemble parts without adhesives and with little labor. The trick to ultrasonic welding work is to design the mating parts with a small feature known as an "energy director." This is a small V-shaped feature that will vibrate and melt into the adjoining part, forming a permanent joint. Assistance in part design for ultrasonic welding is available from Branson Ultrasonics (Danbury, CT) and Dukane (St. Charles, IL). For prototype and low-production numbers, adhesives and fasteners may be more convenient. Ultrasonic welding usually comes into the picture with higher production numbers.

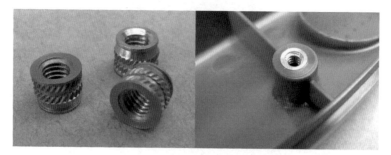

FIGURE 11.13 Threaded inserts.

---

* "SI Inserts for Plastic," Penn Engineering, http://www.pemnet.com/fastening_products/si-inserts-for-plastic.html, (accessed August 11, 2012).

Elements of Injection Molding Style for Medical Device R&D

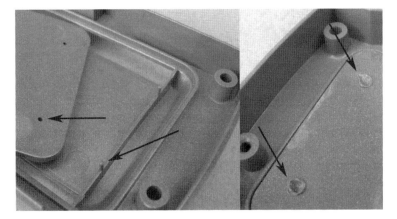

FIGURE 11.14 Heat staking. (Courtesy of T. Kucklick for Novasom, Glen Burnie, MD.)

HEAT STAKING

Heat staking is a simple, cheap reliable, and permanent way to locate and assemble parts. In this example (see Figure 11.14), a filler plate in the bottom of a medical device housing is held in place with heat-staked pegs. In prototype numbers, these can be peened over with an adjustable heat soldering iron. In production, these were staked with an ultrasonic welder.

INTERFERENCE PRESS FIT BOSSES

Another simple and easy-to-mold assembly feature is a cruciform interference press-fit boss. This boss is driven into a drafted hollow boss, which then compresses, locking the assembly together. This method works well with materials that are resistant to stress cracking.

SNAP FITS

Snap fits are relatively easy to design once the basic principles are understood. The first principle is designing the snap fit tab with sufficient flexibility. The second principle is understanding how to design the part and the "pass-though core" that forms the undercut feature of the snap fit (see Figures 11.15 and 11.16). A number of excellent references on the subject of snap fits are included in "Resources" at the end of the chapter. It is important to design the snap fit feature with sufficient draft (3 degrees) to prevent the A and B sides of the mold sliding against each other.

ADHESIVES

The subject of adhesives is handled in Chapter 2 of this book. A special consideration with molded parts and adhesives is molded-in stress. Some plastics such as polycarbonate and polysulfone are especially prone to stress cracking, which can be aggravated by solvent-based adhesives.

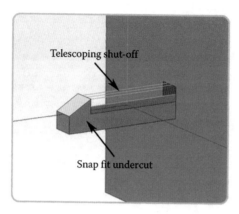

FIGURE 11.15 A telescoping core forming a snap fit clip undercut. (Courtesy of Protomold, Inc., Maple Plain, MN.)

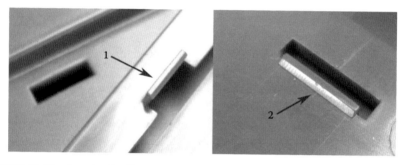

FIGURE 11.16 Snap fit clip (1) and snapped in place (2).

STERILIZATION AND BIOBURDEN

When sterilizing molded parts, it is important to test and know how clean the parts are before they are sterilized. Parts that are prototype molded in a machine shop environment and hand-handled versus parts that are molded in a clean room and double-bagged straight from the press will have vastly different levels of bioburden. These parts will need appropriate cleaning and sterilization dosing to achieve sterility. It is best to make the parts in the cleanest environment possible, and handle them in the cleanest way possible, and to ensure that this cleanliness is consistently maintained.

Parts cleaning can be a costly part of the assembly process. Washing parts to remove oil, particulates, and biological contamination from handling can be time-consuming, and when using a contract manufacturer time literally equals money. Keep the following in mind:

- Always handle parts that will be sterilized with gloved hands. Use nitrile gloves to avoid latex contamination if you have a latex-free product.
- Avoid contamination with silicone oils. Once a part or an assembly area is contaminated with silicone oil it is nearly impossible to eradicate.

- Avoid packaging parts where they can be contaminated with particulates. Avoid packaging that sheds particulates, such as newspaper, corn-based plastic peanuts, or cardboard "peanuts." Use nonshedding packaging like bubble-wrap. Double-bag parts.
- When cleaning parts, the goal is to remove the contamination and get it into the washing medium, and off the parts, not just move the dirt around on the parts.

STERILIZATION EFFECTS ON PLASTICS

One unique consideration for molded plastic medical devices is the effect of sterilization on the material.

The typical methods for sterilizing medical devices are radiation (gamma, e-beam), EtO (ethylene oxide) gas, heat (autoclave, steam), Sterrad® (hydrogen peroxide/gas plasma), and Steris® (peracetic acid). For disposable devices, radiation (gamma, e-beam) and EtO are the most popular methods. For reusable devices, heat and autoclave are the most common. Reusable devices are typically machined from stainless steel or molded from temperature-resistant plastics such as Ultem, PEEK, or polysulfone.

Radiation exacerbates molded-in stress, and therefore it is important to follow good part design practice to avoid sharp corners, stress risers, molded-in stress, bad knit lines, and uneven shrinkage. Radiation can make bad parts even more stiff, brittle, and weaker because of polymer chain scissioning and cross-linking. Other effects of radiation are discoloration (nonradiation-stable polycarbonate turns yellowish) and odor (radiation can attack oil-based plasticizers in PVC).[*]

There are only a few radiation "problem plastics," including PTFE (disintegrates at >4 kGy), acetal, Delrin (suffers embrittlement), and nonstabilized polypropylene (subject to radiation attacks). An attractive feature of acetal is that it is easy to machine, holds up to steam sterilization, and therefore is a popular material for fabricated prototypes. It may find its way, by default, into higher production products where it may no longer be appropriate. For this reason, plan ahead for manufacturing scale-up, not just R&D convenience. These radiation-unfriendly materials may be sterilized using other methods, such as EtO. Plastics containing a benzene ring structure such as styrene, ABS, and PC/ABS tend to be radiation stable. Most elastomers such as TPEs and silicones are stable as well. See Table 11.3.

CHOOSING A BIOCOMPATIBLE MATERIAL

When choosing a material for use in a medical device, the biocompatibility of the material must be taken into consideration, relative to its use in the device. Some materials are now available that are prequalified for medical device use (e.g., Bayer Makrolon® polycarbonate). The duration of contact with the patient (<30 days, implanted) and the type of contact (skin, mucous membrane, bone/dentin, circulating

---

[*] Karl J. Hemmerich, "Polymer Materials Selection for Radiation-sterilized Product," *MD+DI Online* (February 2000), http://www.mddionline.com/article/polymer-materials-selection-radiation-sterilized-products.

TABLE 11.3
Radiation Stability

Radiation Stability	Material	Notes
Excellent	Polyimide, Polyphenylene Sulfide, Styrene acrylonitrile (SAN), Polycarbonate, PC/ABS, Polysulfone, Polyetheneterpthalate (PET), Liquid Crystal Polymer (LCP), Phenolics, Epoxies, Polyester, Polyurethanes, Urethane, Styrenic TPEs	Clear polycarbonates yellow; RS grades available; Polystyrenes tend to be radiation stable
Good/excellent	Polyethylene, Polyvinyl Fluoride (PVF), Polyvinylene Fluoride (PVDF), Polyamides (Nylon), Polyurethane, natural rubber, nitrile,	
Good	Silicone, Acrylics (PMMA), PVC, neoprene	
Poor	Polypropylene (nonstabilized), PTFE (Teflon), FEP, Acetal (Delrin), Butyl rubber	PTFE disintegrates under radiation; Delrin (acetal) becomes brittle

blood) all affect the testing that must be done to meet FDA, CE Mark, and other regulatory requirements. More information on testing for biocompatibility is in Chapter 4.

COLORANTS

When using a colorant, remember that the colorant is part of the plastic and must be tested for biocompatibility in its "as-molded" state. When changing colors, it is possible to retain the biocompatibility qualification if you use a colorant with fewer components than a colorant that is already qualified; however, if a colorant adds a material, then the new colorant compound and plastic will need to be retested. This can have a serious impact on a PMA product, as any change to the product results in a reopening of the PMA file as well as a supplemental application and approval from the FDA. Also, for medical devices the total colorant by weight should not exceed 1%.

OTHER MOLDING METHODS

Silicone Molding

Silicone molding is a type of injection molding that uses thermoset silicone rubber rather than a melted thermoplastic. Silicone is a commonly used material in medical devices with excellent tear resistance, elasticity, and biocompatibility. It is useful in seals, balloons, bladders, o-rings, and many other devices. Silicone is also popular for ovemolding.

RIM Molding

In reaction injection molding (RIM), a two-part thermoset plastic mix is injected into the mold, typically a urethane. RIM is typically used for large housings or short-run parts.

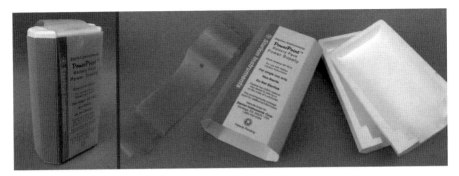

FIGURE 11.17 EPS shell design for disposable surgical battery pack. (Courtesy of T. Kucklick for Starion Instruments, Sunnyvale, CA.)

Foam Molding

Foam molding is for producing larger enclosures. Injecting the plastic melt with gas helps to produce parts with thicker walls (e.g., 0.25 inch or 0.5 inch). This helps to produce large parts at less cost, expense, and weight than solid material parts.

Styrofoam Molding

In Expanded Polystyrene Styrofoam (EPS) molding, Styrofoam pellets are injected into a mold with steam, which expands the pellets into the shape of the mold. The advantage to this method is that the parts are good thermal insulators, shock-absorbing, and inexpensive, and they are commonly used in packaging and insulated containers (see Figure 11.17). EPS molding may be done in a variety of densities and hardnesses.

INSPECTION AND ACCEPTANCE CRITERIA

To get the parts you want, and the ones that will work for their intended purpose, have clear and consistent inspection and acceptance criteria. Know what your critical features are. Inspect the features that matter. Do not spend time (and money) on the ones that do not matter. Having clear acceptance criteria from the beginning will help you build your design history file as the development program moves from R&D to pilot production without having to reconstruct or backfill this information. Do not subject the parts to overtolerance. Make parts that are as accurate as they need to be but no more. Tighter tolerances where they are not required equal unnecessary cost.

GLOSSARY

"A" and "B" Side: The "A" side of a tool is the "cavity" and the "B" side is the "core." Typically the "A" side forms the outer cosmetic surface of the part, and the "B" side forms the noncosmetic inside, the surface where the ejector pins push the part out of the mold. A tool is designed so that the part will release from the "A" side and hold on to the "B" side, so that it can be cleanly ejected by the ejector pins. Sometimes a part is textured to get a part to hold preferentially to the "B" side.

Clean Room Molding: Molding in a clean room with electrically driven presses to reduce particulates and bioburden.

Fastening and Joining: There are several methods of joining parts, including ultrasonic welding, heat staking, threaded inserts, fasteners, adhesives, and interference fit deformable bosses.

Flash: Melted plastic leaking from the mold cavity at the parting line and forming a thin projection of material from the part that must be trimmed off. This is usually a sign of tool wear.

Gate: The gate is where plastic is injected into the mold. Types of gates include edge (or side) gate, post gate, tunnel, or "submarine" gate, and hot tip.

Insert Molding: Insert molding is where plastic is molded around another item. An example of insert molding is the molding of a hub around a metal trocar rod. If a part is insert molded over another plastic part, the melt temperature of the plastic being molded over the base part must be lower than that of the base part to avoid melting or distorting the base part. One way to avoid this is to overmold to the base part using a nonthermoplastic method such as with liquid silicone injection.

Mold Analysis: Analysis software that helps predict how a molded part will fill and any potential problems that will need to be addressed. A commonly used package is Moldflow (Autodesk, Sausalito, CA).

Mold Release: A lubricant sprayed into the mold to prevent parts from sticking in the mold. Any mold release residue must be washed off the part before assembly.

Master Unit Die (MUD) Base: A type of preengineered mold. Preengineered molds may be less expensive than a fully custom tool.

Nominal Wall Thickness: The wall thickness that is appropriate for the material being molded. For best results, the wall thickness should be consistent and not have areas that are significantly thicker or thinner than the nominal wall.

Parting Line: The surface where the two halves of the mold come together. This can be "straight" where the mold halves meet at one flat surface, or "stepped" where the tool faces include a complex surface. Stepped parting lines add to the cost of the tool, and may require ongoing maintenance.

Side Action or Side Pull: A cam (mechanical) or hydraulically operated part of the mold that forms a feature not possible to make in a simple straight pull mold. Examples of features made with side actions are holes perpendicular to the parting line, sides of the part requiring zero draft, and undercuts.

Sink Marks: This is a cosmetic defect in which a local area is thicker that the nominal wall, resulting in a sink mark or a dimple. Careful attention to consistent nominal wall thickness can help avoid sink marks.

Sprue: The sprue is the extra plastic in the runner of an edge gate or post gate molded part. This excess plastic needs to be trimmed off. The scrap plastic is typically reground and recycled.

Steel Safe: Steel safe is allowing enough extra material in a mold to adjust the size of a feature, if needed. When planning for steel safe critical features, remember that the mold is a negative of the part. A positive feature like a rib is formed by a cavity and can be made larger, by removing material, but not smaller, and a hole is formed by a core and can be made smaller, but not larger. Adding material to a mold by welding is possible but it is risky and expensive. Allowing for steel safe features is part of the strategy when optimizing the final production part.

Tool, Single-cavity and Multicavity: A single-cavity tool is typically the simplest and least expensive in terms of tooling cost. Multiple cavity tools are more expensive upfront; however, the per-part cost can be lower as it can produce more parts per hour of molding machine time. Another type of multicavity tool is a "family mold" in which the components of an assembly are produced together in one tool. This can be less expensive than having a dedicated tool for each part.

Tooling, "Hard": Mold tooling made from mold-grade tool steel. A well-designed and constructed hard tool is capable of producing millions of parts. Typical materials for "hard" tools are P-20 steel, stainless steel, and other hardened tool steels.

Tooling, "Soft": Mold tooling made from a soft and easy-to-machine material like aluminum. Soft tools are typically good for less than 1000 parts; however, with good part and mold design, some soft tools can produce many more parts.

Weld Line, Knit Line: Knit lines occur when two flow fronts join together in the mold. This is typically when plastic flows around a hole feature in the part, as this requires the plastic to flow around a core that forms the hole. Knit lines may be a cosmetic problem or may weaken the part.

RESOURCES

REFERENCES: PRINT

Bonenberger, Paul. *The First Snap Fit Handbook.* Munich, Germany: Hanser, 2000.

Campo, E. Alfredo. *The Complete Part Design Handbook: For Injection Molding of Thermoplastics.* Munich, Germany: Hanser, 2006.

CDROMWJT Associates. *Injection Mold Tooling Standards: A Guide for Specifying, Purchasing and Qualifying Injection Molds.* CDROM ISBN: 0936994118, 1993. "Designed to be incorporated into a company's documentation, this will guide both experienced and new-to-plastics processors through the maze of specifying, purchasing, and qualifying injection molds." The Society of Plastics Engineering, www.4spe.org.

Erhard, Gunter. *Designing with Plastics.* Munich, Germany: Hanser, 2006.

Malloy, Robert A. *Plastic Part Design for Injection Molding.* Munich, Germany: Hanser.

Rothheiser, Jordan. *Joining of Plastics: Handbook for Designers and Engineers.* Munich, Germany: Hanser, 1994.

Tres, Paul A. *Designing Plastic Parts for Assembly*, 6th ed. Munich, Germany: Hanser, 2000.

REFERENCES: ONLINE

Modern Plastic Encyclopedia (http://www.modplas.com/worldencyclopedia/search) has extensive information on injection molding plastics, additives, manufacturers, and trade names.

The Society of Plastics Engineering (www.4spe.org) has extensive resources available on plastic molding and materials.

ACKNOWLEDGMENTS

The assistance of Brad Cleveland and Protomold with the contribution of tables and figures for this chapter are gratefully acknowledged. Protomold (http://www.protomold.com) publishes a series of useful design tips and offers a molding "sample cube" that illustrates good and not-so-good molding practices.

Section III

Methods for Medical Device R&D

12 Clinical Observation
How to Be Welcome (or at Least Tolerated) in the Operating Room and Laboratory

Theodore R. Kucklick

CONTENTS

Getting into the Operating Room as an Observer 243
Value of OR Observation in Medical Device Innovation 244
Putting Observations to Work 245
Help in Gaining Access 245
Operating Room Etiquette Primer (for the OR Visitor) 245
Labs and Courses 247
Other Cautions: OR and Lab Safety 248
    Radiation 248
    Sharps and Radiofrequency 248
OR Access Training Credentials 248
Conclusion 249
Resources 249
    References: Credentialing 249
    References: Observation 250
    Vendors: Credentialing 250
Acknowledgments 250

GETTING INTO THE OPERATING ROOM AS AN OBSERVER

Dr. Lanny Johnson, inventor of the arthroscopic shaver, stated in a talk at the 2008 Arthroscopy Association of North America (AANA) national meeting, "The foundation of business is innovation, and its foundation in medicine is clinical observation." Where does observation for medical device take place? The most important place is in the hospital or surgery center operating room, seeing actual procedures. Another is in the wet lab (animal and cadaver, and bench).

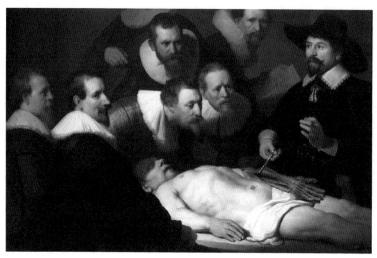

The Anatomy Lesson of Dr. Tulp, by Rembrandt van Rijn

The problem with operating rooms (OR) is they are inaccessible to the average person, and for very good reasons. This is a place where life and death decisions are made, liability risks are high, and dedicated, busy people are working together, sometimes at high speed, operating by strict rules that they do not have time to explain to an outsider. The facility and the surgical team simply cannot afford to have someone in the room who does not know how to follow sterile procedure, patient privacy regulations, and myriad other written and unwritten rules. Where does one begin to learn some of these rules and gain access to the OR?

VALUE OF OR OBSERVATION IN MEDICAL DEVICE INNOVATION

The typical medical device company has their interface with the customers in the OR by way of their sales force and clinical specialists. These are the "boots on the ground" who are in the OR every day dealing with the realities of how medical devices are used. In a typical scenario, these sales reps feed information to their counterparts in the sales and marketing departments and these observations finally filter (sometimes second- and third-hand) to design and engineering. In medical device start-ups, the information filters to the designers through the company's scientific advisory board (SAB).

Medical device companies can help themselves by giving designers, engineers, and product managers the opportunity to see their products used in the hands of actual users in everyday real-life situations on actual patients. Some companies do this. Others can improve. Some engineers who are expected to design medical devices to be used in the OR have never seen the surgical devices they design actually used in the OR. Current best practices in design include design input based on the observation of customer and clinical needs. There are case studies and publications available on how to do this. One example of a formal application of observation and "voice-of-the-customer" methodology is the design of the Harmonic Focus ultrasonic forceps by Ethicon Endosurgery (Cincinnati, OH).[*] Other innovations can come from observation. The Cannuflow Extravastat® technology and EntreVu® portal cannula for reducing fluid extravasation during shoulder arthroscopy procedures originated as the result of a clinical observation in the OR of an unaddressed problem.

When all parties, from the sales representative, to marketing, to the designer, are knowledgeable of the end user's and patient's needs, devices can be designed and produced that are more usable, more innovative, and easier for the rep to sell. If a sales rep cannot sell the product because of a defect in its usability that could have been avoided through clinical observation, it does not matter how innovative a product may be, it is not likely to be successful.

PUTTING OBSERVATIONS TO WORK

The Stanford Biodesign Fellowship Program provides an example of how clinical observations are put to work. The program uses a system of observation to teach the development of medical device innovation. Fellows are assigned to work in Stanford Hospital as surgical technicians for the summer before the start of the program. They are to keep a detailed notebook of their observations, paying special attention to what does and does not work, while keeping an eye out for "high-quality problems." These "bug lists" of hundreds of problems are compiled and ranked. Out of this process comes a short list of important problems that can be solved with an innovative medical device. These become the basis of thesis projects for the Biodesign Fellowship teams. This is a method that you can use to collect and leverage your clinical observations.[†]

HELP IN GAINING ACCESS

A surgical sales representative who works in the area of your surgical specialty is one of the people who can help you get into an OR (provided they do not have a competitive or ethical conflict). This person can help orient you to the local rules and possibly "sponsor" your entry into an OR to do your clinical observation. A supportive surgeon or surgical physician's assistant (PA), or a member of your scientific advisory board (SAB) also might be able to sponsor you into the OR is. Remember that access as an observer in the OR is by invitation only, and you must know the proper decorum and protocol ahead of time to avoid embarrassing or dangerous mistakes.

OPERATING ROOM ETIQUETTE PRIMER (FOR THE OR VISITOR)

Lynne Bass, RN, is medical director, Bascom Surgery Center, San Jose, CA. Lynne has been especially helpful to me in understanding some of the rules of the OR (and diligent in letting me know of any of my infractions). Lynne put together a very

---

[*] Strategyn, Inc. "Case Study: Creating the Ethicon Endo-Surgery HK105 Harmonic Surgical Tool" (2009), http://chrislawer.blogs.com/files/eescasestudy.pdf.
[†] "Innovators Workbench," Stanford Biodesign, http://innovation.stanford.edu/bdn/index.jsp.

helpful basic primer on OR etiquette. Lynne says, "I taught medical students and reps coming into the OR years ago. The primer was partially born as a result of that experience."

1. Do not go into the OR until the patient is prepped and draped.
2. Make certain that your head and facial hair is completely covered with proper attire.
3. Keep your hands behind your back. (DO NOT TOUCH ANYTHING!)
4. Stand away (four feet) from the surgical (sterile) field. This includes the back table, mayo tray, and the draped surgical field.
5. Stand two to three feet away from any member of the surgical team (those fully attired in sterile surgical garb).
6. If pictures are consented to be taken, do not lean over the sterile field with your camera.
7. Hold conversation to a minimum. Ask a team member if you can ask them a question. It may not be appropriate to initiate conversation at particular times during the surgical procedure. Be sensitive to challenges the surgeon or surgical team may be experiencing.
8. Do not open sterile items requested by the team. That is the circulating nurse's responsibility. Hand the product to the nurse for them to open.
9. Be respectful of the employee lounge. Do not linger there. Food and space is budgeted for the employees.
10. Update your shot records (immunization) records and have a copy available.

Be especially aware of the sterile field. *Never* get between the sterile field and sterile instruments or the gowned team. The sterile field is from the draping on the OR table up, three feet in all directions and two feet from a gowned OR team. *Never* reach, lean, or point over the back table. Skin can shed from your hands or arms on to the sterile instruments and cause contamination. If you need to point at things in the sterile field in a technical support role, an inexpensive laser pointer can help.

Wear flat, comfortable shoes (no heels) and socks. You will need to either put on shoe covers or wear provided shoes or sandals (e.g., in many ORs outside the United States). Borrow training or procedure videos for prior review so you have a sense of what to expect in the room and during the procedure. When you put on scrubs, tuck in the shirt to help prevent shedding dead skin on to your scrub pants and the floor.

Do *not* enter the OR without a surgical mask. Most facilities have "redline" areas outside of the actual OR where scrubs, booties, caps, and masks are required. Be aware of these areas. If you do not know *ask*. If you cannot ask, always *observe*.

Even though you may not have thought of them since high school or college, immunization records can be important. Some facilities do not require them; however, some require shot records before you can enter their OR. If a facility does require your shot records, they need to be complete and up to date, including proof of newer shots like Hepatitis B. Find out the requirements *well ahead of time*. The morning you are set to walk in the OR is *not* the time to find out you need this.

Get permission from the facility and the patient *before* taking any pictures in the OR. Federal Health Insurance Portability and Accountability Act (HIPAA) Privacy regulations on this are strict. The facility can get in a lot of trouble for violating these guidelines. Do not retain copies of medical information with identifiable patient names.*

Do not use devices that do not have Food and Drug Administration (FDA) clearance (exempt, 510[k] or Investigational Device Exemption [IDE]) or institutional review board (IRB) approval from the facility. Do not use devices that do not have validated sterilization or that contain materials for which you do not have valid biocompatibility data. Again, you are a guest. You have a strict ethical responsibility to avoid doing anything that puts the patient, the surgeon, or the facility at risk. Some facilities have strict rules for bringing any new products into the OR. Check with the facility's materials management.

Do not take used or "red bag" contaminated disposable devices out of the OR. It may be tempting to take your product back with you for evaluation. Unless you have an approved protocol in place with the facility to do this, don't.

Each facility has its own variation of these rules and may even add a few of their own. Many facilities allow reps and observers to change into scrubs in the surgeon locker room. Others do not. Some have a place to secure valuables (wallets, purses) others do not. You may need to take a small bag to keep your street clothes and wallet with you. Again, check on what you can do *ahead of time* and be flexible to adjust to the local customs.

If you are observing surgeries in another country, be sure to orient yourself to the customs, culture, and conventions of that location. These may be very different from what you are used to in the United States.

LABS AND COURSES

If you have the opportunity to do so, offer to help with a surgical skills lab for your company. This can be invaluable experience. Depending on the location—whether a dedicated facility, university, or trade show setting—each lab has its own protocol, ranging from how specimens are handled to how representatives from industry may interact with the surgeon attendees. You need to be aware and respectful of the fact that there may be sponsoring companies involved.

At cadaver lab courses, such as those held at the Orthopedic Learning Center (OLC; Rosemont, IL), attendees are given a detailed orientation to the Occupational Safety and Health Administration (OSHA) regulations that apply to the cadaver wet lab at the beginning of the course. These regulations are given for the safety of the attendees and staff and to prevent biological contamination of the non–wet lab areas of the facility. If you attend a course like the OLC, be sure to arrive in time for this important orientation information and carefully follow the safety rules. Also, be sure to follow rules on how to clearly identify yourself as an industry representative.

Remember that you are a guest in the lab, and the specimens at these labs are paid for by the surgeon attendees. Do not handle these specimens yourself without the permission of the surgeons at the station attending the course, and the course directors.

---

* For more information, see "Health Information Privacy," U.S. Department of Health and Human Services, http://www.hhs.gov/ocr/hipaa.

Another place to gain experience in clinical observation is in the preclinical animal lab. If you have the opportunity, offer to help assist in these studies as well. Depending on the study, many of the same sterile field rules apply.

OTHER CAUTIONS: OR AND LAB SAFETY

RADIATION

Some OR situations involve specific safety precautions when working around high magnetic fields (e.g., magnetic resonance imaging [MRI])[*], radiation, or lasers. In the case of MRI, metal objects—including small objects like paperclips, jewelry, and pens—can be dangerous. Take the time to become oriented to safety procedures. Working around radiation (e.g., a C-arm fluoroscope in an orthopedic trauma, hip arthroscopy, or cardiology procedure) requires the wearing of a lead apron and thyroid shield for protection.[†] Working around lasers requires laser-safe eye protection for the wavelength of laser being used. Lasers are not always visible, and an unseen stray laser beam can cause permanent eye damage in a fraction of a second.[‡] Problems can be avoided with proper training, orientation, and preparation.

SHARPS AND RADIOFREQUENCY

In the OR, and particularly in hands-on wet labs, safety in handling sharps is essential. It is important not to stab yourself with needles or scalpels, or inadvertently stab your lab partner. This seems obvious, but when your attention is consumed by conducting a particularly interesting (or challenging) experiment, these obvious cautions can be overlooked. Be sure to dispose of sharps in sharps buckets (*not* regular trash!). Keep sharps segregated in a basin during a wet lab session. It is easy for a scalpel or needle to find its way under a cord or gauze and to cause an accidental stab injury or a possible blood-borne pathogen infection (e.g., hepatitis, tetanus,). Be sure to clean up and dispose of all sharps in a sharps bucket after the lab is concluded.

Radiofrequency (RF) devices (monopolar Bovie cutters, monopolar and bipolar RF ablation devices) must be handled with care. Monopolar RF cutters are exceptionally efficient at cutting tissue and can cause deep and painful electrical burns if not handled carefully. Bipolar devices can cause RF burns even of you are not connected to a ground pad.

OR ACCESS TRAINING CREDENTIALS

OR access by persons without basic training has become restricted. Since 2007 the Association of periOperative Registered Nurses (AORN) and the American College

---

[*] Frank G. Shellock, MRIsafety.com, http://www.mrisafety.com, (accessed August 12, 2012).
[†] IAEA "Staff Radiation Protection," https://www.rpop.iaea.org/RPOP/RPoP/Content/InformationFor/HealthProfessionals/4_InterventionalRadiology/fluoroscopy-operating-theatres/fluoroscopy-staff-protection.htm (accessed August 12, 2012).
[‡] Suresh M. Brahmavar, Ph.D., Fred Hetzel, Ph.D., "Medical Lasers: Quality Control, Safety Standards, and Regulations," October 2001, http://www.aapm.org/pubs/reports/rpt_73.pdf (accessed August 12, 2012).

Clinical Observation

of Surgeons (ACS) have begun to formulate rules and guidance on credentialing for industry representatives in ORs and to allow access only to those with proper basic training credentials. Online training materials are now available for a fee for sales representatives who work in the OR. A course available from the AORN is listed in the Resources at the end of this chapter. There are also now a number of vendor credentialing programs. Many hospitals now require that you be registered with a credentialing program before you can access the OR. Some hospitals also require this even if you simply plan to meet with a surgeon at their hospital office. Some of these credentialing programs include VendorMate, REPtrax, and Status Blue. These programs check the following:

- Criminal background
- That the individual is not on the Office of the Inspector General's (OIG) List of Excluded Individuals/Entities
- Proof of vaccination history
- Infection control training
- Vendor orientation sessions
- HIPAA policy compliance
- Proof of current product liability insurance with limits acceptable to the hospital
- Proof of general liability insurance

This process can be time-consuming and may require paying a fee to the credentialing company. It is important to know the policies of the facility before you arrive.

Notes on insurance: Product liability and general liability are two separate policies. Be sure your company carries both. Also, some facilities may require that you add the hospital as a "named insured." You medical device product liability insurance broker can help you with this process.

CONCLUSION

This chapter highlighted a few of the most important guidelines for gaining access and observing proper protocol as an invited guest to clinical observation to inform your design and engineering thinking. Remember, if you have the privilege to be invited into an OR, knowing and observing OR customs, manners, and etiquette can mean the difference between being considered a welcome guest or becoming an ejected pest.

RESOURCES

REFERENCES: CREDENTIALING

AORN Healthstream OR Protocol Certificate Course (http://www.healthstream.com/Products/STS/RepDirect/orProtocol.htm). "HealthStream has partnered with the Association of periOperative Registered Nurses (AORN) to distribute AORN's OR Protocol course to prepare healthcare industry sales representatives for visiting operating rooms at healthcare facilities. Upon successful completion, certificates of credit and a wallet card are awarded for presentation to healthcare facilities as documentation of training. AORN

OR Protocol is designed to award continuing education (CEU) credits for sales professionals and award contact hours for nurses. To maintain certification, a biannual renewal course is required for AORN OR Protocol."

Rogers, Jim R. "Sales Representative Credentialing . . . at What Price?" *Orthoknow* (February 2010), http://www.aimedsales.com/pdf/orthoknow0210.pdf.

References: Observation

Bettencourt, Lance, and Anthony W. Ulwick. "The Customer-Centered Innovation Map." *Harvard Business Review* 86, no. 5. (May 2008).

Ulwick, Anthony W. "Turn Customer Input into Innovation." *Harvard Business Review* 80, no. 1. (January 2002).

———. *What Customers Want*. New York: McGraw-Hill, 2005.

Vendors: Credentialing

Health Industry Representatives Association
http://www.hira.org

Independent Medical Distributors Association
http://www.imda.org

REPtrax
http://www.reptrax.com

Status Blue
http://www.status-blue.com

Vendormate
http://www.vendormate.com

ACKNOWLEDGMENTS

The assistance of Lynne Bass, Robert Bruce, and Lee Fagot in the preparation of this article is gratefully acknowledged.

13 ABCs of NDAs

Theodore R. Kucklick

CONTENTS

Documenting Your Invention: Keeping a Lab Notebook 252
Value of the NDA 253
    Case Example 253
    When Not to Sign an NDA 254
    Who Will Not Sign an NDA 255
    Who Should Sign an NDA 255
Presenting Ideas for Evaluation 256
Read and Heed 256
Who Are You Dealing With? 257
One More NDA Term: Noncircumvention 257
Signing an NDA as an Employee 258
Conclusion 258
Glossary of Typical Terms and Provisions of an NDA 259
Resources 261
Acknowledgment 261
Endnote 261

"If you wish another to keep your secret, first keep it to yourself."

—Seneca

Flossing your teeth can be tedious work, it takes self-discipline, but it helps ensure that you have a smile on your face down the road—sort of like nondisclosure agreements (NDAs). Just like floss, these agreements come in a variety of flavors, and used diligently, they will help you keep a smile on your face down the road, instead of regret. The place to get an NDA form is from your intellectual property (IP) or corporate attorney,[*] who should review the NDA, especially if it seems to contain unusual terms.

Two fundamental skills in building and maintaining IP are keeping secrets and maintaining records. Your conception of a unique idea needs to be developed and nurtured, and turned from the seed of an invention to the flower of a valuable innovation. Keeping this seed of an idea protected and secret during this cultivation process is

---

[*] A sample NDA is available at Nolo.com, http://www.nolo.com/legal-encyclopedia/sample-confidentiality-agreement-nda-33343.html.

essential to being able to eventually harvest the rewards of innovation. If carelessly disclosed, your invention idea can go out into the breeze like dandelion seeds. Once out there, anyone may cultivate it and harvest the value, and once it is disclosed, it cannot be retrieved. Patents help protect your innovation after it is developed, when you are marketing or licensing a product and harvesting the profits from your invention. But before this stage, how do you help protect your invention during the critical cultivation phase? This is where you need an NDA. An NDA is a contract in which the parties agree to keep secret any information with potential commercial value.

DOCUMENTING YOUR INVENTION: KEEPING A LAB NOTEBOOK

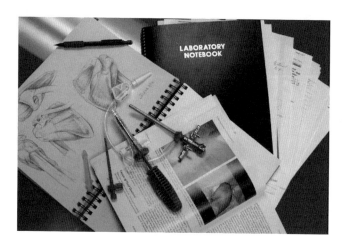

One of the most basic habits innovators must cultivate is that of documenting their work in a timely and systematic way, documenting the date the idea was conceived, and having this witnessed by a person who understands the invention and who is not a co-inventor. The best way to do this is with a lab notebook. These are available from the Scientific Notebook Company (http://www.snco.com/lab.htm) and at some office supply stores. Books are available with stamped serial numbers and company name so that a numbered book can be assigned to a team member. The paper should be of archival quality, with a place for a description, and a place for the inventor and witness to sign. A lab notebook should have numbered pages and a stitched binding. This is to document that work was done in chronological order and that no pages were either removed or inserted after the recorded dates.

Use the notebook to document concepts and experiments, to learn from the data, and to develop solutions. Answers to problems often appear in pieces and need positioning, like puzzle pieces to be arranged into a bigger picture. Generate as many ideas and potential solutions as possible and defer judgment on them. Capture, record, and date these ideas as you generate them. Look at different dimensions of the problem, such as technological matters, ease-of-use issues, how the design affects patients, affordability, clinical utility, and economic impact.

When keeping a notebook, use each page in sequence. Do not leave blank pages. If a page is left blank, a line should be drawn through it to indicate is was not used. Do not use white-out or erase entries. Entries should be made in permanent ink. If an error is made, the item should be struck out with a line. Sketching in entries and diagrams in pencil and then inking them in can help create cleaner entries. If loose items, such as printed charts, journal articles, spreadsheets, computer renderings, and so on, are part of the record, these should be permanently taped into the book. Lab notebooks must be treated as confidential and should not be made accessible to parties who are not covered under NDAs. In the event of a disclosure, a demonstrated lack of care in maintaining secrecy can invalidate a claim for damages.

VALUE OF THE NDA

Because any innovation takes the help, skills, and resources of other people, including investors, vendors, and collaborators, you need to be able to talk to others. In the process of doing so, you will have to reveal your confidential information. It is therefore necessary to get these parties to agree to keep your information confidential.

The basic purpose of an NDA is so that the other party will not reveal your information to others, or run off with your invention, and likewise that you will not run off with the other party's confidential information, either. Remember the old sayings, "loose lips sink ships," "keep it mum, chum," and "the whale that spouts, gets harpooned." It is more important than ever to be diligent about confidential information. There are now many more ways that information can be leaked, whether through conversations, e-mail, and most recently, social media sites, such as Twitter, Facebook, and LinkedIn. Information can leak very quickly and spread very quickly, and it becomes irretrievable once it is posted on the Internet. A common way for information to leak out to third parties and to lose NDA protection is by careless forwarding of e-mail messages. Ensure that if confidential information is sent by e-mail, that the person receiving it has a need for the information, that the information is marked as confidential, that it is only for the use of the recipient, and that it is not to be forwarded without prior authorization.

Be very careful when using the "reply all" feature. I once saw a situation in which a company executive, frustrated with what he considered the slow progress of an academic colleague, made an especially disparaging remark, and instead of replying only to the person who sent him the e-mail, hit "reply all." This e-mail message was distributed to the entire team, including the colleague. This careless act destroyed an important research relationship.

Once information is disclosed to a party not covered by an NDA via e-mail, social media, blog, or other means, that person is under no obligation to keep it secret. Also, do not memorialize statements into an e-mail message that you do not want to see made public or have read back to you in a courtroom.

Case Example

A cautionary story I have heard of inadvertent disclosure comes from the renowned surgeon–innovator Rodney Perkins, MD. In a Stanford Biodesign "Innovators

Workbench" interview,* Perkins shares how he conceived of an idea for an "air splint" while he was a surgical resident. It was a great idea. It was cleaner than a wooden splint, it was clear (so one could see a wound), it provided compression, and it was compact. It had all the elements of a great medical device invention. He began to develop the idea, and disclosed it, unprotected by an NDA to a vendor, and in the course of busy life of a surgical resident, forgot about it. Two years later, the product was on the market, and though understandably unhappy, there was little he could do about it. The moral of the story is to be careful of inadvertent or unprotected disclosure of an invention. You likely will need people who have skills that you do not have to take an idea forward and develop it. Take the precaution of putting an NDA *and* a nonuse agreement in place.

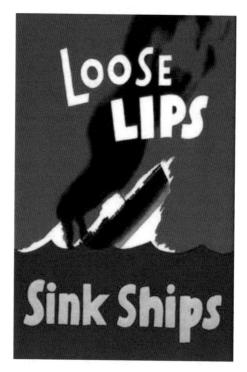

WHEN NOT TO SIGN AN NDA

When considering executing an NDA, the first think to think about is the purpose of your interaction or business relationship. Is it discussing a business opportunity, bringing on an employee, hiring a consultant, or utilizing a vendor? Will confidential

---

* Rodney Perkins, "Innovators Workbench," interview, April 14, 2003, Stanford Biodesign, http://biodesign.stanford .edu/bdn/video/20030414_RodneyPerkins_IWB.jsp. This site includes a number of free Innovators Workbench interviews; they are a goldmine of information and insight on the medical device entrepreneurial process from icons in the medical technology field.

or proprietary information be exchanged, or is the information of a general or public nature? During these times, you will want to have an NDA. But what if you are asking someone for general information, or if someone is asking you for advice? You might want to put an NDA in place if proprietary information might be disclosed, or see whether there is a way to have a discussion without binding yourself to an agreement, while avoiding the disclosure of proprietary information.

Agreeing to an NDA makes you responsible to keep secret and not use the information you are given. If you do not want this potential encumbrance, you might not want to sign the NDA or agree to receive the other party's confidential information.

WHO WILL NOT SIGN AN NDA

There are times when the other party will avoid or refuse to sign an NDA, even if you are disclosing confidential information. One of these times is when you are presenting your idea to a venture capital (VC) firm during a fundraising presentation. You may want to have at least a provisional patent application in place before you make your presentation. This is also the case if you are presenting to an angel investment group (e.g., the Keiretsu Forum or Life Science Angels). These tend to be large groups, and there may be members or guests who are potential competitors; therefore, trying to get an NDA in place would be impractical and having a patent application on file is the best way to be protected.

Some larger companies can be reluctant to sign NDAs with individual inventors or small companies, and if they do, they usually will only allow use of their NDA form. These companies already may be working in the same area that you are and they do not want to have their IP "tainted" or encumbered by your disclosure. Some companies will not even agree to see ideas that "come over the transom" with inventors with whom they do not have a relationship, because they are concerned that they may be sued later if they are already developing a product that parallels an idea brought by an outside inventor.* Medical device companies may be more receptive to ideas that come from surgeons rather than independent inventors.†

WHO SHOULD SIGN AN NDA

Anyone to whom confidential information is disclosed should sign an NDA.‡ If someone is a consultant, and is in a position to contribute inventive content, he or she

---

* For an example of how one major company screens unsolicited inventions, see Johnson & Johnson Consumer Companies, "Disclaimer," INTELLI-IDEAS, http://www.jjconsumerideas.com/idea-submission-process. In their disclaimer, J+J states they will only look at unsolicited ideas with published patent applications and that any such submissions are expressly nonconfidential.
† John McCormick, "Medtronic and Michelson Finally Settle for $1.35 Billion," *Orthopedic and Dental Industry News* (April 25, 2005), http://www.healthpointcapital.com/research/2005/04/25 /medtronic_and_michelson_finally_settle_for_135_billion. An industry–surgeon relationship became especially litigious and expensive between Medtronic and Dr. Gary Michelson, a spine surgeon and prolific medical device inventor.
‡ Apparently, Sabeer Bhatia, founder of Hotmail, collected more than 400 NDAs from anyone who knew of his e-mail start-up, which he eventually sold to Microsoft for $400 million.

needs to sign both an NDA and a patent assignment agreement. For example, a company hired a medical illustrator to do artwork for them. Because this person was "just an artist," the company felt it did not need to obtain an NDA or patent assignment agreement. It turns out that before becoming a medical illustrator, this person was a medical professional in the area the company was working, with considerable experience, and with insight that contributed to a key invention. This led to a rather acrimonious situation when the employer tried to get her to assign the invention to the company after the fact, when they were now aware that the contribution had economic value. Who should sign an NDA? Everyone that receives confidential information.

PRESENTING IDEAS FOR EVALUATION

Do some research and understand the company to which you are presenting. Does the product or idea you are presenting meet a clear strategic need for that company? Companies usually have "shopping lists" of what kinds of products and technologies they are researching. One way to have a better chance at success is to do your study and understand the strategic needs of the company, understand their "shopping list," and present them with something on the list. Too often the inventor would like to rely on the cleverness, novelty, and self-evident brilliance of the invention to make the sale. Presenting your invention is really no different from the mechanics of presenting any product to a prospective customer. There has to be a want and a need on the part of the customer, as well as a compelling value proposition.

When dealing with a company to which you are bringing an invention, you may have to deal with the NIH ("not invented here") factor. Bringing a raw idea to a big company typically has a very small chance of success. To the inventor, this may seem like arrogance (which it in fact may be). Most companies are already fully committed to maintaining what they already have, however, and they are not interested in diverting their resources to help you develop your idea. They have a responsibility to their management and shareholders to allocate their scarce capital to areas where it will get them the best return. They may believe they already have the ideas and resources to develop whatever products they may need. An idea usually needs to be developed to a point at which the company can see the product as one that is just about ready to drop into their salesperson's bag, that their salespeople have the ability and interest in selling, or that is already on the market with demonstrated sales traction. Raw ideas and "projects" usually have limited appeal.

READ AND HEED

Often, NDAs are treated as a formality. They are signed without having been read or without having been looked at very closely. Most NDAs are "plain vanilla," but occasionally a party receiving confidential information will offer a document with the title of NDA, yet embedded in the contract are terms stating that the agreement does "not establish a confidential relationship," or that the receiving party is not obligated to hold the information in confidence, or that they are not assuming any responsibility for any disclosed information. An agreement containing terms like this in fact has the opposite effect of an NDA. Rather than protect your confidential information, it is a waiver of your legal remedy in case of a disclosure or misappropriation.[*]

WHO ARE YOU DEALING WITH?

NDAs are usually understandings between two ethical parties. Before you rely on an NDA to protect confidential information, check the references and reputation of people with whom you intend to have a business relationship. Snakes in the grass do not respect agreements, no matter how well crafted they are. If you get the feeling you are dealing with someone that makes you want to count your fingers after you shake their hand, perhaps you should avoid getting involved with them to begin with.

One such case example was a contractor that did work for a start-up with which I was involved. The contractor was presented an NDA and patent assignment to sign. They said "let me look at it before I sign it." This was a person who was given work to do and came back a few weeks later with their work product. When they came in for their meeting, they claimed to have forgotten their paperwork and promised to bring it in next meeting. After several weeks of this, the company finally demanded that the contractor sign the NDA and assignment papers, or they could not continue as a contractor. At this, the contractor informed the company that they had already filed their own patents and planned to go into competition with them. Because the contracting company was not diligent about getting the agreements signed before disclosing their confidential information, they had little legal recourse.

Snakes in the grass may sometimes use information you disclose under an NDA to do their own patent filings around you. A well-written and properly executed NDA, with a nonuse provision, well-maintained records, and careful lab notebook entries can help protect you in these cases, but be aware that it is time-consuming and expensive to sue for your rights in these cases.

ONE MORE NDA TERM: NONCIRCUMVENTION

A new type of NDA that has developed for companies doing business in places like China is the NNN or "nondisclosure, nonuse, noncircumvention." The typical NDA used in the United States may be useless in countries such as China. In this situation, the standard NDA has a number of deficiencies, including that these agreements usually do not have strong enough nonuse provisions, do not protect against a network of affiliated companies from sharing information, and do not prevent the company from circumvention, (i.e., knocking off your product, selling to your customers, or otherwise bypassing your business relationships). Most NDAs are written to be enforceable in a jurisdiction close and convenient to the disclosing party. When dealing with an entity in another country, you may need to have an agreement stating that the venue is in that country.

---

[*] "Protect Your Secrets: The Non-Disclosure Agreement," http://www.score.org/resources/protect-your-secrets-non-disclosure-agreement (accessed August 12, 2012).

If the violating party is in another country, even if a judgment is obtained against the offending company, with an injunction and damages in your country, these may be unenforceable and uncollectable unless assessed in the country where the offender is located. With increasing globalization, it is important that an NDA have provisions that make the agreement valid and enforceable in the country where you would like to do business.*

SIGNING AN NDA AS AN EMPLOYEE

As an employee, you may be expected to sign an NDA. Often, these NDAs are combined with an IP assignment agreement and sometimes with a noncompete agreement. Under the IP assignment, anything that you invent during the term of employment within the field the company is operating is assigned to the employing company. This is where you may encounter "one-sided" agreements. One onerous example that I have encountered appears as follows:

> If no such list is attached, I represent that there are no such Prior Inventions.
> If, in the course of my Relationship with the Company, I incorporate into a Company product, process or machine a Prior Invention owned by me or in which I have an interest, the Company is hereby granted and shall have a nonexclusive, royalty-free, irrevocable, perpetual, worldwide license (with the right to sublicense) to make, have made, copy, modify, make derivative works of, use, sell and otherwise distribute such Prior Invention as part of or in connection with such product, process or machine.

If this sounds like the old Japanese video game line, "All your base are belong to us," you are about right. As a condition of this NDA, you have to disclose all IP in which you have an interest, and if you do not enumerate it, any inventions not so listed that become incorporated into a product are automatically assigned to the employer.

If you work in California, employees have two rights that are helpful. First, NDAs with automatic assignment clauses are less enforceable in California. Second, Section 2870 of the California Labor Code[1] states that your own work, on own time, at your own place, with your own tools, in a field not related to the employer's business, belongs to you and is not subject to automatic assignment to the employer. Check with an attorney to see what the laws are in your own state or country.

CONCLUSION

There is more to NDA protection that just getting the parties involved to sign a generic agreement. The NDA must have the proper terms and scope to cover what is being disclosed and must include meaningful remedies in the event of a breach. The information disclosed must be documented in a timely way. Information that is expected to be kept confidential must be treated with the care appropriate to confidential information. Appropriate diligence must be taken to document what information

---

* For more information on NNN agreements, see Harris & Moure, China Law Blog, http://www.chinalawblog.com, which publishes details about doing business and protecting IP in China.

was disclosed that is considered confidential. The NDA must be valid and enforceable at the locations where each of the parties does business, especially if one party is in another country.

GLOSSARY OF TYPICAL TERMS AND PROVISIONS OF AN NDA

Damages: This specifies the relief expected for a breach of confidentiality or misappropriation of confidential information. Typically, this is the right to seek an injunction, in which you can demand that the offending party stop using the information or selling products that incorporate the information. Another form of damages is "liquidated damages" or a specified amount of monetary damages expected in case of a breach.

NDA, "One-Way": This agreement covers one party disclosing confidential information to another party, and the other party receiving and not disclosing confidential information.

NDA, "Two-way" or "Mutual" (MNDA): This agreement covers two (or more) parties sharing confidential information. An agreement like this is typically put in place when two companies in the same business are discussing a mutual business opportunity.

Nondisclosure: This means that the party receiving confidential information will not disclose it to a third party and will keep the information confidential.

Nonuse: This term is used to indicate that the receiving party will not make use of the information shared for their own purposes. An NDA will typically have terms of both nondisclosure and nonuse. Nondisclosure without nonuse may leave the receiving party free to appropriate the information and develop it, as long as it is not disclosed outside of the company during the term of the NDA, leaving the party free to use the information for their own purposes when the term of the NDA expires, which may render the NDA practically ineffective. An NDA without a nonuse provision leaves you open to the risk of a company using your information to "patent around" your invention.

Purpose: This describes why you are having a conversation and sharing information to begin with, for example, to collaborate on product development, to evaluate a technology, to explore a business relationship, or as a condition of employment.

Scope: This describes how much information you intend to share and in what area. The NDA should accurately describe the type of information the parties wish to keep secret. The scope will also specify what types of information are not subject to the agreement. Typically, any information that is either publicly known, is arrived at independently by other party, or is made public through disclosure to a third party by the disclosing party, or any information already possessed by the receiving party before the NDA was put in place are not subject to the NDA.

Term: This is the length of time the information is to be kept secret. A typical term is three years. Some NDAs ask for a five-year term, and some ask for 10 years, or an indefinite term. Typically, you want to negotiate the shortest term possible if you are receiving confidential information and should avoid signing an NDA for an indefinite term. Conversely, if you are the disclosing party, you will want to negotiate the longest term possible.

The exception to time limit terms is trade secrets. These should have an indefinite term. A well-known example of a trade secret is the formula for Coca-Cola. True trade secrets are relatively rare.

Maintaining records: This is the real "flossing" part of maintaining an NDA. When information is disclosed under an NDA, it is good practice (or spelled out in the NDA) to keep an accurate record of the information disclosed, to keep a record of it on file with the NDA, and to communicate a list of the information that was disclosed to the other party. Follow-up meetings, or communication by phone or e-mail, to obtain a written agreement representing an accurate record of the information that was disclosed under the agreement are needed for thorough recordkeeping. This can be a tedious, but essential, part of maintaining an enforceable NDA, and it is a step that often is skipped.

It is important to ensure that any information, written or transmitted in any fashion, such as photos or verbal communication, are documented in writing and clearly labeled as "Confidential." It also is important to be diligent about requesting the return of any confidential information and materials after the need to have the materials has passed or after the relationship has terminated. Keeping records and control of information in a timely way is essential to being able to handle these materials properly and being able to later demonstrate that confidential materials were handled in a confidential way. If it is later shown that confidential materials are not handled with due care, the NDA may be found unenforceable.

Ensure that you keep your NDAs current with any parties with whom you maintain an ongoing relationship. Keep a file for NDAs, as well as records of correspondence, such as e-mails and presentations, and keep track of the expiration date of the NDAs, especially if you maintain several NDAs with a number of parties. Here an old Chinese proverb applies: "the faintest ink is better than the strongest memory." You may want to put an alarm in your electronic calendar reminding you of an impending expiration at least 60 days in advance.

The value of clear recordkeeping was demonstrated to me when I had to spend a few days being deposed for a patent infringement suit for a company for which I once worked. Lab notebooks, pictures, and lots of other long-forgotten ephemera relating to projects that I had worked on several years before were vacuumed up by the legal discovery process, and now I was being questioned, with a video camera running, and a stenographer recording my every "and" and "um" everything I could remember about this pile of paperwork laid out in front of me. It gave me an appreciation for the value of clear records that are able to hold up under scrutiny.

When you are working on something that is exciting, and things are moving quickly, and time is tight, it is easy to get sloppy about good recordkeeping, for example, writing invention disclosures and sketches on scratch paper instead of in a lab notebook, not dating your disclosures, and not having lab notebook entries witnessed, and cannibalizing or tossing out early prototypes. The excitement of the discovery and invention experience may be vivid to you at the time, and you think you will never forget. I guarantee, that seven or eight years later, you will absolutely forget some of the details, even with reminders in front of you. The point is that if you have something worth protecting, it is worth the time and effort to document it and to date the documents. If you really came up with an idea first, you want to be able to produce the evidence to prove it. In the future, you may be relying on the memories of other team members. Even if you think you might remember everything, team members may not, or they may not be as motivated as you are to remember, and they may be the ones that are telling the story, so it is important to have clear documentation.

Venue: This is where a legal case to enforce the NDA would be tried. Usually, you want to have this venue to be as close to your business location as possible or to be one that you know handles IP issues quickly and fairly. Some NDAs will specify that any disputes are resolved through arbitration. Another term will be whether attorneys' fees will be awarded to the winning party in the event of litigation.

RESOURCES

DeMatteis, Bob. *Patent to Profit: Secrets and Strategies for the Successful Inventor*. Garden City Park, NY: Square One Publishers, 2005.

ACKNOWLEDGMENT

The assistance of Paul Backofen, Esq., of Crockett and Crockett, LLP, Laguna Hills, CA, in preparing this article is gratefully acknowledged.

Note: *This article is for general information purposes only and is not intended as legal advice. If you need specific information regarding your particular legal situation, seek the assistance of a qualified attorney.*

ENDNOTE

1. Section 2870 of the Code states:
    (a) Any provision in an employment agreement which provides that an employee shall assign, or offer to assign, any of his or her rights in an invention to his or her employer shall not apply to an invention that the employee developed entirely on his or her own time without using the employer's equipment, supplies, facilities, or trade secret information except for those inventions that either:
        (1) Relate at the time of conception or reduction to practice of the invention to the employer's business, or actual or demonstrably anticipated research or development of the employer; or
        (2) Result from any work performed by the employee for the employer.
    (b) To the extent a provision in an employment agreement purports to require an employee to assign an invention otherwise excluded from being required to be assigned under subdivision (a), the provision is against the public policy of this state and is unenforceable.

14 Intellectual Property Strategy for Med-Tech Start-Ups*

Ryan H. Flax

CONTENTS

What Intellectual Property Rights Should a Medical Device–Technology Business Be Concerned About? 264
    Introduction 264
    Where to Start 264
Patents: What Is a Patent and What Is an Invention? 266
Protect Your R&D 269
    Planning for Inventing 269
        Starting a Patent Program 270
        Internal Business Concerns 271
        Working Well with Others 275
    Patenting 275
        Considering Your Options 275
        Pulling the Patent "Trigger" 276
    Foreign Filing 278
    Internal IP Controls 278
        Committees 278
        Getting the Corporate Team Involved 279
What Are Trademarks and Why Do They Matter? 281
Trade Secrets 282
Watch Out for Others' Property 284
    State-of-the-Art Study 284
    Noninfringement Study 284
    Validity Study 285
    Designing around Patents 285
Make Money with Your Patents 286
    Identifying Your Intellectual Property 286
    Enforcing Patents 289

---

* Certain case law cites in this chapter have been provided by Dickstein Shapiro LLP, *Patents, Trademarks, Copyrights, and Trade Secrets: An Introduction to Intellectual Property for In-House Counsel*, 3rd. ed., prepared for the Association of Corporate Counsel (2008).

Licensing Your Technology 291
Conclusion 291
About the Author 292
Endnotes 292

WHAT INTELLECTUAL PROPERTY RIGHTS SHOULD A MEDICAL DEVICE–TECHNOLOGY BUSINESS BE CONCERNED ABOUT?

INTRODUCTION

For small to midsize businesses whose products are based primarily on technology, it may seem an insurmountable task to even begin thinking about what intellectual property (IP) means to the business, why it is important, and how to try to get their hands around it to harness its power for the business. Doing so, however, is an absolute must for the start-up for several reasons. First, you do not want to start your business by stepping on the toes of other companies that are sophisticated in the ways of IP and who will most likely make your company pay dearly for doing so. Second, you want to be ready to bank your own IP rights and start cashing in on them or at least keep others from treading on the fruits of your hard work. In many companies, particularly small to medium (and even very large) medical device–technology companies, the bulk of their value is in their IP.

IP refers to a group of property rights, including patents, copyrights, trademarks, and trade secrets. Other rights are also included, such as trade dress, mask works, unfair competition, and publicity rights. The particular kinds of IP that you care about will depend on the nature of your company and the marketplace in which your company competes, which for medical device–technology companies is typically patents, trademarks, and trade secrets. These IP rights are the focus of this chapter. And, of these three, patents will receive the lion's share of attention as the most important.

WHERE TO START

Once you have created your business and taken care of the corporate necessities relating to that creation, you need to start planning for IP concerns and you will likely need someone in-house to manage this. As a medical technology company, you likely have devoted a significant portion of your focus to research and development (R&D) and have some concrete plans for new products or sellable technology that will be the business of your company. Your in-house IP management will work with your R&D department, your corporate management, and your other in-house and outside counsel to take care of your IP needs. For an average manufacturing enterprise with significant R&D, the following in-house IP services are necessary:

- Establishing an IP plan for the company that includes handling the company's inventions, trade secrets, and trademarks, how to deal with competitors' IP, and how to use IP for the company's advantage
- Recordkeeping to document the company's inventions and trade secrets

Intellectual Property Strategy for Med-Tech Start-Ups

- Evaluating R&D to determine its economic importance and whether to file patent applications or maintain technology as a trade secret
- Managing the preparation and prosecution of patent and trademark applications
- Establishing policies for and dealing with unsolicited invention disclosures from outside the company
- Managing the payment of patent maintenance fees, annuities, and taxes in the various patent offices
- Creating a portfolio of the company's current trademarks and service marks
- Instituting a program for registering trade- and service marks in the United States and abroad, for keeping them in force, and for policing them
- Establishing internal IP committees to meet periodically to determine necessary actions in patent and trademark matters

Who will handle all of these IP services (and more)? Probably your in-house IP counsel and staff, which likely will be a part of your general counsel's office or general legal department, if you have one. Companies that have in-house IP counsel, however, will almost definitely rely on outside counsel for services such as furnishing opinions on IP matters, litigation and dispute resolution, and patent and trademark prosecution. The management of outside counsel will likely be a major focus of the in-house IP counsel.

Supervision of the IP counsel and staff by the general counsel provides centralized control of the company's overall IP and related general law portfolios, which coordinates IP and other legal work in view of general business goals. Furthermore, IP matters frequently affect larger policy issues and having IP counsel centralized in the main law department keeps the entire company's legal team working together.

Some companies want their in-house IP counsel to be independent of those who make the inventions to ensure that the attorneys can exercise independent judgment. For example, having in-house IP counsel make independent appraisals of the advisability of filing an application for a patent or trademark registration provides considerable advantage. Such independence is facilitated by having in-house IP counsel as members of the legal department. Associating with other corporate lawyers also benefits in-house IP counsel professionally; the exchange of ideas between IP attorneys and general counsel increases the knowledge of both. General counsel (and management) can gain a sharper understanding of IP issues affecting broader corporate strategy.

For the most part, companies that have general law departments, but locate patent counsel in research or engineering divisions, obtain cooperation between the two without formal arrangements. For example, in-house IP counsel may at times be engaged in contract, tax, or other matters not directly related to research and development. In such instances, he or she may report directly to the party concerned with the tangential legal issue, while keeping the vice president of R&D advised. An arrangement that may be especially satisfactory is to have an experienced IP attorney in the legal department who acts as a liaison with the patent department located in the research division. In that way, the general counsel can be kept up-to-date on all relevant developments, such as important proceedings in the U.S. Patent and Trademark Office (often abbreviated as USPTO or PTO).

The chief IP counsel should be responsible for the overall direction of the company's IP activities, including the filing of applications, the acquisition, disposition, and licensing of patents and trademarks, handling and supervising infringement matters, and developing and maintaining contacts with relevant government agencies, customers, professional associations, and outside IP counsel. In addition, the chief IP counsel generally has other duties and responsibilities related to the overall administration of the company's IP operation. Some of these are best left to lower-level members of the in-house IP staff to handle. The chief IP counsel assumes a functional responsibility of these direct responsibilities to advise, inform, and assist other departments that become involved in patent, licensing, and trademark matters.

PATENTS: WHAT IS A PATENT AND WHAT IS AN INVENTION?

Patents and inventions are related terms and ideas, but they do not mean the same thing, and the words are not interchangeable. An invention, in layman's terms, is a discovery or creation of something new (whether patentable or not), but legally speaking, inventions are what patents allow their owners to exclude others from practicing.*, 1 A patent is a legal document that basically creates a contract with the government whereby the inventor discloses his invention to the world in exchange for a limited right to exclude others from making, using, selling, offering for sale, or importing (as shorthand, we will call all this "making and using") the invention during the patent term.† Once the patent expires (typically on the 20th anniversary of its filing date), the invention may be used freely by anyone. Interestingly, a patent does not give its owner the right to *practice* the invention itself, only to *exclude* others from doing so. Even though one may get a patent for an invention, the use of the patentable invention can still be blocked by other patents that possibly are owned by others.

In the United States, to be patentable, the invention must be

- *New*, also called the novelty requirement. The invention must not already be in the "prior art," that is, publicly known or used in a single source, in exactly the way the invention is claimed (more on claims later) in the patent, before the first filing of an application for the invention.‡, 2
- *Nonobvious*, even if the invention is likely novel, it is not patentable if it would have been obvious to a person having ordinary skill in the relevant art at the time of the first application for the invention, based on a single reference, a modified single reference, or combined prior art§
- *Useful*, meaning that the invention has a practical application—it has been said that anything under the sun is patentable.

Although we have explained the concept of what a patent is, how do you read and understand a patent (assuming you understand the science involved)? It will help to

---

* U.S. Patent Act, 35 U.S.C. § 101, September 16, 2011.
† U.S. Patent Act, 35 U.S.C. § 271, September 16, 2011.
‡ U.S. Patent Act, 35 U.S.C. § 102, September 16, 2011.
§ U.S. Patent Act, 35 U.S.C. § 103, September 16, 2011.

Intellectual Property Strategy for Med-Tech Start-Ups 267

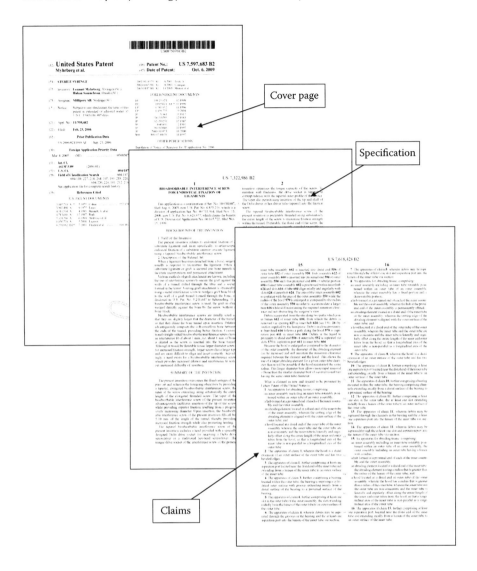

understand what parts make up a typical patent. There must always be a specification and claims and drawings usually accompany the specification.

A patent's specification is a description of the invention in sufficient detail to establish that the inventor actually invented what he claims as the invention and so that those of skill in the relevant field can make and use the invention.* Furthermore, the inventor has an obligation not to hold back his best mode of making or using the invention (e.g., as a trade secret) and this must be disclosed in the specification.[3] The specification may include examples of different preferred or alternative embodiments of the invention and could include experiments illustrating that the invention

---

* U.S. Patent Act, 35 U.S.C. § 112(1), September 16, 2011.

actually has been reduced to practice. Any drawings of the invention, its embodiments, or its components (or any other illustrations needed to explain the invention) accompany and are considered a part of the specification.

At the end of the specification will be at least one and usually many sentences called claims. The claims of the patent actually define what the invention is and what the patent holder has a right to exclude others from making and using (this is the part where patent attorneys earn their money). Typically, the claims look like a bunch of legalese and for good reason—if they are not drafted with care, the patent will not be worth all the time and money the company has invested in what it thinks is its invention. Claims can be directed to structures, methods, and structures made by specific methods. There are two types of claims: independent and dependent. The independent claims stand on their own and are the broadest claims. Dependent claims refer back to one or more other claims, incorporating subject matter by reference, and then add further limitations. You may hear that word, "limitation," when discussing what patent claims cover. A limitation can be set forth in claims as a term, clause, or phrase that defines a feature of the invention that must be embodied by an infringing device or method and there will be one or more limitations in a patent's claim(s).

Patents result from patent applications that, in the United States, are filed with the USPTO in the name of one or more original and true inventors.[*] Two or more persons may jointly conceive of an invention, in which case all of the inventors must apply for the patent. The jointly named inventors do not have to make their respective contribution together, at the same place, or at the same time. Usually, the inventors will execute an assignment of ownership of the invention, the patent application, and any related patent applications to their employer company at the same time the application is filed as a duty and condition of their employment.

Patent applications are almost always prepared by an attorney, with input from the inventor(s). If outside counsel is engaged to prepare the application, they will most likely work to some degree with the in-house counsel of the inventor's company to ensure that the details of the application are correct and that the application satisfies the goals of the company–client. A typical U.S. patent application can be drafted and filed by an outside counsel from anywhere between $5,000 and $8,500 (this cost can be much higher and does not include prosecution to patent grant), depending on the complexity of the case and prior work done by the in-house team.[†] Costs usually can be reduced by providing the outside counsel with as much and as detailed information about the invention as possible at the outset of the matter, so that it takes less time and effort for the outside counsel to shape the information into a patent application.

Once filed with the USPTO, applications are assigned to a patent examiner who will issue a report (commonly referred to as an "office action") to the patent applicant, setting forth the results of the examination of the application in view of the filing requirements and prior art. Typically, the examiner rejects some or all of the patent claims as lacking novelty, being obvious, failing in view of the specification disclosure

---

[*] With the recent amendments to the U.S. Patent Act, under 35 U.S.C. § 118, patent applications can now be filed by the assignee of an invention or an entity to which an inventor is obligated to assign.

[†] American Intellectual Property Law Association, *Report of the Economic Survey* (2011).

Intellectual Property Strategy for Med-Tech Start-Ups

requirements (e.g., being overly broad), or for informalities (being indefinite). This almost-inevitable rejection is all part of the normal process and should not be taken personally. The applicant–inventor (via his attorney), however, may respond with arguments refuting the examiner's findings or amending the claims in view of the rejection.* Once the patent examiner is satisfied that the claims are patentable, they are allowed and a patent is granted. The prosecution to grant usually takes between three and five years.[4]

Before filing a regular utility application, which will undergo this examination process, it may be desirable to file a "provisional" patent application, which acts as a placeholder to secure what is called an "effective" filing date for a later-filed regular utility application.† This placeholder function is important in fields of rapidly evolving technology and in cases in which a company may not be sure what new technology is worth pursuing. The placeholder provides a year to make the decision whether to follow up with a nonprovisional, regular utility–type patent application. The provisional also costs a lot less ($220 for a large entity) than a regular patent application (more than $1,250 for a large entity) because the USPTO fees are low and the requirements for a provisional application are less rigorous than those for a regular application because there will be no examination of the case—no claims are required (but are recommended in view of international IP concerns). Filing a provisional, however, allows the applicant to use the terms "patent pending" on related products.‡ To be proper, a provisional patent application requires only a description of the invention sufficient to enable a skilled person to practice it, an identification of at least one of the inventors, and the prescribed fee. Advantageously, the time before conversion of the provisional application to a regular patent application does not count toward the 20-year term of the utility patent.

PROTECT YOUR R&D

PLANNING FOR INVENTING

If technology and IP are the most important assets of your medical start-up or small technology company, which is likely if you are reading this chapter, then you need to implement a plan for controlling the development and maintenance of your IP portfolio. This will be a key to your company's ability to attract investment dollars and to viably compete with other (potentially more established) companies in the same field that are likely using IP as a strategic part of their business model. Utilizing IP in an ad hoc way is not a plan.

A patent portfolio can be used offensively and defensively by a medical device company. Used offensively, the company can control who uses technology, which may mean that it can charge more for its products and improve its brand and market position, while potentially limiting its competition. The company may choose to

---

* Such arguments or amendments will influence the interpretation of the patent's claims if it is ever litigated, so care must be taken during prosecution.
† Priority to a provisional may be claimed under 35 U.S.C. § 119(e); an "effective filing date" can be established by claiming priority to earlier, related utility applications.
‡ Use of "patent pending" in a deceptive way, on a product not related to the application, opens the party up to fines or damages.

license its technology either for a royalty or in some cross-licensing scheme that enables the company to enter markets otherwise off limits or to ward off litigation. Defensively, having a patent portfolio may insulate the company from infringement accusations by competitors who know that they may well be infringing the company's IP and vulnerable to infringement action. Conversely, not having a patent portfolio may make the company a soft target for infringement accusations, which, even if defensible, could be devastatingly costly to defend for a start-up company with no war chest.* Also, IP assets have transactional value as well, which is supremely useful to small companies open to being acquired by big companies.†

So, you have been convinced that your company needs to get serious about IP and you want a serious patent program, but where do you start? From the initial creation of your medical device–technology start-up company, you should consider adopting an aggressive IP strategy to create a strong IP portfolio. It is easier to create a program at the beginning of a company's existence when all plans and goals are new, but it is never too late.

Starting a Patent Program

Creating a patent program is the most difficult and time-consuming part of implementing an IP strategy. Instituting a new patent program from scratch will likely take many weeks or months. The program may be phased in to address the more urgent areas first and may consist of the following steps:

1. Conduct a baseline *audit* to determine what patents and patent applications the company has and what third-party (e.g., government, university, other companies) relationships exist that affect inventions.
2. Determine what company patent rights are perceived as important to the company. These will include patent rights that are used or projected to be used in your business (but also include those that are sure to be useful to your competitors). You may find that patent rights exist for discontinued products or on inventions that may not be important to the company business.
3. Establish a long-term program and a budget; have these approved by management. Identify how many new patent applications you think you will file annually and account for the related prosecution costs. How much of a staff will you need to run a program based on these numbers?
4. Establish confidentiality agreements and disclosure and publication review guidelines so the company will not unintentionally lose patent rights (or disclose trade secrets).
5. Have all new employees sign invention disclosure and assignment agreements as a condition to employment and before starting work.
6. Set up a Patent Committee, which will be responsible for reviewing invention disclosures and deciding what technology should be patented.

---

* Patents and a good target for infringement may allow investors to back your litigation for a piece of the damages.
† Johnson & Johnson acquired Cordis Corporation and Cook primarily because of their know-how and IP covering cardiac stent technology, likewise with Abbott Laboratories' acquisition of Guidant's vascular business group.

7. Prepare and file patent applications, maintain patent application prosecution, and pay outstanding maintenance fees and annuities on important patents and patent applications. Revival *may* be available for lapsed patent applications and issued patents.
8. Institute the patent program for the long term. This includes having all patent applications entered in a docket system for tracking prosecution and maintenance due dates. Computerized docket systems are preferred and are available from a variety of vendors. Patent annuity payment services are also available.
9. Have company founders, employees, consultants, and any relevant third parties agree to assign IP rights to the company and sign any new agreements as a condition to receiving a raise, bonus, or promotion.

All employees should receive training on the company's policies and procedures regarding inventions. For researchers, engineers, and other employees who are likely to be inventors, as well as mangers, the training should be more extensive, covering basic principles of patentability and the employee's responsibilities to the company regarding reporting and recording inventions. In addition, managers should be trained on their responsibilities under the company's policies and procedures and on interactions with the patent committee. This more extensive training should be conducted by a patent lawyer.

Internal Business Concerns

For an effective patent program, the company must adopt and follow appropriate policies and procedures for managing inventions, which, generally, will address the handling of inventions and patents (and publications) from before the conception of the invention until the patent expiration. This should include establishment of an entity (usually a patent committee) responsible for overseeing employee invention agreements, handling disclosure of inventions outside the company, documentation of new developments, filing for and maintaining patents, and clearance of new products in view of potential patent infringement.

The use of proper and adequate employment agreements is essential to a functioning patent program. In the United States, absent an agreement otherwise, the owner of an invention is the inventor himself (contrast with copyright law, which provides for shop rights conferring ownership to an employer). With some important exceptions, a company employee who makes an invention, rather than the company, will own the invention and all of the patent rights associated with it, even if the employee uses company resources or facilities, or makes the invention while on the job. The exceptions include the following:

- Employed-to-invent. One exception is an employee who has been specifically employed to invent and is therefore obligated to transfer ownership to the company.* This could include research scientists and engineers whose

---

* United States v. Dubilier Condenser Corp., 289 U.S. 178 (1933); Standard Parts Co. v. Peck, 264 U.S. 52 (1924).

specific job responsibilities are to develop new product ideas.* On the other hand, if the employee is hired in a general technical position, he will retain his inventions.
- Fiduciary duty. Another exception is an employee who has a fiduciary duty to the company. This typically includes the officers of the company and may include other employees who are highly important to the company. An employee with a fiduciary duty may be required to transfer ownership of an invention to the company.
- Shop rights. Under the "shop rights doctrine," a company whose employee makes an invention using the company's time or resources may have a non-exclusive, nontransferable, royalty-free *license* to use the invention under any patent that issues.† But this shop right is not ownership and does not entitle the company to participate in procurement, enforcement, or licensing of the patent. However, the shop right survives the employee's termination and may be transferred to a third party along with the entire business.‡

It is best for the company to have its employees enter into agreements requiring disclosure of inventions to the company and assignment of the rights in those inventions to the company (such contracts are governed by state law). Typically, these agreements will require the employee to assign to the company all of his rights to any invention made in the course of employment or on his own time, but in the company's area of interest, as well as require the employee to participate and assist in the patenting process. In some circumstances, it may be reasonable to extend the agreement to inventions conceived during employment and reduced to practice after employment. It is more likely a court will uphold an employment agreement if it is reasonable.§

An invention assignment agreement is a contract and requires consideration, which is usually the employment itself when the agreement is signed before or upon starting work. If the invention assignment agreement is obtained later or is changed for an existing employee, some additional consideration should be given to the employee, such as a raise, bonus, or promotion—mere continued employment is not adequate in some states. As part of executing the invention assignment agreement, the employee should be advised of the company's policies and procedures on inventions. Upon termination of employment, as a part of the postemployment–termination procedures, the employee should receive a copy of his signed invention assignment agreement, be remind of his duties under it, and should sign an acknowledgment that he has received a copy.

Reporting of inventions to the company should be required as soon as possible after their conception so that patent protection can be pursued in a timely manner, if desired. The reporting of inventions should be the employees' responsibility and also the responsibility of the their managers who are aware of the work being performed. Managers can be trained to recognize when an invention is sufficiently developed to

---

* Stranco, Inc. v. Atlantes Chem. Sys., 15 U.S.P.Q.2d 1704, 1716 (S.D. Tex. 1990), affirmed 960 F.2d 156 (Fed. Cir. 1992).
† Wommack v. Durham Pecan Co., 715 F.2d 962 (5th Cir. 1983).
‡ Lane & Bodley Co. v. Locke, 150 U.S. 193 (1893); California E. Lab. v. Gould, 896 F.2d 400 (9th Cir. 1990); Neon Signal Devices v. Alpha-Claude Neon Corp., 54 F.2d 793 (W.D. Pa. 1931).
§ Armorlite Lens Co. v. Campbell, 340 F. Supp. 273 (S.D. Cal. 1972).

Intellectual Property Strategy for Med-Tech Start-Ups 273

report it to the company. A formal Invention Disclosure Form should be used as an invention record for gathering the information needed for the company to consider the merits of the invention and to highlight any potential bars to patentability. The Invention Disclosure Form will play an important role when the patent application is to be drafted because it will include a description of the invention, its proposed advantages and features, a listing of related art, and attached copies of lab notebooks. The key information for this form is provided in a bulleted list.

Employees who may make inventions should keep records of their work on a daily basis to document the conception of inventions, development of the inventions, and their reduction to practice. The U.S. patent system presently grants a patent to the *first-to-invent* (the rest of the world grants to the first-to-file) so documentation of conception and diligence to reduction to practice is important, for now.[5] The records should be complete, made in the ordinary course of the work, and permanent.

Proper recordkeeping under the patent program should preferably include at least the following:

- Use of bound notebooks
- Legible writing
- Use of permanent, dark ink
- Timely entry of information
- Identification of errors with an explanation
- Crossing out of errors, without obliterating or erasing corrections
- Entering the information in chronological order
- Not leaving blank space on a page
- Using every page
- Not allowing the employees to take the books away from the office
- Signing and dating each page at the end of each day
- Having each page promptly witnessed and dated, preferably by two people who understand the information but who are not inventors
- Having the witnesses sign under the statement "Read and understood by"

Such records are often now kept electronically, but a problem with electronic records is that it is hard to verify with certainty *when* they were produced, that they have not been *altered*, and what "version" a witness reviewed. When using electronic records, they should be printed out, signed and witnessed, and then preserved in a manner resistant to alteration. Keeping notebooks properly and timely requires work and discipline on the part of the employee. Some companies motivate their employees to keep these records by making it part of their performance review.

As discussed, the lab notebook is just the first step. Once an inventor or manager believes a technology is ready for patenting, an Invention Disclosure Form should be prepared and submitted to the Patent Committee for review. The Form should include the following information:

- A title for the invention.
- A listing of the names, residence or mailing addresses, contact telephone numbers, e-mail addresses, and citizenships of each inventor.

- A brief description of the invention explaining (a) generally, the purpose and objects of the invention; (b) prior constructions or methods of performing the function of the invention; (c) the disadvantages of these old constructions and/or methods; (d) how the construction operation and/or preparation of the invention changes, adds to, and/or improves over what has been done before; (e) the advantages of these differences in the invention; (f) any unexpected results of the invention; (g) the best known construction, operation, and/or preparation of the invention, and any alternates; (h) if jointly invented, what contribution was made by each inventor; and, finally, (i) the relative value of the invention. The brief description should also provide sketches, prints, photos, and other illustrations if possible, as well as attach any reports or other documents related to the invention.
- Identify the conception of the invention by indicating (a) the date of first drawings and where they can be found; (b) the date of first written description and where it can be found; (c) the date of first disclosure to others (oral or written) and to whom; and (d) the date of first disclosure to others outside the company (oral or written), to whom, and for what purpose.
- Identify the first actual reduction to practice (construction of the complete device or performance of the process of the invention) by date, if any prototypes are made, by whom, where the prototype can be found.
- Denote, if any experiments have been performed on the invention or in its development, when it was performed, who witnessed the experiments, and the results.
- Explain whether the invention part of a joint venture with a third party (not the company) or developed under a government contract? If so, provide the details.
- Has the invention been sold or offered for sale? If so, when, to whom?
- Has the invention been used (publicly)? If so, when? Describe this fully. Describe plans to use it in the future.
- Identify any publications (articles, sales literature, internet postings, etc.), patents, or patent applications relating specifically to the invention and also, as background, those most closely relating to its technology generally.

After the disclosure is completed, it should be signed and dated by the inventor(s) and then read, signed, and dated by two witnesses. Then submit the form to the Patent Committee so that it can decide whether a patent should be pursued or whether the technology should be maintained as a trade secret, whether the invention needs further development, or whether moving forward with the technology has no value at all.

Under the new Patent Act (as amended by the America Invents Act signed into law on September 16, 2011; effective in relevant part on March 16, 2013) a new importance is placed on public disclosure of technology—a public policy of the U.S. patent system being the dissemination of knowledge. Publication of inventions can be a defensive strategy for a company as doing so can create "prior art" for competitors' patent applications. Public disclosures are not, however, prior art for one's own patent applications if made within a year of the application's effective filing date in the USPTO. In view of this one-year grace period, it is wise for a company to encourage, but carefully control, the publications by its R&D group.

Working Well with Others

Another element of the patent program is the handling of the disclosure and development of inventions between the company and third parties. Often, in joint ventures between companies or dealings with customers or vendors, companies share information and before or during the relationship, either party may independently develop relevant inventions or may do so jointly.[*] Information to be disclosed and inventions developed by the company should be reviewed prior to disclosure to third parties to ensure that disclosure will not adversely affect patent rights.

The company's patent policy should specify the involvement of in-house counsel at the onset of such dealings—appropriate agreements should be put in place before such disclosure or development, including an initial nondisclosure agreement and a more extensive agreement detailing, for example: (1) the parties' respective ownership of inventions and subsequent patents; (2) their responsibilities for disclosure or documentation of inventions independently or jointly made; (3) the parties' responsibilities for procurement, maintenance, and enforcement of patents made independently or jointly; (4) warranties and indemnification; and (5) duties to keep confidential. It is not uncommon for disputes to arise long after companies initiate such dealings as to whether inventions are jointly made and patents should be jointly owned, so this is an important aspect of any such agreement. Without a confidentiality obligation, the patentability of the invention may be adversely affected by such a disclosure. This impact attaches immediately in some foreign countries.

The confidentiality period should preferably extend at least until the invention has been published by the company through a patent (or patent application) publication or other publication controlled by your company. Typically, the authorized use of the information should be limited to the business purpose for which the company disclosed it. Further measures may be warranted in some cases to protect the information, such as a contractual obligation specific to the handling and return of the information, a limitation as to which employees are allowed access, or technical measures to prevent reverse engineering of any product samples that may be disclosed. Such disclosures may occur in either direction. When the company is receiving information, it may be desirable to minimize the company's obligations of confidentiality and nonuse of the other party's technical or business information.

PATENTING

Considering Your Options

The subject matter that may be patented has been interpreted to be "anything under the sun that is made by man."[†,6] What may not be patented has been identified by the

---

[*] U.S. Patent Act, 35 U.S.C. § 102, September 16, 2011 (effective in relevant part on March 16, 2013) encourages joint-research projects and agreements between parties and removes from the realm of "prior art" some such joint-research work.
[†] Diamond v. Chakrabarty, 447 U.S. 303 (1980).

Supreme Court as "laws of nature, natural phenomena, and abstract ideas."[*] It should be noted, however, that business methods and medical procedures are not patentable in some foreign countries.[†]

Almost never will a company file a patent application for every invention it creates. The decision to do so will be based on the costs versus the benefits of filing. The costs include the monetary expense (as discussed already, these can reach the tens of thousands of dollars), the time required of the prosecution process (three to five years, typically), and the mandatory disclosure of the invention to the public (loss of trade secret).

In making this decision, the company should consider whether the invention relates to a company profit center—does it relate to the core business of the company? If the invention does relate directly to a company profit center, consider whether the scope and timing of patent rights will provide a sufficient advantage in the marketplace—meaning, will the invention be broad enough and viable enough to keep up with the market's technology so as to provide meaningful value and protection for the company? It is important for corporate decision makers not to be "blinded" by their love of a technology. The technology is supposed to fit the company's business plans—it can be somewhat dangerous, especially for start-ups, to bend your business plans around a technology just for the sake of its "neatness" and a hope that it will generate profits.

Benefits are the right to exclude conferred by the patent and the improved value having the patent may bring to the company. Another benefit of filing a patent application is that it can establish prior art against patent applications filed later, such as by the company's competitors, which can prevent a competitor from making the same invention and patenting it. Patent applications are published 18 months after their filing, which helps in this creation of prior art. Another benefit of patenting is the value (in money, status, or cross-licensed technology) that may be received from patent sale or licensing. Furthermore, when confronted by a competitor that itself holds patents and accuses your start-up of infringing, it may be to your advantage to assert your own patents against the competitor. Doing so will neuter much of the competitor's litigation strategy and improves your chances of success—but you need patents first to be able to do this.

Pulling the Patent "Trigger"

Once the company decides that it wants patent protection for an invention, a good (but not mandatory) next step is to conduct a patentability study to assess the likely patentability of the invention and scope of the exclusive rights to be had. This study should be conducted through an in-house or outside patent lawyer.[7] Such an investigation allows the company to evaluate whether the likely patent coverage is worth the expense before incurring the large part of the costs and the results can also be used to focus the application on the patentable aspects of the invention, which will again save costs and shorten prosecution time. Also, the company should consider

---

[*] Diamond v. Diehr, 450 U.S. 175, 185 (1981); Bilski v. Kappos, 130 S. Ct. 3218 (2010).
[†] Susan L. DeBlasio, *Patents on Medical Procedures and the Physician Profiteer*, accessed September 19, 2004, http://library.findlaw.com/2004 /Sep/19/133572.html.

examining the availability of patent rights in foreign countries as well as in the United States if they do business internationally (or intend to).

If the company decides to proceed after reviewing the patentability opinion, it is best to have a patent lawyer prepare a patent application, which will be reviewed by the inventors for accuracy and completeness. It is possible to patent your inventions yourself, but this is akin to giving yourself a haircut or doing your own dental work—it might work out, but is not recommended.

Once the attorney has drafted the patent application and it has been approved by the inventors, the inventors must execute a declaration (an oath) that they are the actual inventors and that they believe the invention is patentable.* At this time, they should also execute an assignment of the invention to the company. Some time (usually many months) after the application with all the related papers and fees are filed with the USPTO, the examination process begins.

There are different types of patent applications, including utility patents, design patents, and plant patents. Typically a medical device or technology company is not concerned with design patents, which cover the aesthetic, nonfunctional aspects of inventions, or plant patents. You are likely more familiar with utility patents, which cover device and method inventions. As discussed, for utility inventions, a provisional patent application can initially be filed as an inexpensive placeholder for a filing date and to give the company time to consider whether a full patent should be applied for.

Another type of patent application you may hear about is a divisional patent application, which is a follow-up application based on a prior filed utility patent application; it becomes necessary when the claims have been restricted and divided by the examiner because they are directed to separate inventions and not all claims are prosecuted and allowed, but are desired to be pursued. Similarly, a continuation application is similar to a divisional, but it is used when different claim scope is desired, not necessarily in response to claim restrictions in the parent case. Both divisional and continuation applications use the same specification as their parent patent and are accorded the parent case's filing date in relation to the prior art, over which the claims must be patentable. A continuation-in-part (CIP) is another type of application also spawned from a parent case, but adding some previously undisclosed subject matter to the specification or claims. A CIP application is accorded a filing date based on the first application disclosure of the claimed subject matter, which may be that of the parent case or the actual filing date of the CIP.

Patent applications should normally be filed before public use or disclosure of the invention and before offering it for sale, each of which can destroy patentability. The United States has a grace period of one year after such events to file, but most other countries have no grace period. Also, filing promptly will establish an earlier filing date with respect to prior art and can enhance the company's position should a USPTO priority adjudication between different inventors with respective applications occur.[8] The company's patent lawyer should consider the information provided in the Invention Disclosure Form or other record of invention in determining the critical dates for filing.

---

* U.S. Patent Act, 35 U.S.C. § 111, September 16, 2011.

FOREIGN FILING

There are differences in the patent (and other IP) laws of the U.S. and foreign countries, so if your company does business internationally or has significant foreign competitors, you should consider a global IP strategy and consult with outside counsel in formulating the strategy. Foreign patent filing and prosecution can be expensive and the cost can multiply based on the number of foreign countries of interest.

Most foreign countries, unlike the traditional practice in the United States, have a "first-to-file" system, which gives rights to patent filers on a first-come-first-served basis without regard to priority in inventorship.[9] Also, most foreign countries have strict disclosure rules that foreclose patent rights after public disclosure (the U.S. law is not so strict). These two factors make what your company does in the United States very important. First, if you are interested in foreign rights, you must consider filing as early as possible. Second, you should keep your invention(s) confidential until you file for a patent. Third, you must consider simultaneous filing of your U.S. case with foreign cases.

One way to work within the system and potentially save costs and buy time is to file a Patent Cooperation Treaty (PCT) application based on your U.S. patent application, which can later be converted into one or several foreign national applications. A PCT application can be filed within a year of your U.S. filing (including your U.S. provisional filing). PCT applications are sometimes called "international applications" because the filing date is recognized in most industrial nations; however, the PCT application cannot mature into an enforceable patent. To obtain enforceable patent rights, an applicant must proceed to individual national filings based on the PCT application.

INTERNAL IP CONTROLS

Committees

Patent and trademark committees are often used by companies to help shape the company's IP policies and to review and evaluate possible related courses of action. These are usually standing committees that meet regularly. The most common arrangement for carrying out IP committee operations is a single committee that considers both domestic and overseas patent and trademark matters.

Members of a patent committee can include executives such as the chief IP counsel and the various vice presidents for R&D and marketing, divisional managers, the head of the international division, and staff members of departments involved in patent projects. Membership is not required, however, and companies can decide who best can make the determinations relating to its IP goals and strategies.

The most common IP committee activity is screening and evaluating proposed and pending patent and trademark applications. Other activities include shaping overall patent policies; presenting issues to senior management regarding IP; establishing guidelines on licensing, interference, and settlement of IP matters; setting the terms and conditions under which licenses will be offered; evaluating strategies and the impact of compliance with IP policies of industrial organizations and government agencies; locating and dealing with infringers and collecting licensing or litigation damages money; determining the need to continue the maintenance of pending applications or issued patents; determining awards for worthwhile employee patent suggestions and inventions; reviewing domestic patent applications for possible foreign filings; and controlling the dissemination of possible trade secrets.

Getting the Corporate Team Involved

Invention Rewards

Most companies have systems for rewarding employees that invent. Invention awards programs are generally made available to all regular employees should they have a patentable idea; however, the members of research and engineering staffs are usually the principal beneficiaries.

There are reasons some companies choose not to pay cash awards to company inventors. One is that not all valuable ideas are patentable. Ideas that may result in innovation range from clearly unpatentable ones to ones that become the subject of as much protection effort as possible. The value of these ideas, however, may have no relation to their patentability. Also, it is often difficult to distribute cash rewards fairly. Most successful projects are the result of a team effort, and it can be difficult to allocate credit without injustice. And because projects are usually assigned, cash awards for successful outcomes could depend more on the assignments than on the skill of the individual, and such awards can engender ill will among employees.

For the most part, cash awards are token payments (e.g., $1,000 at patent filing and again at issue) that are not intended to correspond in value to the idea or patent. They are intended primarily to encourage inventors to bring their ideas to the attention of management (e.g., via invention disclosures). Companies that pay fixed awards for employee patents generally provide for each inventor. Some companies that reward inventors make awards according to an estimate of the invention's worth. Some companies that grant no immediate cash reward for filing or issuance of a patent pay the inventor if the patent is sold or licensed. An award program also may provide that when an employee's patent is combined with other patents to form a product or process, any income from licensing or sale is placed in a fund according to each inventor's share.

Other than cash awards to employee–inventors, ways to recognize the employee's contribution include trophies, of sorts, publicity releases and congratulatory letters, public or corporate presentations to the employee, or publications in a company newspaper or on an annually updated commemorative plaque. Such practices may seem a bit stingy, however, and perhaps are better combined with some financial incentive.

Reporting on Innovation

Companies usually provide senior management with IP reports on a regular (monthly or quarterly) basis to update on the status of pending and pipeline IP matters. In some instances, periodic reports are supplemented by an annual summary of IP activities, including reporting on patent and trademark litigation, new patents filed for, and new patents granted. Financial reports also can be included to identify the value of IP in profits made on patented technology, licenses granted, or new IP acquired.

Additionally, more informal reporting can be made. For example, senior management can be informed of general patent progress through periodic (e.g., luncheon) meetings with the in-house IP counsel.

Senior management's interest usually governs the topics included in most patent reports and this interest usually increases proportionally with the value and profits IP brings the company. Senior executives often note that their primary desire is to be advised of patent problems involving company policy and requiring a decision on their part, or that bears on the strength of the company's patent position or competitive position relating to current and projected processes and products.

Kinds of patent information to be reported to the senior management can include the following:

- U.S. and foreign patent protection on company products
- Company products or projects dominated by others' patents
- Patent protection available for projected products or operations
- Potential infringement litigation by or against the company
- Instances of infringement of company patents
- The status of any pending patent litigation involving the company
- Data on patents issued to other companies
- Changes in patent or trademark laws
- Licenses extended to other companies or obtained by the company
- The company's participation in industry organizations and its impact on patent rights
- Progress of important patent applications
- Analyses of the strength of the company's and competitions' patents
- A listing of upcoming patent expiration dates

Key technical personnel should also be kept informed of important IP information. Patents issued to other competitive companies is the most common type of information supplied to technical personnel by IP in-house counsel. Some companies keep their technical staff advised on other companies' new methods or products that might lead to patentable ideas. In any event, companies should provide technical personnel with guidance on the importance of patents, requirements for patentability, and the role played by the patent department.

Corporate IP staff stays current with invention progress by frequently communicating with members of the research staff who are working on potentially patentable innovations. IP staff should attend research meetings or committee meetings of technical and production personnel. If the company has enough invention activity, each member of the patent staff is generally assigned to serve as a liaison with a particular research group.

Frequent contact can help with the most common problem encountered by patent counsel—that is, getting inventors to keep an adequate log of an invention development and document supporting data necessary for preparing a patent application. It is important for IP counsel to instill in R&D staff an appreciation of the nature of potentially patentable inventions and of the need to maintain complete, signed, dated, and witnessed records.[10]

Another difficulty that some companies may encounter includes avoiding the premature public disclosure of a potential invention when the item represents a potential commercial product. R&D and sales staff generally like to submit new products to selected customers for evaluation and feedback before freezing a product design, and the marketing division is naturally anxious to get new products on the market. Although in the U.S. companies are allowed one year following the first publication, public use, or offer for sale (generally, public disclosure) in which to file a patent application, there is no such grace period in many other countries. The best practice is to file a patent application before any other disclosure anywhere, and it is best not to get that one-year clock ticking (provisional patent applications come in handy in these circumstances).

WHAT ARE TRADEMARKS AND WHY DO THEY MATTER?

A trademark is any word, name, symbol, device, or any combination of these, which identifies goods (or services in the case of a service mark) in a way to distinguish them from the goods of others. They are protectable under federal law, state law, and common law. Trade names and trade dress (two other ways to identify products and services) exist on their own, but they also may function as a form of trademark. A well-known medical trademark is Tylenol®. The power of this mark is its instant recognizablility to consumers, which makes it very valuable to McNeil PPC (a Johnson & Johnson company), the company that markets the product.

Under common law, mere use of a mark provides protection commensurate in scope to the extent of the mark's use—usually geographically limited. Federal registration of the mark with the USPTO affords additional rights. Registration with the USPTO on the Principal Register entitles the owner to use the mark and to exclude use of the trademark by others throughout the United States if it would likely lead to confusion by the public.[*] Registration with the USPTO on the Supplemental Register is for marks that *could* be distinctive, but have not yet become so and affords no exclusive rights, but it will preclude others from obtaining a registration to your mark. The symbol ® is used to give notice that a trademark is federally registered in these ways. The symbols ™ and ℠ are used to give notice that a trademark or service mark is considered by its owner to function as such to indicate the source of the goods or services. State trademark registrations also may be obtained, but they typically provide no more protection than is already available to the trademark owner under common law.

You may have heard of various types of "marks" (see 15 U.S.C. § 1127), including the following:

- Trademark. Any word, name, symbol, or device, or any combination thereof used by a company to identify its products and distinguish them from the products of others. It is usually a word, short phrase, or slogan. However, a product's shape or its packaging, or even a sound, can be a trademark.

---

[*] Lanham Act, 15 U.S.C. § 1057 (2011). Title 15, Chapter 22 of the U.S. Code the Federal law governing trademarks (and unfair competition).

- Service mark. A word, name, symbol, or device, or any combination thereof used to identify and distinguish the services of one entity from those of others. A trademark relates to goods and a service mark relates to services.
- Collective marks. Trademarks and service marks used by the members of a cooperative, an association, or other collective group or organization, including marks known as collective membership marks, indicating membership in a union, an association, or other organization.
- Certification mark. Used to certify regional or other origin, material, mode of manufacture, quality, accuracy, or other characteristics of goods or services or that the work or labor on the goods or services was performed by members of a union or other organization. For instance, the mark "UL" is a certification mark of Underwriters Laboratories, Inc.
- Trade name. Used to identify a business rather than its products. For example, HGS (Human Genome Sciences) or IBM (International Business Machines).
- Trade dress. The total image or overall appearance of a product and can be protected under section 43(a) of the Lanham Act* or under common law if it is distinctive and nonfunctional, such as a unique way of packaging a product.

Trademarks are important to medical device technology start-up companies for the same reasons they are important to any other business—that is, they enable your customers to recognize your products and business. Constant policing of trademarks is necessary to keep them protected, which means that counterfeiters and infringers must be discovered and dealt with immediately for fear of losing your trademark rights. This is also important to maintain the goodwill you create for your company by using your trademarks, which ultimately can be very valuable.

TRADE SECRETS

Trade secret law is the flipside of patent law. It provides protection for any information that is not generally known or used by others and is of value to the owner for that reason, so long as the owner reasonably maintains it as a secret. Contrast this with a patent, which requires full disclosure to the public. The knowledge and experience of a company's employees relating to the company's business matters, such as technical designs, customer and vendor information, and manufacturing processes, usually has significant value. Use of this information can yield improved product performance or manufacturing efficiencies that greatly enhance the company's competitiveness. A trade secret can be information of any type, including, for example, a formula, pattern, compilation, program, device, method, technique, or process, that is actually or potentially valuable to its owner and not readily available to or ascertainable by the public. Some common types of trade secrets include the following:

---

* Lanham Act, 15 U.S.C. § 1125(a) (2011).

- Data compilations like customer lists
- Designs and blueprints
- Algorithms and other computer-implemented programs
- Instructional methods
- Manufacturing processes and techniques
- Business strategies and plans, marketing plans
- Financial information
- Personnel records
- Training manuals
- Ingredients
- R&D information

Trade secret protection is different from patents and trademarks in that it solely arises under state common law and statutes, which differ state-to-state, but usually resemble the Uniform Trade Secrets Act and the Economic Espionage Act of 1996 (18 U.S.C. §§ 1831–1839).* Whether or not information is protectable under the patent laws, by using reasonable efforts to keep the information confidential, the company can protect it under trade secret law. These reasonable efforts can include limiting access to the information, requiring confidentiality agreements for access, marking documents or things "confidential," and keeping the information under "lock and key." But trade secrets are protected only from misappropriation (i.e., stealing) from the owner by others. Thus, if a person obtains the information by independent development, or from another, lawful source, the owner's trade secret rights will not preclude that person from using it or disclosing it.

It is often a difficult decision whether to seek patent protection for innovation or to keep it a trade secret. The decision can turn on the technology and the rate at which it evolves, the likelihood that competitors could lawfully gain the secret knowledge, and the value of any patent that could be obtained. Consider what is possibly the most famous trade secret—the Coke recipe—if it were patentable at some point (more than 100 years ago) and a patent was applied for and granted, by now any patent would have long expired and anyone who wanted to could use that recipe and make the very same soft drink as the Coca-Cola Company. Because it has been kept as a trade secret, however, we can only guess at the ingredients, and this provides value for the company. Other considerations that help in making a decision on whether to keep information a trade secret include the following:

- Whether the secret is patentable
- Whether the information can be kept a secret
- Whether the secret relates to a manufacturing process rather than to a product, which could be reverse engineered
- Whether related technology has been patented or the subject of a patent application

---

* The lack of a Federal trade secret law means that most trade secret litigation will take place in the state courts.

WATCH OUT FOR OTHERS' PROPERTY

Patent infringement problems most typically arise for a company after it has already started marketing an (allegedly) infringing product. At that point, the infringement can result in serious consequences, including litigation costs, retooling costs, distraction of employees to deal with the matter, adverse customer relations, perhaps the loss of the entire product line, and, finally, damages (which can be trebled in some instances, e.g., for willful infringement). A company can take steps to avoid these problems. It is important for the company to be aware of its new manufacturing processes and product designs and clear them from infringement concerns early on in the game (i.e., before tooling up and making and selling product), when any necessary changes usually can be carried out more economically. By monitoring new product developments and company invention disclosures, the company can identify significant proposed products and processes that warrant clearance.

STATE-OF-THE-ART STUDY

A "state-of-the-art" study can be conducted during product development to find existing patents and publications for similar technology. This study can provide information on what others have invented when confronted with similar problems. It also will identify, early in the design process, any existing patents to be avoided or designed around. Any necessary design changes can likely be made at this stage efficiently and at low cost. This is generally the first step in product "clearance."

NONINFRINGEMENT STUDY

Once a product or service is sufficiently developed to a final functional configuration, the company should conduct a patent noninfringement study and obtain a noninfringement opinion from outside counsel so that the company can move forward with a well-reasoned understanding that it is free to do so in view of other's property rights. This should be done before launching the new product or service into the market. If the study reveals infringement issues, they may be correctible at this stage. Also, in the event the product or service is later found to infringe a patent, having the noninfringement opinion can help avoid any award of enhanced damages for willful infringement, which could be up to three times the amount of compensatory damages,[*,11] as well as any award of attorneys' fees to the patentee.[†] The noninfringement opinion should

- Be in writing and rendered by a competent patent lawyer;
- Include a claim construction based on the intrinsic record (i.e., the claims, specification, and prosecution history);

---

[*] U.S. Patent Act, 35 U.S.C. § 284, September 16, 2011.
[†] U.S. Patent Act, 35 U.S.C. § 285, September 16, 2011.

- Include a comparison of the interpreted claims of the patent with the company's product and include reasons why the product does not come within the scope of the patent claims; and
- Be rendered before commencement of manufacturing and marketing activity.

If the company makes changes to the design of the product after the infringement opinion is rendered, a supplemental opinion should be obtained. If it turns out that the most reasonable answer is that the company's product will likely infringe the patent, the patent should be investigated for invalidity and a separate opinion should be rendered. If this again results in bad news for the company, and it appears that the patent is valid and likely infringed, the company has a business decision to make: Is it cheaper (or even possible) to redesign the product so that it does not infringe (design around the patent) or proceed with going to market on the chance that the patent will not be enforced or that the product's profits will so outweigh the possible damages as to make it worthwhile. Another alternative is to seek a license from the patent owner.

Validity Study

As discussed, if an infringement issue is discovered and the product cannot be modified to avoid the patent without rendering the product inferior or uncompetitive, the validity of the patent claims can be analyzed. U.S. patents are entitled to a presumption that they are valid, however, so the burden is on the party seeking to invalidate the patent to prove by *clear and convincing* evidence (between a mere *preponderance of the evidence* standard and the criminal-law *beyond a reasonable doubt* standard) that the claims are invalid. For this reason, it is usually more difficult to defend a patent infringement claim based on invalidity than noninfringement.

The most common basis for invalidating a patent is prior art that was not considered by the USPTO in examining the patent's application (but there are other ways, too, such as lack of enablement). Thus, the invalidity study should include a search specifically for such additional prior art and the opinion should explain why that prior art anticipates or renders obvious the patent's claimed subject matter. The invalidity search often extends beyond the records of the USPTO or even U.S. patents to other patent collections that may not yet have been searched, such as those at the European Patent Office and the Japanese Patent Office. Publications should be searched as well, as they can also be used to invalidate claims.

Designing around Patents

"Designing around" a patent means to configure a product or process so that it does not infringe the patent. Because a product or process infringes a patent only if it includes all of the elements of any one of the patent's claims in exactly the way claimed (or, in some instances, using equivalent means) a "design around" can succeed if it eliminates at least one element in each of the patent's claims.

Often, the same element can be identified for many, if not all, of the claims in a patent since the independent claims recite subject matter carried throughout the other dependent claims. The changed element does not have to be a novel one or the one that bestowed patentability on the claims, but it can be one that is old in the art. Sometimes avoiding use of the element is simple. Other times, extensive effort is required to develop an alternative approach while still maintaining a commercially acceptable product.

MAKE MONEY WITH YOUR PATENTS

IDENTIFYING YOUR INTELLECTUAL PROPERTY

The purpose of having IP is to make money with it, but to do that, you have to first know what you have and your position in the world of IP. A necessary first task is to identify what IP exists using an IP audit. An IP audit should answer the following three questions:

- What is the economic and strategic value of the company's IP and what is its character and scope?
- Does the company have clear title to the IP?
- Does the company have potential liability for infringing the IP rights of others?

First, consider the general nature of the company. Different types of companies require different focus during IP audits. For example, a start-up medical device company may require a more in-depth investigation than a cement manufacturer. Companies that market consumer products may require a closer look into trademarks and design patents than other companies. Chemical and pharmaceutical companies may have important trade secrets and know-how. The audit should develop lists of the IP holdings, such as the following:

- A list of all U.S. and foreign patents, patent applications, including with a brief description of the products, processes, or information covered thereby or subject thereto, and (where applicable) the corresponding grant or application filing dates
- A list of registered trademarks and service marks, trademark and service mark registration applications, unregistered but used trademarks/service marks, including with a brief description of the goods or services covered thereby or subject thereto, and (where applicable) the corresponding registration grant and/or application dates
- A list of registered and unregistered copyrights
- A list of trade secrets currently held by the company, including a brief description of the products, processes, or information covered thereby or subject thereto
- A list of all IP licenses, other technical assistance agreements, confidentiality agreements, and technology development grants

The sources for this information should include the company patent counsel, company marketing and engineering personnel, and independent outside sources, the company's marketing materials, catalogs, web sites, and other related material. The best place to start, however, is with the company personnel who have been dealing with the IP. They likely can lead you to records as well as to any outside lawyers involved with the IP who also will have information. Talk to all these people about the important aspects of the company technology, the important trademarks, and about trade secrets: What *are* the crucial proprietary secret processes and techniques? *Where* are these documented? What steps are actually taken to *safeguard* these key trade secrets?

Much of the information may reside on databases kept by current in-house and outside lawyers. Other public databases can be searched and many are accessible online.[12] The searches can be conducted in the names of the company, key personnel, and licensors. With respect to trade secret protection, a plant or facilities visit might reveal whether appropriate physical security precautions and safeguards are in place.

Other things you should do in the course of the audit include the following:

- Obtain patent maintenance and annuity fee records.
- For patents of special interest, identify all prior art in the company's files. Later, the company may need to determine whether any validity issues would justify further investigation.
- Review all products, marketing, promotional, and packaging materials of the company to determine whether the materials and products have been properly marked with the company's patents.[*]
- Review all products, marketing, promotional, and packaging materials of the company to determine if the company's trademarks have been used properly.
- Obtain copies of all U.S. and foreign trademark registrations and registration applications.
- Review trademark renewal records.
- Obtain results of any trademark searches conducted by or for the company.
- Identify any marks of the company that may have been abandoned.
- Identify all unregistered copyrights.
- Review know-how licenses and other technical assistance agreements, and confidentiality agreements.
- Check employee, consultant, and officer agreements to confirm obligations to assign U.S. and foreign rights.
- Determine whether appropriate confidentiality and noncompete agreements are in place, especially with respect to key personnel.
- Consider the impact of recent arrivals or departures of key personnel.

---

[*] U.S. Patent Act, 35 U.S.C. 287(a), September 16, 2011, was amended under the recently enacted America Invents Act to allow for the "virtual marking" of products by providing a list of covering patents on a website and providing the web address thereto on products or marketing.

- Assess the company's existing procedures for identifying patentable inventions and designs, and for ensuring applications are timely filed. Determine whether the procedures are appropriate and effective under the circumstances.
- Evaluate the adequacy of hiring and exit interviews procedures. Review records for key personnel.
- Evaluate secrecy policies, including physical security, employed by the company.
- Evaluate security policies for computer software and electronic data.
- Evaluate the company's policy for identifying and protecting its copyrights.
- Evaluate the company's policy for avoiding infringement of patents, trademarks, or copyrights and obtain copyright clearance to protect against infringement claims.
- Determine whether the company has recorded ownership assignments (where applicable) for all U.S. and foreign patents and patent applications.
- Obtain copies of all licenses concerning patents, trademarks, copyrights, trade secrets, know-how, or other IP or proprietary products, information, or processes, including expired licenses, held by the company, whether as licensor or licensee, together with a brief description of the products, processes, or information covered thereby or subject thereto.
- Review all records of audits conducted by or against the company pursuant to license agreements or research and development agreements.
- Identify procedures employed by the company for quality control monitoring of licensee use of trademarks.
- Obtain copies of all research and development contracts, agreements, and proposals between the company and any other company or companies.
- Determine whether the company has assigned or granted security interests against any patents or patent applications.
- Review all work-for-hire agreements and consultant contracts.
- Identify all assertions and potential assertions of infringement against the company, and all license offers received by the company, within the last six years, concerning patents, trademarks, copyrights, trade secrets, know-how, or other IP, and the status of any negotiations or correspondence concerning such assertions or license offers.
- Obtain correspondence from the company accusing others of infringing its IP or offering licenses under the company's IP. Consider whether any matters justify further negotiations or litigation.
- Identify any actual litigation involving the company's IP. Identify the current status of any ongoing proceedings or negotiations. Obtain copies of settlement agreements and releases.
- Obtain records of any U.S. trademark opposition or cancellation proceedings, and foreign equivalent proceedings.
- Identify and review all covenants not to sue and indemnification agreements.
- Review press reports.
- Determine whether key technologies and other IP rights have been transferred to one or more government agencies, for example, via U.S. government purpose rights provisions.
- Assess the adequacy of insurance coverage against IP infringement claims.

Intellectual Property Strategy for Med-Tech Start-Ups

ENFORCING PATENTS

One way to stay competitive in the marketplace as well as recoup some value from your IP is to actively police and enforce your patents. If the competition knows that your company has important IP rights and it is made clear that the company is serious about wielding those rights in court, the company, in turn, must be taken seriously. To do this, a company needs intelligence on the products and services of its competitors. Some sources of such intelligence include the following:

- Trade shows
- Websites
- Trade journals
- Patent searches
- Customers and vendors
- Private detectives
- Reverse engineered products
- Competitors' employees[13]

Your patent program should include such intelligence gathering as one of its core functions. Marketing personnel may be a source or pathway to such information, and they should be trained how to gather it properly and report it back.

Once you have information on competitor's products, you may feel that the company's patent rights have been violated by your competitor. At that point, you have a variety of options that you may pursue ranging from offering to license the technology to filing a lawsuit. Before actually filing a complaint, even if you are intent on doing so, it is prudent to carefully, but clearly, warn the alleged infringer of its infringement of the company's patent(s).[14] This warning letter should ask that the competitor *cease and desist* its infringing activities and also warn of the company's intentions to enforce its patent rights. If the alleged infringer fails to cease its infringing use, suit should be filed in a timely fashion to ensure that the company obtains the venue (litigation court) of its choice for trial because the letter likely will open the company up to a declaratory judgment action by the accused infringer.

The accused infringer may file its own lawsuit against the company called a declaratory judgment action, and if it does so before you file suit, it can obtain a venue of its choice for the trial. A declaratory judgment action by an accused infringer seeks the invalidation of your patent and a finding that the patent is not infringed. The alleged infringer must have standing to sue and, generally, anyone who has received a direct threat of enforcement of patent rights has such standing. Even a present licensee who believes the licensed patent is invalid may seek a declaratory judgment challenging the patent's validity.[*]

The two most common forms of remedies awarded for a finding of infringement of a patent are monetary damages and an injunction preventing the defendant from further utilizing the patent—both of these give the patentee a competitive advantage.[†] Monetary

---

[*] MedImmune, Inc. v. Gennentech, Inc., 127 S. Ct. 764 (2007).
[†] Injunctive relief, however, is becoming rare to all those but direct competitors.

damages are typically awarded as a reasonable royalty (based on a hypothetically negotiated license) for the use of the patent or lost profits—the current trend is to focus damages on *exactly* what value the patented invention brings to the infringing product, so if it is a key part, the damages are bigger, and if it is a tangential part, the damages are less. An injunction prohibits the infringer from further use of the patented technology. The Supreme Court held that the factors in determining whether to issue an injunction are as follows: (1) patentee has suffered an irreparable injury; (2) monetary damages would not be able to fully compensate the patent holder's injuries; (3) the balance of hardships between the parties warrants an equitable remedy such as an injunction; and (4) an injunction would not disserve the public's interests.[*] Competition between the parties is important, as is a showing that money alone cannot fully compensate the patent holder.

Besides the Federal courts, the U.S. International Trade Commission (ITC) provides another forum in which to enforce patent rights—here, relating to the importation of infringing things.[†] The ITC cannot impose monetary penalties, but its prohibiting the importation of products that it deems to infringe patent rights is also competitively advantageous for the patent holder. It is common for litigation actions to proceed in the ITC and federal district court at the same time. ITC litigation is usually much faster than litigation in the federal courts.

The cost of patent litigation can vary greatly and generally corresponds to the amount of money that is at issue in the action. A 2011 survey reported typical midrange costs for U.S. patent litigation:[‡]

- Less than $1 million at issue
  To the end of discovery: $350,000
  All costs: $650,000

- $1 to $25 million at issue
  To the end of discovery: $1. 5 million
  All costs: $2.5 million

- More than $25 million at issue
  To the end of discovery: $3 million
  All costs: $5 million

Such costs are likely to continue increasing. Furthermore, other recent developments driving up costs, especially in big-dollar litigations, include electronic discovery (required by the Federal Rules of procedure), the housing of electronic documents in expensive databases using outside vendors, and increased technology in the courtroom driving the need to use electronically created evidence. Litigation is expensive and the costs should be a core factor in deciding the company's course of action. You should consult outside counsel for your realistic chances of success. Success, however, is defined by your business goals. So, if you can get a preliminary injunction to

---

[*] eBay, Inc. v. MercExchange, L.L.C., 126 S. Ct. 1837 (2006).
[†] Tariff Act, 19 U.S.C. § 1337(e) (2011).
[‡] American Intellectual Property Law Association, *Report of the Economic Survey* (2011), available at http://www.aipla.org.

keep a competitive product off market over the course of the litigation (even if you cannot ultimately win a case), maybe that is enough.

LICENSING YOUR TECHNOLOGY

Another option for dealing with a believed infringer is to negotiate a license for the patented technology. If the patent owner is willing to grant a license under commercially acceptable terms, this enables the accused infringer to use the needed patented technology in its products or services. The patent-holding company can use licensing negotiations in other ways besides making money—for example, it can be an avenue to cross-license patents so it may use the technology of its competitors. Licensing can be a sword against accused infringers and a shield against accusing patent holders (this makes having strong IP rights all the more important). You can be sure that larger, more established companies in your field that have larger patent portfolios will be using them against you, so you need to prepare.

Your company's sales and manufacturing executives can initiate the creation of licensing arrangements, including preliminary negotiations. Final negotiations are generally the responsibility of senior corporate management, IP counsel, or the general law department. In some small, specialized industrial products companies, patent licensing can be the responsibility of the president, with the concurrence of the company's chairman.

Regardless of who negotiates a license agreement, the company's legal counsel should enter the picture at an early stage. Counsel's role can range from advising the negotiator to conducting the negotiations. In-house IP counsel should also draft the license agreement, with outside IP counsel usually providing legal guidance in licensing matters. Occasionally, however, the company will assign the task to the general law department. Resident outside licensing specialists may be called on as needed, especially to deal with foreign licenses. In the end, however, as in all IP rights, the license is a business document and is made for business reasons, so the company must ensure it makes sense for this reason.

CONCLUSION

It has been said that without a coherent plan to acquire, manage, and protect IP, a start-up or small company in the high-tech (including medical technology) business will always be, at best, a small company.* The techniques and strategies discussed in this chapter should be considered and discussed by your corporate management, IP counsel, and outside counsel to implement the best plan for your company. Whether dealing with U.S. IP issues or IP issues in foreign countries, surrounding yourself with the most competent staff and hiring those that are experts or have access to experts in areas of interest is essential. A strong in-house IP group and outside counsel for your company can enable you to catch up with and move ahead of your competitors.

---

* Hung H. Bui, *Practical Strategies to Develop an IP Portfolio and Avoid MistakesPertaining to IP for High-Tech Startup and Small Technology Companies* (paper presented at the 6th VACETS Technical International Conference, 2005).

ABOUT THE AUTHOR

Ryan H. Flax is an attorney in the Washington, DC, headquarters of the national law firm Dickstein Shapiro LLP. Mr. Flax's law practice focuses on intellectual property, in particular patent, trademark, and trade secret law. Mr. Flax's patent law practice spans an array of technologies, including medical devices, and includes experience in patent litigation at both the trial court and appellate levels, patent prosecution, counseling and opinion work, and transactional matters. Mr. Flax received his law degree from Southern Methodist University (Dedman) School of Law and has a degree in biology from Wake Forest University. Before becoming an attorney, Mr. Flax was a scientist involved in DNA research for R.J. Reynolds Tobacco, Co. Ryan Flax was a member of the litigation team at Dickstein Shapiro LLP representing Bruce N. Saffran, MD, PhD, in his trial victories against Boston Scientific Corp. and Johnson & Johnson where two juries awarded Dr. Saffran damages totaling about $1 billion relating to a drug-releasing layer used in drug-eluting cardiac stents.

ENDNOTES

1. There are a number of different types of patents, however utility patents are the most common type. They are available for any "new and useful process, machine, manufacture, or composition of matter, or any new and useful improvement thereof." To be patentable, an invention need not be a pioneering discovery, but can be a novel and unobvious improvement on a prior design. Design and plant patents are also available.
2. Section 102 has recently be drastically amended by the America Invents Act, signed into law by President Obama on September 16, 2011. The amendment expands the definition of "prior art" and creates incentive to publish one's work and file quickly for a patent. It also creates incentive for joint-research agreements.
3. As mentioned in endnote 1, the U.S. patent laws have recently been amended. One important amendment to the laws does away with the best mode requirement of 35 U.S.C. § 112 going forward. So, for existing patents, the best mode must be disclosed, but for future patents it need not be.
4. Under a new USPTO procedure (see 37 C.F.R. § 1.102) a patent application's prosecution can be prioritized and expedited so that rather than being taken up in the order it was filed, the application will move to the front of the queue. Such prosecution is intended to be completed in just one year, but only 10,000 such prioritizations will be approved each year.
5. Possibly the most important change to the U.S. Patent Act by the recent amendments is the switch of the U.S. system to a *first-inventor-to-file* system. The new system is effective for patents filed as of March 16, 2013. At this point, it will be more important to document to whom and when the invention has been disclosed than the diligent work that went into development. However, scientific best practices still require a detailed lab notebook.
6. This "anything under the sun" doctrine has received considerable attention recently as the courts try to sort out patent eligibility. For example, software and biotech patents have been particularly scrutinized and, on occasion, found ineligible and, at other times, eligible for patent. Patents are not available for abstract ideas.
7. The USPTO website (http://www.uspto.gov) is a good source of prior art information as well as the rules for prosecuting a patent application (*Manual for Patent Examination Procedure* and Title 37 of the Code of Federal Regulations). Another good source is Google Patents (http://www.google.com/patents), where Google provides access to U.S. patents and published patent applications by familiar word searching.

8. With the implementation of the newly amended Patent Act, interferences will be discontinued and replaced by derivation proceedings, which will be used to establish whether a prior patent or application's disclosed/claimed invention was derived from the inventor of a subsequently filed application.
9. With the enactment of the new Patent Act on September 16, 2011, the United States has somewhat harmonized its patent laws with those of most foreign, industrialized nations. The United States has moved to a *first-inventor-to-file* (meaning that the first filer gets the patent, with certain exceptions). The United States has also expanded the definition of "prior art" to include foreign-filed patents and publications.
10. Although the new Patent Act does away with interference practice where prior invention and diligence toward reduction to practice is key evidence, it remains a good idea to continue the practice of documenting invention conception and development because this documentation is very useful to attorneys charged with drafting patent applications and may be useful in litigation some day, either to defend against charges of infringement or to establish the patentee's work at inventing.
11. Under the newly amended Patent Act (see 35 U.S.C. § 298), the failure of an infringer to obtain the advice of counsel, for example, by getting an opinion letter, with respect to any alleged infringement cannot be used to prove willful infringement or intent to induce infringement by another. An opinion can be used by the accused infringer to establish lack of willfulness and lack of intent to induce infringement, but doing so typically implicates waiver of attorney-client privilege to a degree.
12. See the U.S. Patent and Trademark Office website, http://www.uspto.gov, for searchable online records for patent inventors and owners and for trademark registrations and applications. The Google Patents website, http://www.google.com/patents, is a good search engine to find U.S. patents. On the U.S. Copyright Office website, http://www.copyright.gov, U.S. copyright registrations can be searched. See Thomson & Thomson for trademark matters. See ESpaceNet, http://www.espacenet.com, a useful, if cumbersome, site for non-U.S. patents. See National IP Offices and the World Intellectual Property Organization (WIPO) for records that can be searched, many of them online. See Westlaw or Lexis searching for patent and trademark information.
13. Be very careful dealing with a competitor's employees, however. This practice, while potentially fruitful, can open you up to litigation for tortious interference or misappropriation of trade secrets if the competitor's employees are under a duty of confidentiality.
14. Before sending this letter, an infringement opinion should be obtained from outside counsel so that the company can assert that its belief of infringement is reasonable and founded in facts. This can prevent sanctions against the company for bringing a lawsuit in the event there is no infringement.

15 Regulatory Affairs
Medical Devices

Thomas Wehman

CONTENTS

Introduction 296
   Regulatory Requirements Are Enforced by Law 296
   Make Regulatory Affairs Cost-Effective 296
   Regulatory Requirements Improve Device Safety and Effectiveness 297
   Regulatory Affairs Requires Good Judgment 297
FDA Overview and Authority 298
   Important FDA Jurisdiction Acts, History, and Assistance 298
   Online Assistance 299
Basics: Short Discussion of Establishment Registration, Device
Submissions, Device Listing, and Device Classification 299
   Establishment Registration 299
   Device Listing 299
   Device Classification 300
   Device Functional Classification 301
   510(k) Premarket Notification 301
   Substantial Equivalence 302
   Premarket Approval Submission 302
   Investigational Device Exemption and Supporting Studies 303
   Third-Party Submission Review by Accredited Parties 304
   Importing into the United States 304
      Initial Importers 304
   Exporting Devices 305
      Certificates for Foreign Government 305
   Additional Regulations by Different States 305
Special Considerations 306
   Exemptions from 510(k) and GMP Requirements 306
      Class I Devices 306
      Class II Devices 306
   Special 510(k) 306
   Abbreviated 510(k) 307
   De Novo 308
   Product Development Protocol 308
   Humanitarian Use Device/Humanitarian Device Exemption 309

Good Quality and Procedural Practices 309
  Quality System Regulations 309
  Quality System Inspection Technique 310
  Good Clinical Practice 310
  Good Laboratory Practices... 311
    Regulations... 311
  Preclinical Studies.. 311
Summary of Title 21 of the Code of Federal Regulations, Parts 800 to 1299,
for Medical Devices.. 311
  Part 800: General Requirements 311
  Part 801: Labeling.. 312
  Part 803: Medical Device Reporting (MDR).. 313
  Part 806: Medical Devices: Reports of Corrections and Removals 314
  Part 807: Establishment Registration and Device Listing for Manufacturer
  and Individual Importers of Devices.. 314
  Part 808: Exemptions from Federal Preemption of State and Local Medical
  Device Requirements 316
  Part 809: In Vitro Diagnostic Products for Human Use............................... 316
  Part 810: Medical Device Recall Authority 317
  Part 812: Investigational Device Exemptions 318
  Part 820: Quality System Regulation... 324
  Part 821: Medical Device Tracking Requirements 326
  Part 822: Postmarket Surveillance 327
  Part 860: Medical Device Classification Procedures 329
  Part 861: Procedures for Performance Standards Development 330
  Parts 862 to 1050... 330
Abbreviations 331
  International and National Standard Abbreviations 331
  Regulatory Abbreviations... 331
About the Author... 332

INTRODUCTION

REGULATORY REQUIREMENTS ARE ENFORCED BY LAW

The first rule of regulatory affairs is that it is based on regulation—that is, it is a legal obligation. From a business point of view, it is expense, and it does contribute to the cost of doing business. Thus, for the sake of maintaining a profitable business while still providing for necessary safety and effectiveness of a medical device, regulatory affairs must be a well-planned function and not just improvised as the need arises. For a medical device start-up company, regulatory affairs strategy and implementation must be addressed from the very beginning.

MAKE REGULATORY AFFAIRS COST-EFFECTIVE

The discussion in this chapter focuses on meeting all regulatory needs for a company in a cost-effective fashion. The emphasis on cost-effectiveness leads to the second rule of regulatory affairs: More is not better. Good regulatory control requires good documentation, but it does not require an ever-growing set of instructions and procedures. Adherence to documented procedures is of paramount importance. Thus, if documents become too complex or too numerous, adherence may suffer.

The Medical Device User Fee and Modernization Act of October 2002 increased the cost of doing business for any company wishing to sell medical devices in the United States by imposing device submission fees. The fees, as of May 2005, which underscore the need for good device development and regulation planning, are listed in the following table:

Submission Type	Standard Fee	Small-Business Fee
Premarket approval (PMA)	$206,811	$78,588
180-day PMA supplement	$44,464	$16,896
510(k)	$3,480	$2,784

REGULATORY REQUIREMENTS IMPROVE DEVICE SAFETY AND EFFECTIVENESS

Medical device regulations were implemented and are enforced to ensure that the best possible safety and effectiveness will be obtained from a Food and Drug Administration (FDA)-cleared or -approved device. It is the company's management responsibility to provide continued safety and effectiveness after a device is released for sale by employing a good-quality validation and reliability program. The U.S. FDA Quality System Regulation (QSR) is described in the "Summary of Title 21 of the Code of Federal Regulations (CFR), Part 820: Good Manufacturing Practices" section of this chapter. Similar international quality systems (ISO 9000), specifically for medical devices (ISO 13485), are beyond the scope of this chapter.

REGULATORY AFFAIRS REQUIRES GOOD JUDGMENT

Immediately following the text in each section is a short list of bullet points of what was covered. The intent of these lists is to enable the reader to quickly visualize the essence of each regulation. The goal of this chapter is to make the reader aware of requirements and options so that he or she can speak knowledgeably with regulatory affairs professionals in order to exercise good judgment. Only study, training, and experience will lead to a full grasp of regulatory complexity in order to exercise good judgment.

- Regulations are enforced by law.
- More documentation is not always better.
- Adhering to all regulations does not guarantee that there will not be any adverse events, but it will lessen the likelihood of punitive damages.
- FDA medical device regulations were implemented to ensure safety and effectiveness.
- Start regulatory affairs strategies immediately after funding of company.

FDA OVERVIEW AND AUTHORITY

The FDA is composed of six different centers and two offices:

Centers

- Center for Food Safety and Applied Nutrition (CFSAN)
- Center for Drug Evaluation and Research (CDER)
- Center for Devices and Radiological Health (CDRH)
- Center for Biologics Evaluation and Research (CBER)
- Center for Veterinary Medicine (CVR)
- National Center for Toxicological Research (NCTR)

Offices

- Office of the Commissioner (OC)
- Office of Regulatory Affairs (ORA)

The division that deals with medical devices is CDRH. If a device has some other component, such as drugs or biological products, the FDA decides which is the primary mode of action and assigns review responsibility accordingly.

IMPORTANT FDA JURISDICTION ACTS, HISTORY, AND ASSISTANCE

FDA reorganization 1930: There was a sweeping expansion of FDA to include coverage of new drugs, devices, and cosmetics. Also, the FDA was given increased court jurisdiction.

The Federal Food, Drug and Cosmetics Act (FD&C) of 1938: The FDA was expanded to regulate cosmetics and therapeutic devices and additional regulation of food and drugs.

The Medical Device Amendments of 1976: Added provisions governing device and facility registration and listing, classifications, premarket notification (510(k)), premarket approval (PMA), investigational device exemption (IDE), good manufacturing practice (GMP), medical device reports (MDR), and other controls. This expansion was so extensive that over time devices are referred to as preamendment or postamendment.

The Safe Medical Devices Act of 1990: Comprehensive changes to include device recall, preproduction design validation, expanding authority to surgical hospitals and nursing homes, and establishing biological divisions to include devices that contain drugs and biological products (CBER).

FDA Export Reform and Enhancement Act of 1996: Substantially reduces many regulatory obstacles for exporting unapproved drugs, biologics, and devices.

1997 FDA Modernization Act (FDAMA): Significantly reduced time frame and work required for clinical studies, clearances, approvals, and device manufacture and design requirements.

2002 Medical Device User Fee Modernization Act (MDUFMA): Instigated user fees for device submissions, third-party inspections, reprocessed single-use devices, and other provisions.

ONLINE ASSISTANCE

Division of Small Manufacturers, International and Consumer Assistance (DSMICA): This is a special group within the FDA that was set up to answer questions from the medical device industry. It can be contacted via its website at http://www.fda.gov/cdrh/dsmamain.html.

International regulations: To obtain medical regulations for other countries listed in *International Organizations and Foreign Government Agencies*, go to http://www.fda.gov/oia/agencies.htm.

The FDA has multiple divisions to ensure health and safety for food, drugs, and devices. There are multiple levels of device classification to meet different levels of risk.

There have been many FDA amendments and acts to improve safety and reduce regulatory obstacles.

BASICS: SHORT DISCUSSION OF ESTABLISHMENT REGISTRATION, DEVICE SUBMISSIONS, DEVICE LISTING, AND DEVICE CLASSIFICATION*

ESTABLISHMENT REGISTRATION

Establishments involved in the production and distribution of medical devices intended for marketing or leasing (commercial distribution) in the United States are required to register with the FDA. Registration provides the FDA with the location of medical device manufacturing facilities and importers. No registration fee is required. An establishment means any place of business under one management at one physical location at which a device is manufactured, assembled, or otherwise processed for commercial distribution. The owner or operator of the establishment is responsible for registration. Owner or operator means the corporation, subsidiary, affiliated company, partnership, or proprietor directly responsible for the activities of the registering establishment.

DEVICE LISTING

Most medical device establishments required to register with the FDA must list the devices they have in commercial distribution, including devices produced exclusively for export. This process is a means of keeping the FDA advised of the generic

---

* 21 C.F.R. §§ 800–1299. See additional details in the section "Summary of Title 21 of the Code of Federal Regulations, Parts 800 to 1299, for Medical Devices" (some of the text in this and following sections are taken directly from 21 CFR).

categories of devices an establishment is marketing. Each generic category is represented by a separate classification regulation found in Title 21 of CFR, Parts 862 to 892, or by an FDA-assigned device name. Each regulation number or device name is associated with one or more product codes. Regulation numbers with more than one product code identify the product in further detail. For example, "Manual Surgical Instruments for General Use," 21 CFR 878.4800, contains several product codes, including GAB (disposable suturing needle), GDX (scalpel), HTD (forceps), and HRQ (hemostat).

Listing of a medical device is not approval of the establishment or a device by the FDA. Unless exempt, a premarket clearance (510(k)) or PMA is required before a device can be marketed or placed into commercial distribution in the United States. No listing fee is required.

Device Classification

The FDA has established classifications for approximately 1700 different generic types of devices and grouped them into 16 medical specialties, referred to as panels. Each of these generic types of devices is assigned to one of three regulatory classes based on the level of control necessary to ensure the safety and effectiveness of the device. The three classes and the requirements that apply to them are as follows:

1. Class I: General Controls
    a. With exemptions
    b. Without exemptions
2. Class II: General and Special Controls
    a. With exemptions
    b. Without exemptions
3. Class III: General Controls and Premarket Approval

The class to which your device is assigned determines, among other things, the type of premarketing submission or application required for FDA clearance to market. If your device is classified as Class I or II, and if it is not exempt, a 510(k) will be required for marketing. All devices classified as exempt are subject to the limitations on exemptions. Limitations of device exemptions are covered under 21 CFR xxx.9, where xxx refers to Parts 862–892. For Class III devices, a PMA application will be required unless the device is a preamendments device (on the market before the passage of the medical device amendments in 1976, or substantially equivalent [SE] to such a device) and the device has not been designated a PMA. In that case, a 510(k) will be the route to market.

Device classification depends on the *intended use* of the device and also upon *indications for use*. For example, a scalpel's intended use is to cut tissue. A subset of intended use arises when a more specialized indication is added in the device's labeling, such as "for making incisions in the cornea." Indications for use can be found in the device's labeling, but they may also be conveyed orally during sale of the product. A discussion of the meaning of intended use is contained in *Premarket Notification Review Program K86-3*.

In addition, classification is risk based—that is, the risk the device poses to the patient or the user is a major factor in the class it is assigned. Class I includes devices with the lowest risk, and Class III includes those with the greatest risk.

DEVICE FUNCTIONAL CLASSIFICATION

As mentioned, the FDA has established classifications for more than 1700 types of devices and has categorized them into 16 medical specialties, referred to as panels. Experts from the different panels are often called on to review regulatory requirements or rulings for specific devices. Panel numbers and panels are as follows:

- 868 Anesthesiology
- 870 Cardiovascular
- 862 Clinical Chemistry and Clinical Toxicology
- 872 Dental
- 874 Ear, Nose, and Throat
- 876 Gastroenterology and Urology
- 878 General and Plastic Surgery
- 880 General Hospital and Personal Use
- 864 Hematology and Pathology
- 866 Immunology and Microbiology
- 882 Neurology
- 884 Obstetrical and Gynecological
- 886 Ophthalmic
- 888 Orthopedic
- 890 Physical Medicine
- 892 Radiology

510(k) PREMARKET NOTIFICATION

The designation 510(k) refers to section 510(k) of the 1976 Medical Device Amendment Act.

Each company that wants to market Class I, II, and some III devices intended for human use in the United States must submit a 510(k) to the FDA at least 90 days before marketing unless the device is exempt from 510(k) requirements. There is no 510(k) form, but instead a format for the submission is described in 21 CFR 807.

A 510(k) is a premarketing submission made to the FDA to demonstrate that the device to be marketed is as safe and effective as—that is, SE—to a legally marketed device that is not subject to PMA. Applicants must compare their 510(k) device to one or more similar devices currently on the U.S. market and make and support their substantial equivalency claims. A legally marketed device is a device that was legally marketed before May 28, 1976 (preamendments device), a device that has been reclassified from Class III to Class II or I, a device that has been found to be SE to such a device through the 510(k) process, or a device established through the evaluation of automatic Class III definition. The legally marketed device to which equivalence is drawn is known as the predicate device.

Applicants must submit descriptive data and, when necessary, performance data to establish that their device is SE to a predicate device. Again, the data in a 510(k) is to show comparability (i.e., SE) of a new device to a predicate device. The data need not show superiority to the predicate device.

SUBSTANTIAL EQUIVALENCE

Unlike PMA, which requires demonstration of reasonable safety and effectiveness, 510(k) requires demonstration of SE. SE means that the new device is as safe and effective as the predicate device.

A device is SE if, in comparison to a predicate device, it

- Has the same intended use as the predicate device *and*
- Has the same technological characteristics as the predicate device *or*
- Has different technological characteristics that do not raise new questions of safety and effectiveness, and the sponsor demonstrates that the device is as safe and effective as the legally marketed device. A claim of SE does not mean the new and predicate devices must be identical. SE is established with respect to intended use, design, energy used or delivered, materials, performance, safety, effectiveness, labeling, biocompatibility, standards, and other applicable characteristics. Detailed information on how the FDA determines substantial equivalence can be found in the *Premarket Notification Review Program 6/30/86 (K86-3)* blue book memorandum.

Until the applicant receives an order declaring a device SE and a 501(k) clearance, he may not proceed to market the device. Once the device is determined to be SE, it can then be marketed in the United States. If the FDA determines that a device is *not* SE, the applicant may resubmit another 510(k) with new data, file a reclassification petition, or submit a PMA application. The SE determination is usually made within 90 days and is made based on the information submitted by the applicant.

PREMARKET APPROVAL SUBMISSION

PMA is the FDA process of scientific and regulatory review to evaluate the safety and effectiveness of Class III medical devices. Class III devices are those that support or sustain human life, are of substantial importance in preventing impairment of human health, or that present a potential, unreasonable risk of illness or injury. Because of the level of risk associated with Class III devices, the FDA has determined that general and special controls alone are insufficient to ensure the safety and effectiveness of Class III devices. Please note that some Class III preamendment devices may require a Class III 510(k). See the "Historical Background" section for additional information.

A PMA is the most stringent type of device marketing application required by the FDA. The applicant must receive FDA approval of its PMA application before marketing the device. PMA approval is based on a determination by the FDA that the PMA contains sufficient valid scientific evidence to ensure that the device is safe and effective for its intended use. An approved PMA is, in effect, a private license granting the applicant (or owner) permission to market the device.

The PMA applicant is usually the person who owns the rights, or otherwise has authorized access, to the data and other information to be submitted in support of FDA approval. This person may be an individual, partnership, corporation, association, scientific or academic establishment, government agency or organizational unit, or other legal entity. The applicant is often the inventor or developer and ultimately the manufacturer.

FDA regulations provide 180 days to review the PMA and make a determination. In reality, the review time is normally longer. Before approving or denying a PMA, the appropriate FDA advisory committee may review the PMA at a public meeting and provide the FDA with the committee's recommendation on whether the FDA should approve the submission. After the FDA notifies the applicant that the PMA has been approved or denied, a notice is published on the Internet (1) announcing the data on which the decision is based and (2) providing interested persons an opportunity to petition the FDA within 30 days for reconsideration of the decision.

The regulation governing premarket approval is located in 21 CFR 814, "Premarket Approval." A Class III device that fails to meet PMA requirements is considered to be adulterated under Section 501(f) of the FD&C Act and cannot be marketed.

INVESTIGATIONAL DEVICE EXEMPTION AND SUPPORTING STUDIES

An IDE allows the investigational device to be used in a clinical study to collect safety and effectiveness data required to support a PMA application or a premarket notification (510[k]) submission to the FDA. Clinical studies are most often conducted to support a PMA. Only a small percentage of 510(k)s require clinical data to support the application. Investigational use also includes clinical evaluation of certain modifications or new intended uses of legally marketed devices. All clinical evaluations of investigational devices, unless exempt, must have an approved IDE *before* the study is initiated, either from an institutional review board (IRB) for a nonsignificant risk device or an IRB and the FDA for a significant risk device.

Clinical evaluation of devices that have not been cleared for marketing requires the following:

- An IDE approved by an IRB. If the study involves a significant risk device, the IDE must also be approved by the FDA.
- Informed consent from all patients.
- Labeling for investigational use only.
- Monitoring of the study.
- Required records and reports.

An approved IDE permits a device to be shipped lawfully for the purpose of conducting investigations of the device without complying with other requirements of the FD&C that would apply to devices in commercial distribution. Sponsors need not submit a PMA or premarket notification 510(k), register their establishment, or list the device while the device is under investigation. Sponsors of IDEs are also exempt from the QSR except for the requirements for design control.

THIRD-PARTY SUBMISSION REVIEW BY ACCREDITED PARTIES

The purpose of the Accredited Persons Program is to conduct the initial review of 510(k)s for selected low- to moderate-risk devices to reduce workload and backlog. Thus, it enables the FDA to use its scientific review resources for higher-risk devices, while maintaining a high degree of confidence in the review of low- to moderate-risk devices, and it provides manufacturers of eligible devices an alternative review process that may yield more rapid 510(k) decisions.

Specifically, an accredited person may not review any Class III device, or Class II devices that are permanently implantable, life supporting, life sustaining, or for which clinical data are required. The FDA also sets limits on the number of Class II devices that may be ineligible for accredited person review because clinical data are required.

On September 23, 1998, the FDA published a list of persons accredited to conduct 510(k) reviews for certain devices, which is available at http://www.fda.gov/cdrh/thirdparty. Accredited persons were eligible to begin reviewing applications after they successfully completed a training session. On November 21, 1998, the agency began accepting 510(k) reviews from accredited persons and terminated the Third Party Review Pilot Program that began on August 1, 1996.

IMPORTING INTO THE UNITED STATES

Foreign manufacturers must meet applicable U.S. medical device regulations to import devices into the United States, even if the product is authorized for marketing in another country. These requirements include registration of establishment, listing of devices, manufacturing in accordance with the quality system regulation, medical device reporting (MDR) of adverse events, and premarket notification 510(k) or PMA, if applicable. In addition, the foreign manufacturers must designate a U.S. agent. As with domestic manufacturers, foreign manufacturing sites are subject to FDA inspection.

Initial Importers

An initial importer is any importer who furthers the marketing of a device from a foreign manufacturer to the person who makes the final delivery or sale of the device to the ultimate consumer or user, but who does not repackage or otherwise change the container, wrapper, or labeling of the device or device package. The initial importer of the device must register its establishment with the FDA. Registration information, including the registration form FDA-2891, can be found under "Establishment Registration" on the FDA website.

Initial importers are also subject to MDR under 21 CFR 803, "Reports of Corrections and Removals" under 21 CFR 806, and "Medical Device Tracking" under 21 CFR 821, if applicable. Under the MDR regulations, importers are required to report incidents in which a device may have caused or contributed to a death or serious injury, as well as report certain malfunctions. The importers must maintain an MDR event file for each adverse event. All product complaints (MDR and non-MDR events) must be forwarded to the manufacturer. Under medical device tracking requirements, certain devices must be tracked through the distribution chain.

EXPORTING DEVICES

Any medical device that is legally cleared or approved by the FDA in the United States may be exported anywhere in the world without prior FDA notification or approval. The export provisions of the FD&C only apply to unapproved devices. For a device to be legally in commercial distribution in the United States, the following requirements must be met:

- The manufacturing facility must be registered with the FDA on Form FDA-2891.
- The device must be listed on Form FDA-2892 with the FDA.
- The device must have a cleared premarket notification 510(k) or premarket approval unless exempted by regulation, or if the device was on the market before May 28, 1976 (before the medical device amendments to the FD&C).
- The device must meet the labeling requirements of 21 CFR 801 and 809, if applicable.
- The device must be manufactured in accordance with the QSR of 21 CFR 820 (also known as GMPs), unless exempted by regulation.

In addition, the U.S. exporter must comply with the laws of the importing country.

Certificates for Foreign Government

Although the FDA does not place any restrictions on the export of these devices, certain countries may require written certification that a firm or its devices are in compliance with U.S. law. In such instances, the FDA will accommodate U.S. firms by providing a certificate for foreign government (CFG). These export certifications were formerly referred to as a certificate for products for export or certificate of free sale. The CFG is a self-certification process that is used to speed the processing of requests. Original certificates will be provided on special counterfeit-resistant paper with an embossed gold foil seal.

As of May 2005, CDRH requires an initial fee of $175 per certificate and $15 per certificate for additional certificates issued for the same products in the same letter of request.

ADDITIONAL REGULATIONS BY DIFFERENT STATES

Each state should be contacted for its specific medical regulations; here is an example for California's FDB:

> The Food and Drug Branch (FDB) mission is to protect and improve the health of all California residents by ensuring that foods, drugs, medical devices, cosmetics, and certain other consumer products are safe and are not adulterated, misbranded, or falsely advertised, and that drugs and medical devices are effective.

- They accomplish their mission through sound investigations and inspections, based on valid scientific principles and specific legal authority, and effective industry and consumer education.
- They strive to regulate fairly and without unduly burdening California businesses.
- They do this by helping businesses understand the public health basis for regulatory requirements, encouraging businesses to voluntarily correct deficiencies, and uniformly enforcing regulatory requirements to prevent unfair competition.
- This success is crucial to the health of California residents and the economic vitality of the industries we regulate.

This discussion on basics applies to all medical devices and medical device companies in the United States.

SPECIAL CONSIDERATIONS

EXEMPTIONS FROM 510(K) AND GMP REQUIREMENTS

Class I Devices

The FDA has exempted almost all Class I devices with the exception of reserved devices from the premarket notification requirement, including those devices that were exempted by final regulation published in the *Federal Registers* of December 7, 1994, and January 16, 1996. It is important to confirm the exempt status and any limitations that apply with 21 CFR 862 to 892.

If a manufacturer's device falls into a generic category of exempted Class I devices, a premarket notification application and FDA clearance is not required before marketing the device in the United States. These manufacturers, however, are required to register their establishment by submitting Form FDA 2891, "Initial Registration of Device Establishment," and to list the generic category or classification name of the device by submitting Form FDA 2892, "Device Listing."

Class II Devices

The FDA has also published a list of Class II (special controls) devices, subject to certain limitations, that are now exempt from the premarket notification requirements under the FDAMA. The FDA believes that these exemptions will relieve manufacturers from the need to submit premarket notification submissions for these devices and will enable the FDA to redirect the resources that would be spent on reviewing such submissions to more significant public health issues. The FDA is taking this action to meet a requirement of the Modernization Act. Class II devices are annotated II. Please note that Class II devices are *not* exempt from GMP requirements.

SPECIAL 510(K)

Because design control requirements are now in effect and require the manufacturer to conduct verification and validation studies of a type that have traditionally been included in 510(k) submissions, the agency believes that it may be appropriate to forgo a detailed review of the underlying data normally required in 510(k)s. For this reason, the FDA is allowing an alternative to the traditional method of demonstrating substantial equivalence for certain device modifications. For these well-defined modifications, the agency believes that the rigorous design control procedure requirements produce highly reliable results that can form, in addition to the other 510(k) content requirements, a basis for the substantial equivalence determination. Under the QSR, data that are generated as a result of the design control procedures must be maintained by the manufacturer and be available for FDA inspection.

For a Special 510(k) submission, a manufacturer should refer to 21 CFR 807.81(a)(3) and the FDA guidance document entitled "Deciding When to Submit a 510(k) for a Change to an Existing Device" to decide whether a device modification may be implemented without submission of a new 510(k). If a new 510(k) is needed for the modification, and if the modification does not affect the intended use of the device or alter the fundamental scientific technology of the device, then summary information that results from the design control process can serve as the basis for clearing the application.

Thus, a manufacturer who is intending to modify his or her own legally marketed device will conduct the risk analysis and the necessary verification and validation activities to demonstrate that the design outputs of the modified device meet the design input requirements. Once the manufacturer has ensured the satisfactory completion of this process, a "Special 510(k): Device Modification" form may be submitted. Although the basic content requirements of the 510(k) (21 CFR 807.87) will remain the same, this type of submission should also reference the already cleared 510(k) number and contain a declaration of conformity with design control requirements. Refer to http://www.fda.gov/cdrh/ode/parad510.html for the contents of a "Special 510(k): Device Modification" form with a declaration of conformity to design controls.

ABBREVIATED 510(K)

Device manufacturers may choose to submit an abbreviated 510(k) when (1) guidance documents exist, (2) a special control has been established, or (3) the FDA has recognized a relevant consensus standard. An abbreviated 510(k) submission must include the required elements identified in 21 CFR 807.87. In addition, manufacturers submitting an abbreviated 510(k) that relies on a guidance document or special controls should include a summary report that describes how the guidance document or special controls were used during device development and testing. The summary report should include information regarding the manufacturer's efforts to conform to the guidance document or special controls and should outline any deviations. Persons submitting an abbreviated 510(k) that relies on a recognized standard should provide the necessary information and a declaration of conformity to the recognized standard. Such persons should also refer to the agency's guidance entitled "Guidance on the Recognition and Use of Consensus Standards." Although abbreviated submissions will compete with traditional 510(k) submissions, it is anticipated that their review will be more efficient than that of traditional submissions.

In an abbreviated 510(k), a manufacturer will also have the option of using a third party to assess conformance with the recognized standard. Under this scenario, the third party will perform a conformance assessment to the standard for the device manufacturer and should provide the manufacturer with a statement to this effect. Like a special 510(k), the application should include a declaration of conformity signed by the manufacturer, and the statement from the third party should be maintained in the device master record (DMR) pursuant to the QSR. Responsibility for conformance with the recognized standard, however, rests with the manufacturer, not the third party.

The incentive for manufacturers to elect to provide summary reports on the use of guidance documents or special controls or declarations of conformity to recognized standards will be an expedited review of their submissions.

DE NOVO

This provision, which is referred to as the evaluation of automatic Class III designation provision (also known as *de novo* or risk-based classification), is intended to apply to low-risk products that have been classified as Class III because they were found not substantially equivalent (NSE) to any identifiable predicate device.

Under this provision, within 30 days of receiving an NSE determination (which places the device into Class III), the person receiving the classification order may request that a risk-based classification determination be made for the device. The request must provide a description of the device and detailed information and reasons for any recommended classification. FDA will then classify the device.

Not later than 60 days after the date of the submission of such a request, the FDA must make a classification determination by written order, placing the device into one of the three statutory device classes. A device placed into Class I or II in this written order can then be commercially distributed. A device classified into Class III may not be marketed based on the classification order and will require an approved PMA or completed product development protocol (PDP) before commercial distribution can commence. Any clinical studies performed with a Class III device must be performed in accordance with an IDE. A device classified into Class I or II under this provision becomes a predicate device for future premarket notification submissions, which means that any manufacturer may show that a new device is SE to this predicate.

PRODUCT DEVELOPMENT PROTOCOL

In the PDP method for gaining marketing approval, the clinical evaluation of a device and the development of necessary information for marketing approval are merged into one regulatory mechanism. Ideal candidates for the PDP process are those devices in which the technology is well established in industry. The PDP process provides the manufacturer with the advantage of predictability once the agreement has been reached with the FDA.

The PDP allows a sponsor to come to early agreement with the FDA as to what would be done to demonstrate the safety and effectiveness of a new device. Early interaction in the development cycle of a device allows a sponsor to address the concerns of the FDA before expensive and time-consuming resources are expended.

The PDP is essentially a contract that describes the agreed-upon details of design and development activities, the outputs of these activities, and acceptance criteria for these outputs. It establishes reporting milestones that convey important data to the FDA as they are generated, where they can be reviewed and responded to in a timely manner. The sponsor would be able to execute its PDP at its own pace, keeping the FDA informed of its progress with these milestone reports. A PDP that has been declared completed by the FDA is considered to have an approved premarket approval.

HUMANITARIAN USE DEVICE/HUMANITARIAN DEVICE EXEMPTION

The regulation provides for the submission of a humanitarian device exemption (HDE) application, which is similar in both form and content to a premarket approval application, but it is exempt from the effectiveness requirements of a PMA. An HDE application is not required to contain the results of scientifically valid clinical investigations demonstrating that the device is effective for its intended purpose. The application, however, must contain sufficient information for the FDA to determine that the device does not pose an unreasonable or significant risk of illness or injury and that the probable benefit to health outweighs the risk of injury or illness from its use, taking into account the probable risks and benefits of currently available devices or alternative forms of treatment. Additionally, the applicant must demonstrate that no comparable devices are available to treat or diagnose the disease or condition and that they could not otherwise bring the device to market.

An approved HDE authorizes marketing of the humanitarian use device (HUD). However, an HUD may only be used after IRB approval has been obtained for the use of the device for the FDA-approved indication. The labeling for an HUD must state that the device is an HUD and that although the device is authorized by federal law, the effectiveness of the device for the specific indication has not been demonstrated.

The above discussion on special considerations and methodology applies only in exceptional circumstances.

GOOD QUALITY AND PROCEDURAL PRACTICES

QUALITY SYSTEM REGULATIONS

The current GMP (or sometimes referred to as cGMP) requirements set forth in the QSR require that domestic or foreign manufacturers have a quality system for the design, manufacture, packaging, labeling, storage, installation, and servicing of finished medical devices intended for commercial distribution in the United States. The regulation requires that various specifications and controls be established for devices; that devices be designed under a quality system to meet these specifications; that devices be manufactured under a quality system; that finished devices meet these specifications; that devices be correctly installed, checked, and serviced; that quality data be analyzed to identify and correct quality problems; and that complaints be processed.

Thus, the QSR helps ensure that medical devices are safe and effective for their intended use. The FDA monitors device problem data and inspects the operations and records of device developers and manufacturers to determine compliance with the GMP requirements in the QSR. The QSR is contained in Title 21 CFR 820. The "Good Manufacturing Practice (GMP)/Quality System Regulation" page has a link to the *Medical Device Quality Systems Manual: A Small Entity Compliance Guide*, which details the requirements of the new QSR and provides detailed guidance in the following areas.

QUALITY SYSTEM INSPECTION TECHNIQUE

The Quality System Inspection Technique (QSIT) guide was prepared by the ORA and the CDRH. It provides guidance to the FDA field staff for inspecting medical device manufacturers against the Quality System Regulation (21 CFR 820) and related regulations. It serves as a guide for a company to prepare for a site inspection by the FDA. Field investigators may conduct an efficient and effective comprehensive inspection using this guidance material, which will help them focus on key elements of a firm's quality system.

This process for inspections is based on a top-down approach to inspecting. The subsystem approach is designed to provide the key objectives that can help determine a firm's state of compliance. The process was designed to account for the time constraints placed on field investigators when performing device quality system inspections.

GOOD CLINICAL PRACTICE

Good clinical practice (GCP) is a standard for the design, conduct, performance, monitoring, auditing, recording, analysis, and reporting of clinical trials. It is composed of the regulations and requirements that must be complied with while conducting a clinical study. Specifically, these regulations apply to the manufacturers, sponsors, clinical investigators, institutional review boards, and medical devices. The primary regulations that govern the conduct of clinical studies are included in 21 CFR:

21 CFR 812, "Investigational Device Exemptions," covers the procedures for the conduct of clinical studies with medical devices, including application, responsibilities of sponsors and investigators, labeling, records, and reports.
21 CFR 50, "Protection of Human Subjects," provides the requirements and general elements of informed consent.
21 CFR 56, "Institutional Review Boards," covers the procedures and responsibilities for an IRB that approves clinical investigations protocols.
21 CFR 54, "Financial Disclosure by Clinical Investigators," covers the disclosure of financial compensation to clinical investigators that are part of the FDA's assessment of the reliability of the clinical data.
21 CFR 820 Subpart C, "Design Controls of the Quality System Regulation," provides the requirement for procedures to control the design of the device to ensure that the specified design requirements are met.

GOOD LABORATORY PRACTICES

Good laboratory practices (GLP) under 21 CFR 58 apply to nonclinical laboratory studies (safety studies) that are intended to support applications for research and marketing permits, including IDE and PMA applications. Compliance with this part is intended to ensure the quality and integrity of safety data obtained from studies such as animal studies submitted to the FDA.

If information on nonclinical laboratory studies is provided in the IDE application as part of the report of prior investigations, a statement that all such studies have been conducted in compliance with applicable requirements in the good laboratory practice regulations in Part 58 must be provided. If any study was not conducted in compliance with the GLP regulations, a brief statement of the reason for the noncompliance must be provided.

Regulations

21 CFR 58, "Good Laboratory Practice for Nonclinical Laboratory Studies," http://www.accessdata.fda.gov/scripts/cdrh/cfdocs/cfcfr/showCFR.cfm/CFRPart = 58.

PRECLINICAL STUDIES

Preclinical studies are conducted primarily for safety purposes, although they can show effectiveness in a nonclinical setting. There are two major categories of preclinical studies: in vitro (bench top) and in vivo (animal model or cadavers). In vitro studies can utilize excised tissue and organs, or just use simulated equipment to demonstrate effects. In vivo studies may either be GLP or non-GLP.

There is a third type of study, which is not utilized very often but is still allowed to demonstrate safety: non-IDE, outside-the-U.S. human studies. As may be seen from the introductory section, every country has its own regulatory requirements.

This section is the most important for demonstrating that a device has been designed to be effective and safe. It also describes procedures that will ensure continued good quality, reliability, and cost-effectiveness (good quality is free).

SUMMARY OF TITLE 21 OF THE CODE OF FEDERAL REGULATIONS, PARTS 800 TO 1299, FOR MEDICAL DEVICES

Note: This summary is intended only as an overview because only highlights of the sections have been discussed. Answers to specific questions and detailed information should be obtained directly from Title 21 of the CFR, or online at http://www.fda.gov/cdrh.

PART 800: GENERAL REQUIREMENTS

This part of the CFR describes requirements for specific medical devices (Subpart B) and administrative practices and procedures (Subpart C).

Subpart A: Reserved for the FDA's future use
Subpart B: Requirements for specific medical devices

1. Contact lens solutions
2. Patient examination gloves and surgical gloves, sample plans and test method for leakage defects (due to great demand for examination and surgical gloves)

Subpart C: Administrative practices and procedures
Administrative detention of device that is considered altered or mishandled during an FDA audit:
1. A written detention order is given that the devices are not used, moved, or tampered with during the detention period (maximum 20 days unless extended). A detention order may be appealed and a hearing requested. Records of the detention order and the release must be retained by the company for at least 2 years.

PART 801: LABELING

Subpart A: General provisions
1. Name and place of business or manufacturer, packer, or distributor. The name shall be qualified by a phrase that describes the connection with the device, such as "manufactured for," "distributed by," or any other expression of the facts.
2. Similar phrases may be used, such as "indication" or "intended for" to describe the intended use. *Caution*: Any representation of a device to be used for something other than its approved intended use, including misleading statements, is considered misbranding and may result in recall and fines.
3. Directions must be adequate so that a layman can use a device safely and for the purpose for which it was intended, even though the device is intended to be used by a skilled practitioner.
4. Misleading statements can be considered misbranding, a serious offense.
5. Labeling must be readable. This requirement, as anyone who has struggled to read the fine print on a label can attest, is difficult to fulfill because of all the information that sometimes is required to be added to the labeling. The simplest way to meet this requirement is to have a package insert.
6. For distribution in the Commonwealth of Puerto Rico, labels must be in Spanish.
7. The label that is most prominent in an over-the-counter device must display the principal feature of the device in bold.
8. The most prominent part of the label must report the contents of the package.

Subpart B: Reserved
Subpart C: Labeling requirements for over-the-counter devices
1. The panel to be displayed, the principal display panel, must be large enough to accommodate all mandatory information.

Regulatory Affairs

2. The most prominent part of the label must have a statement of identity.
3. There must be a declaration of net quantity of contents.
4. The label must contain a warning if the device contains any ozone-depleting substances.

Subpart D: Exemption from adequate direction for use
Specific direction for use may be exempted from placement on a label if the device requires a unique skill set for use, such as a physician, dentist, or any other licensed practitioner. In that case, the following wording must be applied to the label: "Caution: Federal law restricts this device to sale by or on the order of a healthcare professional (physician, dentist, etc.)."

Subpart E: Other exemptions
Medical devices, processing, labeling, or repackaging exemptions are discussed.

Subparts F and G: Reserved

Subpart H: Special requirements for specific devices
Requirements for impact resistant lenses, maximum levels of ozone and chlorofluorocarbon propellants, hearing aids, menstrual tampons, latex, and natural rubber products are discussed.

PART 803: MEDICAL DEVICE REPORTING (MDR)

Subpart A: General procedures
1. Device user facilities, importers, and manufacturers must report to the FDA deaths and serious injuries to which a device has or may have caused or contributed. Also, files must be established and maintained for adverse events, including device malfunctions. Specific follow-up and summary reports must be submitted to the FDA.
2. These reports must be available to the public.
3. Reports must follow the instructions and format outlined in CFR Sections 803.10 through 803.11. Further instructions concerning reports are contained in CFR Sections 803.12 through 803.19.

Subpart B: Generally applicable requirements for individual adverse event reports
1. Medwatch forms described in Section 803.20 must be used, including reporting codes in CFR Section 803.21.
2. User facilities must submit an MDR report to device manufacture and the FDA within 10 days.
3. Importers must submit reports to the manufacturer and the FDA within 30 days.
4. Manufacturers are required to submit MDR reports to the FDA within 30 days.
5. Manufacturers are required to submit MDRs within 5 days if there are indications (e.g., trend analysis) that necessitate remedial action or if the FDA has made a written request for a 5-day reporting.

Subpart C: User facility reporting requirements
1. The user facility has 10 days to report to the FDA on Form 3500A.
2. Detailed information in Form 3500A is described in CFR Section 803.32 for individual adverse event report data elements.
3. Annual reports must be written and submitted to the FDA.

Subpart D: Importer reporting requirements
1. Importer must file FDA Form 3500A within 30 days of the event.
2. Detailed information needed for Form 3500A is given in CFR Section 803.42.

Subpart E: Manufacturer reporting requirements
1. Manufacturers must file Form 3500A within 30 days.
2. Detailed information is given in CFR Section 803.52.
3. Reports, which require 5 days for notification, are described in Subpart B above.
4. A manufacturer must submit an annual baseline report on FDA Form 3417 or its electronic equivalent.
5. Supplemental reports must be submitted if information was not known or was not available when the initial report was written.
6. Foreign manufacturer: Every foreign manufacturer must designate a U.S. agent to be responsible for reporting MDRs. The manufacturer has 5 days to report a change of the designated agent.

PART 806: MEDICAL DEVICES: REPORTS OF CORRECTIONS AND REMOVALS

Subpart A: General provisions
1. Manufacturers and importers must maintain records of all corrections and removals whether they are required to be reported to the FDA or not.
2. Exemptions to reporting requirements that may improve the performance or quality but do not reduce risk to health are listed below:
   - Market withdrawals
   - Routine servicing
   - Stock recoveries

Subpart B: Reports and records
1. Information to be reported is described in Section 806.10 of CFR.
2. Detailed records must be kept of all corrections and removals that need not be reported to the FDA, as well as those that must be reported.
3. All reports that were submitted to the FDA are available to the public after personnel and trade secret information is removed.

PART 807: ESTABLISHMENT REGISTRATION AND DEVICE LISTING FOR MANUFACTURER AND INDIVIDUAL IMPORTERS OF DEVICES

Note: Only frequently addressed definitions are listed here. See CFR 807 for additional definitions.

Regulatory Affairs

Subpart A: General provisions
1. **Commercial distribution**: Distribution of any device intended for human use.
2. **Establishment**: Place of business under one management at one general physical location at which a device is manufactured, assembled, or processed.
3. **Manufacturer**: Place where preparation, propagation, compounding, assembly, processing or repackaging, importation, or initiation of specification for manufacturing of a device occurs.
4. **Official correspondent**: Person designated by operator of establishment to correspond with the FDA.
5. **Classification name**: Term used by panel to describe the device.
6. **510(k) summary**: Summary of information regarding safety and effectiveness of device described in 510(k).
7. **510(k) statement**: Statement made in 510(k) that all safety and effectiveness data will be made available within 30 days of the request.

Subpart B: Procedure for device establishment
1. All owners or operators of an establishment, which is not designated exempt (see Subpart B below), engaged in the manufacture of a device intended for human use shall register with the FDA, Form 2891. Annual registration is done with Form 2891A.
2. Listing must be within 30 days of the time of first manufacture, repackaging of the final device design.
3. Initial listing of each device for sale must be done on a separate Form 2892 sheet.
4. Exact information required for registration may be seen in CFR Section 807.35.
5. See Sections 807.26 through 807.37 for discussions on amendments, updating, notification, and inspection of registrations.
6. Establishment or device registration does not in any way denote approval or clearance of the establishment or products.

Subpart C: Registration procedure for foreign device establishments
1. An establishment within any foreign country engaged in manufacturing a medical device for sale in the United States must register with the FDA. All information shall be in English.
2. All imported devices must be listed with the FDA. All information shall be in English.
3. Each foreign establishment must appoint a U.S. agent who maintains a place of business in the United States. Any changes in agent must be reported within 10 days to the FDA.
4. All imported devices must go through appropriate FDA regulation clearances or approvals before sale in the United States.
5. This restriction does not apply to devices imported for investigative use (IDE; see CFR 812).

Subpart D: Exemptions
   Subcontractors, veterinary devices, general-purpose chemical and laboratory equipment, licensed practitioners, and others are exempted per CFR Section 807.65.

Subpart E: Premarket notification procedure (510[k])
1. All devices that require a premarket notification must have one submitted 90 days prior to introduction of it is for commercial distribution. Commercial distribution or sale cannot start until the FDA clears the premarket notification.
2. A device is exempt from premarket notification if it
   - Is listed by the FDA as an exempt device classification
   - Was in commercial distribution before May 28, 1976
   - Requires a premarket approval (PMA)
3. A list of information required in a premarket notification submission is given in CFR Section 807.87. The format of a premarket submission, the content and format of 510(k) summary, and the 510(k) statement are given in Sections 807.90, 807.92, and 807.93, respectively, or can be found on the FDA website.
4. Substantial equivalence to a device already cleared for sale must be demonstrated. Confidentiality of information can be obtained.
5. Any representation that the FDA has approved a 510(k) cleared device is considered misbranding.
6. After the premarket notification is reviewed, the FDA can
   - Issue an order that the device is SE and clear it
   - Issue an order that it is NSE
   - Request additional information
   - Advise the applicant that a 510(k) is not necessary

Part 808: Exemptions from Federal Preemption of State and Local Medical Device Requirements

Subpart A: General provisions
   This section contains special provisions governing the regulation of devices by states and localities.

Subpart B: Exemption procedures
   An exemption may only be granted for a requirement that has been enacted by a state.

Subpart C: Listing of specific state and local exemptions
   See CFR Section 808.53 for specific exemptions for different states.

Part 809: In Vitro Diagnostic Products for Human Use

Subpart A: General provision
1. In vitro diagnostic products are the reagents, instruments, and systems intended for use in the diagnosis of disease or other conditions.
2. Product class relates to all products intended for use for a particular determination with common or related use.

Subpart B: Labeling
1. Labels shall in general state proprietary name and intended use, name and place of business or manufacture, and a warning statement: "For in vitro diagnostic use."
2. Labels for reagents shall also state quantity, concentration of reactive ingredients, source for biological material, date of manufacture and required storage conditions, expiration date, lot number, and statement of an observable alteration or degradation of the product.
3. For additional required label information, see CFR 809.10.

Subpart C: Requirements for manufacturers and producers
1. In vitro diagnostic products shall be manufactured in accordance with the good manufacturing practice requirements found in the section on Part 820 in this chapter.
2. Analyzed specific reagents (ASRs) are restricted to be sold to
   - In vitro diagnostic manufacturers
   - Clinical laboratories
   - Facilities where sample testing is performed in a laboratory, using screening tests recognized by the Food and Drug Administration

PART 810: MEDICAL DEVICE RECALL AUTHORITY

Subpart A: General provisions (definitions)
1. **Cease distribution and notification strategy or mandatory recall strategy:** A planned, specific course of action to be taken by the person named in a cease distribution and notification order or in a mandatory recall order.
2. **Consignee:** Any person or firm that has received, purchased, or used a device that is subject to a cease distribution.
3. **Correction:** Repair, modification, adjustment, relabeling, destruction, or inspection (including patient monitoring) of a device, without its physical removal from its point of use to some other location.
4. **Device user facility:** A hospital, ambulatory surgical facility, nursing home, or outpatient treatment or diagnostic facility that is not a physician's office.
5. **Health professionals:** Practitioners that have a role in using a device for human use.
6. **Reasonable probability:** That it is more likely than not that an event will occur.
7. **Serious, adverse health consequence:** Any significant adverse experience.
8. **Recall:** The correction or removal of a device for human use in cases in which the FDA finds that there is a reasonable probability that the device would cause serious, adverse health consequences, or death.
9. **Removal:** The physical removal of a device from its point of use to some other location.

Subpart B: Mandatory medical device recall procedures
Cease distribution and notification order
If, after providing the appropriate person with an opportunity to consult with the agency, the FDA finds that there is a reasonable probability that a device intended for human use would cause serious adverse health consequences or death, the agency may issue a cease distribution and notification order.
Regulatory hearing
1. Any request for a regulatory hearing shall be submitted in writing to the agency employee identified in the order within the time frame specified by the FDA.
2. In lieu of requesting a regulatory hearing under 810.11, the person named in a cease distribution and notification order may submit a written request to the FDA asking that the order be modified or vacated.
3. If a person named in a cease distribution and notification order does not request a regulatory hearing or submit a request for agency review of the order, the FDA shall amend the order to require such a recall.

Cease distribution notification or mandatory recall strategy
The person named in a cease distribution and notification order issued under paragraph 810.10 CFR shall comply with the order and develop a recall strategy that meets all requirements of this section.

Communications concerning a cease distribution and notification or mandatory recall order
1. The person named in a cease distribution and notification order may request termination of the order by submitting a written request to the FDA.
2. The agency will make available to the public in the weekly *FDA Enforcement Report* a descriptive listing of each new mandatory recall.

PART 812: INVESTIGATIONAL DEVICE EXEMPTIONS

Subpart A: General provisions
1. The purpose of this part is to encourage the discovery and development of useful devices intended for human use.
2. This part applies to all clinical investigations of a device to determine safety and effectiveness.
3. An investigation of a device, other than a significant risk device, may be started by obtaining IRB approval.
4. A brief explanation of why the device is not a significant risk device must be presented to the IRB.

Definitions
1. **Custom device:** A device that necessarily deviates from devices generally available or from an applicable performance standard or premarket approval requirement and is not offered for commercial distribution through labeling or advertising.

2. **Implant:** A device that is placed into a surgically or naturally formed cavity of the human body.
3. **Institution:** A person, other than an individual, who engages in the conduct of research on subjects or in the delivery of medical services.
4. **Institutional review board (IRB):** Any board, committee, or other group formally designated by an institution to review biomedical research involving subjects and established, operated, and functioning in conformance with CFR 56.
5. **Investigator:** An individual who actually conducts a clinical investigation, that is, under whose immediate direction the test article is administered or dispensed.
6. **Principal investigator:** An individual who is responsible for designing and coordinating all studies conducted by investigators.
7. **Monitor:** An individual designated by a sponsor or contract research organization to oversee the progress of an investigation.
8. **Noninvasive:** One that does not by design or intention penetrate or pierce the skin, mucous membranes, or body.
9. **Significant risk device:** Investigational device that is intended as an implant, is purported or represented to be for use in supporting or sustaining human life, or presents a potential for serious risk to the health, safety, or welfare of a subject.
10. **Sponsor:** A person who initiates a study, but who does not actually conduct the investigation.
11. **Sponsor-investigator:** An individual who both initiates and actually conducts an investigation.
12. **Transitional device:** A device subject to Section 520(1) of the Act, that is, a device that the FDA considered to be a new drug or an antibiotic drug before May 28, 1976.
13. **Unanticipated adverse device effect:** Any serious adverse effect on health or safety, or any life-threatening problem or death caused by, or associated with, a device, or a death that was not previously identified in nature, severity, or degree of incidence in the investigational plan.

Labeling and promotion
1. An investigational device or its immediate package shall bear a label with the following information: the name and place of business and "CAUTION: Investigational device. Limited by Federal (or United States) law to investigational use."
2. Devices for animal research shall bear the label "CAUTION: Device for investigational use in laboratory animals or other tests that do not involve human subjects."
3. A sponsor, investigator, or any person acting for or on behalf of a sponsor or investigator shall not
   - Promote or test market an investigational device until after the FDA has approved the device for commercial distribution

- Commercialize an investigational device by charging the subjects or investigators for a device a price larger than that necessary to recover costs of manufacture, research, development, and handling

Address for IDE correspondence

On the outside wrapper of each submission, the purpose of the submission must be stated. For example, an "IDE application," a "supplemental IDE application," or a "correspondence concerning an IDE (or an IDE application)."

Subpart B: Application and Administrative Action
1. A sponsor shall submit an application to the FDA if the sponsor intends to use a significant risk device in an investigation.
2. A sponsor shall not begin an investigation until the FDA has approved the application.

Investigational plan

The investigational plan shall include, in the following order:
- Protocol
- Risk analysis
- Description of device
- Monitoring procedures
- Consent materials
- IRB information
- Other institutions
- Additional records and reports

Report of prior investigations
1. The report of prior investigations shall include reports of all prior clinical, animal, and laboratory testing of the device and shall be comprehensive and adequate to justify the proposed investigation.
2. The FDA will notify the sponsor in writing of the date it receives an application. An investigation may not begin until 30 days after the FDA receives the application and approves it.

Supplemental applications
1. A sponsor must obtain approval of a supplemental application.
2. A device under clinical investigation may be used in the treatment of patients not in the trial under the provision of a treatment IDE for desperately ill patients.
3. The FDA will not disclose the existence of an IDE unless its existence has previously been publicly disclosed or acknowledged.

Subpart C: Responsibilities of sponsors
1. A sponsor is responsible for selecting qualified investigators and providing them with the information they need to conduct the investigation properly, ensuring proper monitoring of the investigation, ensuring that IRB review and approval are obtained, submitting an IDE application to FDA, and ensuring that any reviewing IRB and the FDA are promptly informed of significant new information.

Regulatory Affairs

2. A sponsor shall not begin an investigation or part of an investigation until both an IRB and the FDA have approved the application or supplemental application relating to the investigation or part of an investigation.
3. A sponsor shall select investigators qualified by training or experience to investigate the device.
4. A sponsor shall ship investigational devices only to qualified investigators participating in the investigation.
5. A sponsor shall obtain a signed agreement from each participating investigator.

Subpart D: IRB review and approval
An IRB shall review and have authority to approve, require modification (to secure approval), or disapprove all investigations.

Subpart E: Responsibilities of investigators
1. An investigator is responsible for ensuring that an investigation is conducted according to the signed agreement, the investigational plan, and applicable FDA regulations, for protecting rights, safety, and welfare, and for the control of devices under investigation.
2. If the FDA has information indicating that an investigator has repeatedly or deliberately failed to comply with the requirements of this part, it will furnish the investigator written notice of the matter.

Subpart F: Reserved

Subpart G: Records and Reports

Records
A participating investigator shall maintain accurate, complete, and current records relating to the investigator's participation in an investigation.

Inspections
A sponsor or an investigator who has authority to grant access to a facility shall permit authorized FDA employees to inspect any establishment.

Reports
An investigator shall prepare and submit any of the following applicable reports in a complete, accurate, and timely manner:
- Unanticipated adverse device effects
- Withdrawal of IRB approval
- Progress
- Deviations from the investigation
- Informed consent from patient
- Final report

This part applies to any Class III medical device whether it is new and has not been classified (automatically Class III) or has been designated Class III by the FDA.

Definitions
1. **Master file:** A reference source that a person submits to the FDA. A master file may contain detailed information on a specific manufacturing

facility, process, methodology, or component used in the manufacture, processing, or packaging of a medical device.
2. **PMA:** Any premarket approval application for a Class III medical device, including all information submitted with or incorporated by reference therein.
3. **PMA amendment:** Information an applicant submits to the FDA to modify a pending PMA or a pending PMA supplement.
4. **PMA supplement:** A supplemental application to an approved PMA.
5. **Thirty-day PMA supplement:** A supplemental application to an approved PMA in accordance with paragraph 814.39(e).
6. **Serious, adverse health consequences:** Any significant adverse experience, including those that may be either life threatening or involve permanent or long-term injuries.
7. **HDE:** A humane device exemption to a premarket approval.

Confidentiality of data and information in a PMA file
A PMA file includes all data and information submitted with the PMA, any IDE incorporated into the PMA, any PMA supplement, any report, any master file, or any other PMA-related submission and is considered confidential.

Research conducted outside the United States
A study conducted outside the United States submitted in support of a PMA and conducted under an IDE shall comply with Part 812 (IDE requirements).

Product development protocol (PDP)
A Class III device for which the FDA has declared a PDP completed under this chapter will be considered to have an approved PMA. (*Note*: PDP was discussed in the "Special Considerations" section of this chapter.)

Subpart B: Premarket approval application (PMA)

Note: This list contains only important items and is not intended to be exhaustive. Additional information may be obtained from the web address at the end of the section.

1. The applicant or an authorized representative shall sign the PMA.
2. A table of contents that specifies the volume and page number for each item referred to in the table.
3. A summary in sufficient detail that the reader may gain a general understanding of the data and information in the application.
4. A general description of the disease or condition the device will diagnose, treat, prevent, cure, or mitigate, including a description of the patient population for which the device is intended.
5. An explanation of how the device functions and the basic scientific concepts that form the basis for the device.
6. A description of existing alternative practices or procedures for diagnosing, treating, preventing, curing, or mitigating the disease or condition.

Regulatory Affairs

7. A brief description of the foreign and U.S. marketing history of the device, if any.
8. An abstract of any information or report described in the PMA.
9. A summary of the nonclinical laboratory studies submitted in the application.
10. A summary of the clinical investigation.
11. Conclusions drawn from the studies.
12. A complete description of the following:
    - The device
    - Each of the functional components
    - The properties of the device
    - The principles of operation
    - The method used
    - Reference to any performance standard
    - Adequate information to demonstrate how the device meets, or justification of any deviation from any performance standards
    - Any deviation from a voluntary standard
    - A section containing results of the nonclinical laboratory studies with the device, including microbiological, toxicological, immunological, and biocompatibility tests
    - A section containing results of the clinical investigations involving human subjects with the device, including clinical protocols, number of investigators, and subjects per investigator
    - A statement with respect to each study that it was conducted in compliance with the institutional review board regulations
    - A statement that each study was conducted in compliance with Part 812 (IDE section) or Part 814 (PMA section) concerning sponsors of clinical investigations and clinical investigators
    - For a PMA supported solely by data from one investigation, a justification showing that data and other information from a single investigator are sufficient
    - A bibliography of all published reports, whether adverse or supportive, known to the applicant
    - One or more samples of the device and its components
    - Copies of all proposed labeling for the device
    - An environmental assessment
    - A financial certification or disclosure statement
    - Periodical updates of the device's pending application

The FDA has issued a PMA guidance document to assist the applicant in the arrangement and content of a PMA. This guidance document is available at http://www.fda.gov/cdrh/dsma/pmaman/front.html.

PMA amendments and resubmitted PMAs
- An applicant may amend a pending PMA or PMA supplement to revise existing information or provide additional information.
- After the FDA's approval of a PMA, an applicant shall submit a PMA supplement for review and approval by the FDA before making a

change affecting the safety or effectiveness of the device for which the applicant has an approved PMA.

Subpart C: FDA action on a PMA
Time frames for reviewing a PMA
Within 180 days of receipt of an application that is accepted for filing, the FDA will review the PMA and, after receiving appropriate FDA advisory committee input, send the applicant a reply.
Subpart D: Administrative review (reserved)
Subpart E: Postapproval requirements
The FDA may require postapproval requirements as part of the PMA approval.
Subpart F: Reserved
Subpart G: Reserved
Subpart H: HDE amendment and resubmitted HDEs
If the FDA requests an HDE applicant to submit an HDE amendment and a written response to the FDA's request is not received within 75 days of the date of the request, the FDA will consider the pending HDE or HDE supplement to be withdrawn voluntarily by the applicant.

PART 820: QUALITY SYSTEM REGULATION

Subpart A: General provision
1. Current good manufacturing practice (cGMP): Requirements are set forth in this Quality System Regulation (QSR). The requirements in this part govern the methods, facilities, and controls used for the design, manufacture, packaging, labeling, storage, installation, and servicing of all finished devices intended for human use.
2. **Foreign manufacturers:** If a manufacturer who offers devices for import into the United Sates refuses to permit or allow the completion of an FDA inspection of the foreign facility for the purpose of determining compliance with cGMP, then the devices manufactured at that facility are considered adulterated under Section 501(h) of the act.
3. **Quality system:** Each manufacturer shall establish and maintain a quality system.

Subpart B: Quality system requirements
Management responsibility
1. Quality policy: Management with executive responsibility shall establish its policy, objectives, and commitments to quality. Management with executive responsibility shall ensure that the quality policy is understood, implemented, and maintained at all levels of the organization. Specifically, the management shall describe the following:
   - Quality policy
   - Organization
   - Responsibility and authority
   - Resources

- Management representative
- Management review
- Quality planning
- Quality system procedures
2. Each manufacturer shall establish a quality audit procedure and perform audits.
3. Each manufacturer shall have sufficient personnel with necessary education to operate the facility.

Subpart C: Design controls
Design controls must include the following:
- Design and development planning
- Design input
- Design review
- Design output
- Design verification
- Design validation
- Design transfer
- Design changes
- Design history file

Subpart D: Document controls
Each manufacturer shall establish and maintain a document control function.

Subpart E: Purchasing controls
Each manufacturer shall establish and maintain a purchasing control function.

Subpart F: Identification and traceability
Each manufacturer shall establish and maintain manufacturing traceability.

Subpart G: Production and process controls
The following information must be in place:
- Instruction documents
- Monitoring and process control
- Compliance with specified reference standards or codes
- The qualification of process and process equipment
- Criteria for workmanship that shall be expressed in documented standards
- Production and process changes
- Environmental control
- Personnel records
- Building records
- Equipment records
- Maintenance schedule
- Inspection records
- Adjustment records
- Manufacturing material description
- Automated processes description
- Control of inspection, measuring, and test equipment
- Process validation records

Subpart H: Acceptance activities
- Receiving, in-process, and finished device acceptance logs must be available.
- Acceptance status records must be complete.

Subpart I: Nonconforming product (NCP)
An NCP shall be controlled and isolated.

Subpart J: Corrective and preventive action (CPA)
CPA procedure records must be up-to-date.

Subpart K: Labeling and packaging control
Control must include the following:
- Label integrity
- Labeling inspection
- Labeling storage
- Labeling operations
- Control number

Subpart L: Handling, storage, distribution, and installation
A procedure must be in place before manufacturing begins.

Subpart M: Records
- Design history file
- Device master record
- Device history record
- Quality system record
- Complaint files

Subpart N: Servicing
If servicing is specified, procedures must be in place.

Subpart O: Statistical techniques
Applicable statistical techniques must be in place to cover:
- Statistical process control
- Sampling plans

PART 821: MEDICAL DEVICE TRACKING REQUIREMENTS

Subpart A: General provisions
- Manufacturer must have a tracking system.
- Manufacturing must define exemptions and variances.
- Serious adverse health consequences must be tracked.
- Life-supporting or life-sustaining device used outside a device user facility must be traceable.

Subpart B: Tracking requirements
A manufacturer of any Class II or III device must track that device in accordance with this part.

A manufacturer of a tracked device shall adopt a method of tracking that allows information to be provided to the FDA within 3 days, with the name, address, and telephone number of the distributor, multiple distributors, or final distributor holding the device for distribution and the location of the device.

Furthermore, within 10 days of a request from the FDA for tracked devices that are intended for use by a single patient over the life of the device, after distribution to or implantation in a patient, the following is required:

1. The lot number, batch number, model number, or serial number of the device
2. The date the device was shipped by the manufacturer
3. The name, address, telephone number, and social security number (if available) of the patient receiving the device
4. The date the device was provided to the patient

Also, a manufacturer of a tracked device shall establish a written standard operating procedure for the collection, maintenance, and auditing of the data.

Subpart C: Additional requirements and responsibilities

A distributor must promptly provide the manufacturer tracking the device with the following information:

- Name and address of the distributor
- Lot number, batch number, model number, or serial number of the device
- Date the device was received
- Person from whom the device was received
- Final distributor, upon sale or other distribution of a tracked device

Subpart D: Records and inspection

Manufacturers, distributors, multiple distributors, and final distributors shall, upon the presentation by an FDA representative of official credentials and the issuance of Form 482, make all records and information required to be collected and maintained under this part, and all records and information related to the events and persons identified in such records, available to FDA personnel. Records under this part shall be maintained for the useful life of each tracked device that is manufactured or distributed.

PART 822: POSTMARKET SURVEILLANCE

Subpart A: General provisions

This part provides procedures and requirements for postmarket surveillance of Class II and III devices that meet any of the following criteria:

1. Failure of the device would be reasonably likely to have serious adverse consequences.
2. The device is intended to be implanted in the human body for more than one year.
3. The device is intended to be used outside a user facility to support or sustain life.

Subpart B: Notification
- The FDA will notify in writing the company that is required to conduct postmarketing surveillance.
- If the company does not agree with the surveillance requirements, a review of the order may be requested.

Subpart C: Postmarket surveillance plan
A plan must be submitted within 30 days of the date you receive the postmarket surveillance order. The submission must include the following:
1. Organizational and administrative information
2. Your name and address
3. Generic and trade names of your device
4. Name and address of the contact person for the submission
5. Table of contents identifying the page numbers for each section of the submission
6. Subscription of the device
7. Product codes and a list of all relevant model numbers
8. Indications for use and claims for the device
9. Postmarket surveillance plan

If the company stops marketing the device subject to postmarket surveillance, it must continue to conduct postmarket surveillance in accordance with its approved plan even if it no longer markets the device.

Subpart D: FDA review and action
The FDA will determine whether the surveillance report is complete and notify the company.

Subpart E: Responsibilities of manufacturers
1. If the company changes ownership, the new owners must continue the surveillance plan.
2. If the company goes out of business, the FDA must be notified within 30 days, and the method by which the surveillance is continued should be discussed with the FDA.
3. If the company stops marketing the device subject to postmarket surveillance, it must continue surveillance in accordance with an approved plan.

Subpart F: Waivers and exemptions
Waivers may be requested for any specific requirement.

Subpart G: Records and reports
All correspondence with your investigators or the FDA must be kept for a minimum of two years, including the following:
1. Signed agreements from each of your investigators
2. Your approved postmarket surveillance plan
3. All data collected and analyses conducted in support of your postmarket surveillance plan
4. Any other records that the FDA requires to be maintained by regulation or by order

Regulatory Affairs

PART 860: MEDICAL DEVICE CLASSIFICATION PROCEDURES

Subpart A: General
1. **Class I:** The class of devices that are subject to only the general controls.
2. **Class II:** The class of devices that are or eventually will be subject to special controls.
3. **Class III:** The class of devices for which premarket approval is or will be required. A device is in Class III if insufficient information exists to determine that general controls are sufficient to provide reasonable assurance of its safety and effectiveness.

The classification panels, in reviewing evidence concerning the safety and effectiveness of a device, will consider the following:
- The persons for whose use the device is represented or intended
- The conditions of use for the device
- The probable benefit to health
- The reliability of the device

Subpart B: Classification
1. This subpart sets forth the procedures for the original classification of distribution before May 28, 1976, or is substantially equivalent to a device that was in commercial distribution before that date. Such a device will be Class I (general controls), Class II (special controls), or Class III (premarket approval) depending on the level of reasonable assurance of the safety and effectiveness of the device.
2. The commissioner refers the device to the appropriate classification panel.
3. To make recommendations to the commissioner on the class of regulatory control (Class I, II, or III) appropriate for the device, the panel reviews the device for safety and effectiveness.
4. Based on its review of evidence of the safety and effectiveness of the device, and applying the definition of each class, the panel submits to the commissioner a recommendation regarding the classification of the device.
5. The commissioner publishes the panel's recommendation in the *Federal Register*.
6. The classification panel will recommend classification into Class III of any implant or life-supporting or life-sustaining device.

Subpart C: Reclassification
Any petition for reclassification of a device shall include the following:
1. A specification of the type of device
2. A statement of the action requested by the petitioner
3. A completed supplemental data sheet applicable to the device
4. A completed classification questionnaire applicable to the device
5. A statement of the basis for disagreement with the present classification
6. A full statement of the reasons why the device should not be classified into its present classification
7. Representative data and information known by the petitioner that are unfavorable to the petitioner's position

8. If the petition is based on new information, a summary of the new information

Note: Consultation with the panel is allowed.

PART 861: PROCEDURES FOR PERFORMANCE STANDARDS DEVELOPMENT

Subpart A: General
1. This part describes the establishment, amendment, and revocation of performance standards applicable to devices intended for human use.
2. The Food and Drub Administration may determine that a performance standard is necessary to provide effectiveness of the device.

In carrying out its duties under this section, the Food and Drug Administration will, to the maximum extent practical:
1. Use personnel, facilities, and other technical support available in other federal agencies
2. Consult with other federal agencies concerned with a standard setting and other nationally or internationally recognized standard-setting entities
3. Invite participation, through conferences, workshops, or other means, by representatives of scientific, professional, industry, or consumer organizations that can make as significant contribution

Any performance standard established under this part will include the following:
1. Performance characteristics of the device
2. The design, construction, components, ingredients, and properties of the device
3. The manufacturing processes
4. Testing of the device
5. The publication of the results of each test
6. Manufacturer's certification to purchasers that the device conforms to the applicable performance standard.

Subpart B: Procedures for Performance Standards Development and Publication
1. The Food and Drug Administration may accept an existing standard, a proposed standard, or a draft standard.
2. The Food and Drug Administration will establish advisory committees to which the proposed regulations may be referred.

PARTS 862 TO 1050

The following parts describe special requirements for the indicated devices:
- 862 Clinical chemistry and clinical toxicology devices
- 864 Hematology and pathology devices
- 866 Immunology and microbiology devices
- 868 Anesthesiology devices
- 870 Cardiovascular devices
- 872 Dental devices

Regulatory Affairs

874	Ear, nose, and throat devices
876	Gastroenterology–urology devices
878	General and plastic surgery devices
880	General hospital and personal use devices
882	Neurological devices
884	Obstetrical and gynecological devices
886	Orthopedic devices
888	Physical medicine devices
890	Radiology devices
892	Banned devices
898	Performance standard for electrode lead wires and patient cables
900	Mammography
1004	Repurchase, repairs, or replacement of electronic products
1005	Importation of electronic products
1010	Performance standards for electronic products: general
1020	Performance standards for ionizing radiation-emitting products
1030	Performance standards for microwave- and radio frequency-emitting products
1040	Performance standards for light-emitting products
1050	Performance standards for sonic, infrasonic, and ultrasonic radiation-emitting products

ABBREVIATIONS

Following are standard and regulatory abbreviations commonly used in medical device R&D.

INTERNATIONAL AND NATIONAL STANDARD ABBREVIATIONS

AAMI	Association for the Advancement of Medical Instrumentation
ANSI	American National Standards Institute
ASTM	American Society for Testing and Materials
CB	Certified body
IEC	International Electrotechnical Commission
ISO	International Organization for Standardization
NBMed	Notified bodies medical devices

REGULATORY ABBREVIATIONS

510(k)	Premarket notification
CADx	Computer-aided diagnosis
CAPA	Corrective action/preventative action
CBER	Center for Biologics Evaluation and Research
CDRH	Center for Devices and Radiological Health
CFR	*Code of Federal Regulations*
cGMP	Current good manufacturing practice
CLIA	Clinical laboratory improvement amendments

CMS	Centers for Medicare and Medicaid Services
DEN	Device experience network
DHF	Design history file
DMR	Device master record
DSMICA	Division of Small Manufacturers, International and Consumer Assistance
FDA	Food and Drug Administration
FOI	Freedom of Information Act
GAO	General Accounting Office
GCP	Good clinical practice
GLP	Good laboratory practice
GMP	Good manufacturing practice
GPO	Government Printing Office
HCFA	Health Care Financing Administration
HDE	Humanitarian device exemption
HUD	Humanitarian use device
ID	Intended use
IDE	Investigational Device Exemption
IFU	Instruction for use
IRB	Investigative review board
IVD	In vitro diagnostics
MAUDE	Manufacturer and user facility device experience
MDR	Medical device report
NSE	Not substantially equivalent
NSR	Nonsignificant risk
OCER	Office of Communication, Education, and Radiation Programs
ODE	Office of Device Evaluation
OIVD	Office of In Vitro Diagnostic Device Evaluation and Safety
OSEL	Office of Science and Engineering Laboratories (formerly OST)
PDP	Product development protocol
PMA	Premarket approval
QSIT	*Guide to Inspections of Quality Systems*
QSR	Quality System Regulation
SE	Substantial equivalence
SMDA	Safe Medical Devices Act
SR	Significant risk

ABOUT THE AUTHOR

Thomas Wehman has held senior operations, quality, and regulatory affairs roles for five medical device start-up companies with successful IPOs. He is an expert in national and international requirements for medical devices, combination drug/devices, and over-the-counter products. He has written many papers on various regulatory, QA, and manufacturing subjects. He received a PhD with honors from Michigan State University in analytical chemistry and his undergraduate degree from Northern Illinois University with honors.

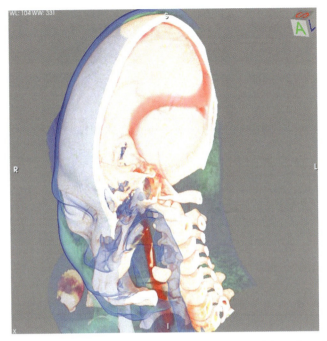

FIGURE 8.7 Digital reconstruction of cranial anatomy from radiology data. (Courtesy of Andrew Swift, CMI.)

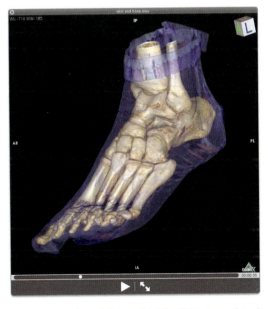

FIGURE 8.5 Osirix reconstruction of foot and ankle. (Courtesy of Andrew Swift, CMI.)

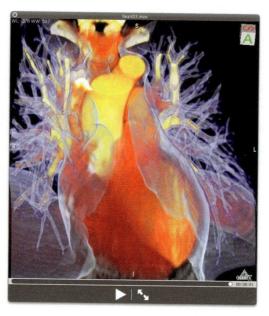

FIGURE 8.6 Image of heart and pulomonary vessels. (Courtesy of Andrew Swift, CMI.)

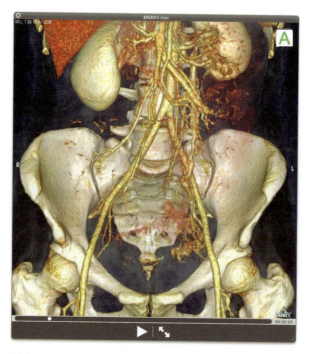

FIGURE 8.8 Digital reconstruction of kidneys and abdominal vasculature from radiology data. (Courtesy of Andrew Swift, CMI.)

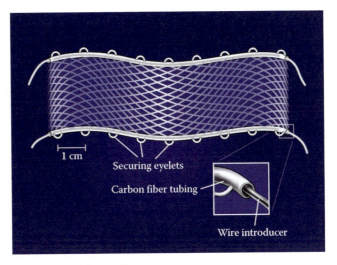

FIGURE 19.1 Conceptual device illustration.

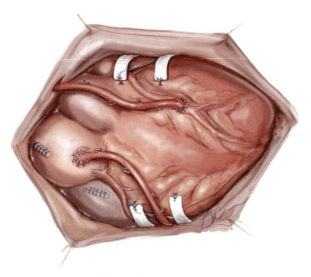

FIGURE 19.4 Surgical planning illustration, step 3.

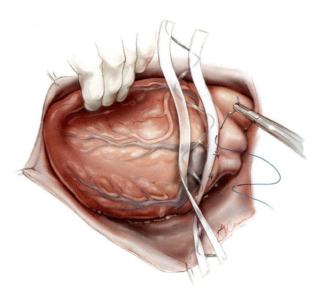

FIGURE 19.2 Surgical planning illustration, step 1.

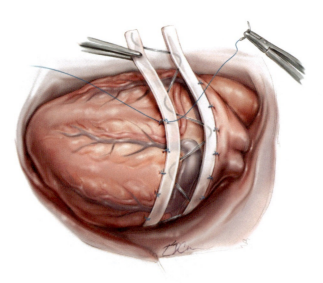

FIGURE 19.3 Surgical planning illustration, step 2.

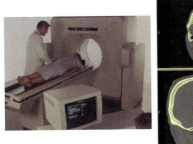 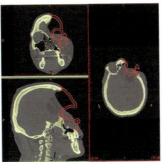 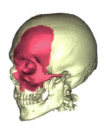

FIGURE 8.9 Process of capturing radiology data for 3D reconstruction and implant production. (Courtesy of Materialise, Leuven, Belgium.)

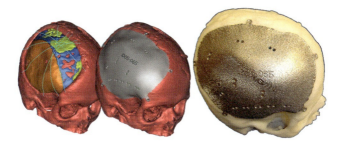

FIGURE 8.4 Titanium skull plate made in direct metal from a 3D digital model derived from patient radiology data. (Courtesy of Materialise Leuven, Belgium and Dr. Jules Poukens, Academic Hospital, Maastricht, Belgium.)

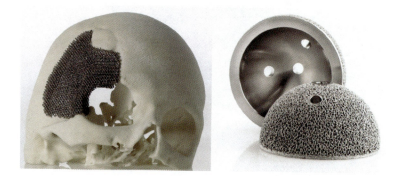

FIGURE 8.13 Complex direct-metal mesh skull plate and acetabular cup implant. (Courtesy of Arcam AB, Mölndal, Sweden.)

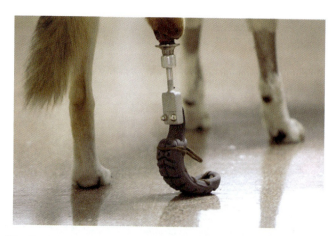

FIGURE 8.17 Cassidy walking on his osseointegrated prosthetic.

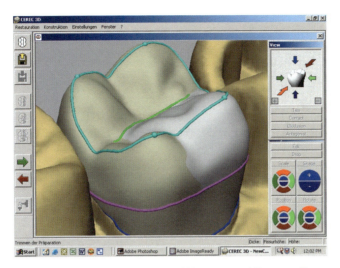

FIGURE 7.9 The CEREC system. (Courtesy of Sirona Dental Systems, Germany.)

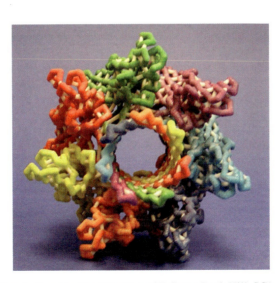

FIGURE 7.3 Hemolysin molecule. (Courtesy of Z Corp., Rock Hill, SC.)

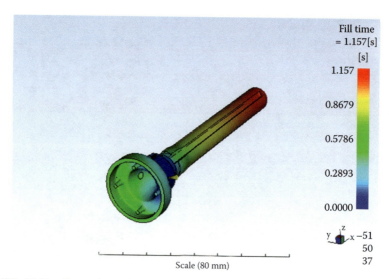

FIGURE 11.11 Screenshot of Moldflow analysis of confidence of fill. (Courtesy of Cannuflow Inc., San Jose, CA.)

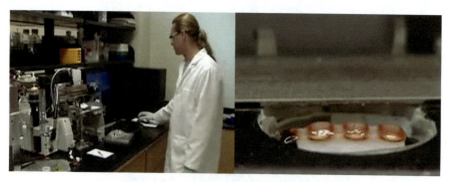

FIGURE 8.19 Printed hydrogel biologic constructs incorporating living cells. (Courtesy of Vladimir Mironov PhD, MUSC, from the *Medical Applications of Rapid Prototyping* [DVD], 2007, SME.)

16 510(k) Reform
The Stakes Are High

Sherrie Conroy

CONTENTS

FDA's Plan of Action 333
Chilling Data 337
Small Companies Suffer 339
Sound System 339
Just One of Many Issues 341
Still More to Come: IOM Recommendations 341
Implementing One Reform 342
Not All Studies Are Created Equal 343
Conclusion 345
About the Author 345
Resources 345

The Food and Drug Administration's (FDA's) ability to implement its plan for rehabilitating the 510(k) process will directly affect the future of U.S. medical technology innovation and U.S. patients' access to treatment. This theme is echoed by a number of industry experts, including AdvaMed's David Nexon, senior executive vice president and head of policy, and Janet Trunzo, executive vice president for technology and regulatory affairs.[*] Nexon, who said AdvaMed was pleased with the way the implementation plan came out compared with the initial set of proposals, also said it was important to put the plan "in the context of American competitiveness and patient access."

FDA'S PLAN OF ACTION

Concerns about the state of the existing 510(k) program have been raised in recent years by parties within and outside the FDA, prompting the review of the program. In January 2011, the FDA issued its "Plan of Action for Implementation of 510(k) and Science Recommendations."[†] The FDA believed the improvements outlined in the report would "foster medical device innovation and enhance patient safety." The

---

[*] "The FDA 510(k) plan: Implementation holds the key to US innovation, patient access to treatment," Sherrie Conroy, January 20, 2011, http://blog.medicaldesign.com/perspectives/2011/01/20/the-fda-510k-plan-implementation-holds-the-key-to-us-innovation-patient-access-to-treatment/.

[†] "CDRH Plan of Action for 510(k) and Science," http://www.fda.gov/AboutFDA/CentersOffices/OfficeofMedicalProductsandTobacco/CDRH/CDRHReports/ucm239448.htm.

agency implemented recommendations, published standard operating procedures (SOPs), and issued new processes outlined in the Plan of Action. The agency has posted updates on the status of planned actions on the *Center for Devices and Radiological Health* (CDRH) website.

The agency completed many of actions in the Plan and undertook several additional efforts to improve its premarket programs. Two items—implementing a unique device identification (UDI) system and developing a Pre-Submission Interactions Guidance—were pushed forward to 2012 and were completed as of July 2012. Five additional items were started in 2011, but are not complete as of publication. These include the following

- Clarify and improve third-party review, which entails posting an SOP to FDA's website
- Developing a standards guidance to clarify the appropriate use of consensus standards
- Issuing a proposed regulation to improve medical device labeling and to clarify the statutory listing requirements for the submission of labeling
- Issuing a proposed regulation to better identify 510(k) transfers of ownership
- Issuing a proposed regulation to clarify the circumstances under which the FDA would rely on clinical studies conducted in and for other countries.

According to the FDA's "CDRH 2012 Strategic Priorities," in 2012, the agency will focus on completing or continuing the work it already started in its four priority areas. In alignment with its four priority areas, CDRH says it will fully implement a total product life cycle approach, enhance communication and transparency, strengthen its workforce and workplace, and facilitate innovation to address unmet public health needs.

The Strategic Priorities document includes time frames associated with each strategy, and specific actions that the FDA will take to meet those goals or make significant progress towards achieving those goals.

In September 2009, the FDA formed the 510(k) Working Group and the Task Force on the Utilization of Science in Regulatory Decision Making committees to "address critical challenges facing the Center for Devices and Radiological Health (CDRH) and [FDA's] external constituencies." The 510(k) Working Group was assigned to evaluate the 510(k) program and explore actions that the CDRH could take to enhance 510(k) decision making. Meanwhile, the Task Force set about making recommendations for how CDRH could incorporate new science into its decision making quickly "in as predictable a manner as is practical." Independently, the Institute of Medicine (IOM) also conducted an evaluation of the 510(k) program. In August 2010, the committees issued their preliminary reports, which were then released for public comment. During the course of this committee process from September 2009 to August 2010, the FDA solicited perspectives for review from two public meetings, three town hall meetings, three open public dockets, and several meetings with stakeholders.

The Plan of Action included four sections of action items: guidance issues, internal and administrative matters, programmatic and regulatory items, and issues to be referred to the IOM. Each section identified the purpose of the action item, a milestone goal, and a date of completion. Starting with March 2011, the Plan of Action outlined the projects that were to be completed throughout the year, including a particularly busy summer of analyzing issues for the IOM report. On April 7 and 8, 2011, public meetings were held to address the action items regarding the issue of additional information about regulated products as well as improving medical device labeling, both of which were outlined in the programmatic and regulatory section.

Eight draft guidances made up the first section of action items that were to be completed in 2011. The 510(k) Modifications Guidance draft to clarify which changes do or do not warrant submission of a new 510(k) and which modifications are eligible for a Special 510(k) was completed July 12, 2011. By August 15, a draft of the Clinical Trial Guidance to improve quality and performance also was issued. The largest guidance item to be drafted was for the 510(k) Paradigm. This guidance, published December 27, 2011, provides greater clarity regarding seven critical issues: when clinical data should be submitted in support of a 510(k); the submission of photographs or schematics for internal FDA use only; the appropriate use of multiple predicates; the criteria for identifying different questions of safety and effectiveness and technological changes that generally raise such questions; resolving discrepancies between the 510(k) flowchart and the Food, Drug, and Cosmetic Act; the characteristics that should be included in the concept of intended use; and the development of 510(k) summaries to ensure that they are accurate and include all required information. In addition to the 510(k) Paradigm Guidance, the Evaluation of Automatic Class III Designation Guidance to streamline the *de novo* classification process was published on September 30. To clarify the appropriate use of consensus standards, the Standards Guidance draft, which was originally to be completed by October 31, 2011, is still being drafted. The draft of the Appeals Guidance to clarify the process for appealing CDRH decisions, including those to rescind a 510(k) was completed on December 27, 2011. The Pre-Submission Interactions Guidance was completed July 13, 2012, to supplement available guidance on pre-IDE (investigational device exemption) meetings and to enhance presubmission interactions between industry and CDRH staff. By the end of 2011, the Product Code Guidance to draft methods to more consistently develop and assign unique product codes was finished.

Internal and administrative matters are broken into five action items: establish a CDRH Science Council, assess CDRH staffing needs, enhance training, leverage external experts, and continue integration and knowledge management. The Center Science Council was established March 31, 2011 to oversee the development of a business process and SOP for determining and implementing an appropriate response to new scientific information. Serving also to promote the development of improved metrics to continuously assess the quality, consistency, and effectiveness of the 510(k) program, the Center Science Council will periodically audit the 510(k) review decisions to assess adequacy, accuracy, and consistency, and it planned to assemble an internal team of clinical trial experts to provide support and advice on clinical trial design for CDRH staff and prospective IDE applicants.

As part of the process to establish the Center Science Council, the FDA posted a council charter to the FDA's website on March 31, 2011 and posted the initial results of the 510(k) audit on June 15. Looking inward, the administration then focused on assessing its staffing needs and enhancing training. A process for identifying, recruiting, retaining, and training needed staff was drafted by July 15, 2011, and steps to develop and implement training on core competencies for new staff were in place August 2011. As part of the emphasis on training and core competencies, the FDA focused the training of CDRH staff and industry on six key issues: the determination of "intended use"; the determination of whether a 510(k) raises "different questions of safety and effectiveness"; the review of 510(k)s that use "multiple predicates"; the development and assignment of product codes; the interpretation of the "least burdensome" principles; and the appropriate use of consensus standards.

To further enhance training efforts, the FDA began to leverage external scientific experts appropriately and efficiently, as well as to assess best practices and develop SOPs for staff engagement with external experts, which were posted to the agency's website on September 15, 2011. The final action item addressed the need to continue integration and knowledge management efforts in the future. An evaluation of methods used to integrate device information into a dynamic format so that it can more readily be used by staff to make regulatory decisions was completed by September 30. This set of action items was slated to be completed in the shortest window of time.

Making up the bulk of the 2011 Plan of Action were items in the programmatic and regulatory section, which consisted of 11 action items, including a pilot program that began on March 31, 2011, to explore the use of an "assurance case" framework for 510(k) submissions and the two items that went up for public discussion on April 7 and 8. The two action items on the public discussion agenda addressed the needs to make device photographs available in a public database without disclosing proprietary information and to develop an online labeling repository. Four action items were slated for completion in June 2011. On June 15, 2011, the FDA posted SOPs on its website to establish a "Notice to Industry Letters" as a standard practice to clarify and more quickly inform stakeholders when the CDRH has changed its regulatory expectations on the basis of new scientific information. By the end of the month, the FDA determined system requirements and selected the platform for a new adverse event database as part of its effort to improve analysis of postmarket information; completed a program assessment of the IDE process; and on July 3, 2011, it issued proposed regulation for a unique device identification (UDI) system.

The adverse event database was created as a tool to enable collection and analysis of postmarket information and to enhance the CDRH's capabilities to support evidence synthesis and quantitative decision making. Assessment of the IDE process is being completed to better characterize the root causes of existing challenges and trends in IDE decision making and to mitigate those challenges when reviewing IDEs. Implementation of the UDI system is meant to permit the rapid and accurate identification of devices, as well as to facilitate and improve adverse event reporting and identification of device-specific problems. Guidance for streamlining and improving efficiencies and predictability in the regulation development process was posted as SOPs to the FDA website on July 31, 2011. More SOPs were posted in September to clarify and improve third-party review by developing a process for regularly evaluating the list of device types eligible for third-party review and to enhance reviewer training. Next, the FDA published results of its multiple predicate analysis conducted to determine the basis for the apparent association between citing more than five predicates and a greater mean rate of adverse event reports. By the end of 2011, the FDA had begun to draft proposed regulation for 510(k) transfer of ownership to improve documentation and to improve medical device labeling by clarifying the statutory listing requirements for the submission of labeling.

In September 2011, the FDA held a public meeting to solicit comments on the recommendations proposed in the Institute of Medicine (IOM) report. The FDA referred seven action items to the IOM. Rescission authority was referred to the IOM for defining the scope and grounds for the exercise of the CDRH's authority to fully or partially rescind a 510(k) clearance. The IOM also addressed the issues of postmarket surveillance authorities and requiring postmarket surveillance studies as a condition of clearance for certain devices, as well as of clarifying when a device should no longer be available for use as a predicate. Clarifying and consolidating regulatory terms was referred to the IOM for review. Specific concepts included in this action item are "indication for use" and "intended use." The IOM covered establishing a Class IIb device and how to develop guidance for defining Class IIb devices for which clinical information, manufacturing information, or, potentially, additional evaluation in the postmarket setting would typically be necessary to support a substantial equivalence determination. Finally, the the IOM was asked to review whether each 510(k) submitter should be required to keep at least one unit of the device under review available for CDRH to access upon request, and to explore whether to pursue a statutory amendment that would provide the agency with the express authority to consider an off-label use when determining the "intended use" of a device.

CHILLING DATA

It is clear that a healthy 510(k) submission process will enhance innovation and global competitiveness of U.S. medical device companies. PricewaterhouseCoopers (PwC) issued a report in February 2011 that found that while the United States is currently number one in medical device innovation, the nation is slipping in all dimensions of leadership. Nexon put that finding in perspective by noting that 10 years ago the United States was the unchallenged leader in medical technology. As of 2012, the United States is the challenged leader. If we do not take effective steps to address the problem, he said, in 10 years we won't be the leader at all. Studies, reports, and experts all say that the FDA, while not the whole problem, plays a crucial role in reversing the trend.

The PwC study found that the United States ranked seven out of nine competitor nations in the speed of regulatory review. Armed with such data, industry has pointed straight at the troubled FDA process as a hindrance to innovation and investment in the medical device space. Moreover, the slow pace of reviews, the changing of reviewers on a submission, and inconsistent requirements cause an undue burden on device companies, especially venture-capital-backed start-up companies. In some cases, such delays have been too costly for these companies, and good products have failed to make it to market.

Another study found that U.S. patients wait on average a full two years longer than their European counterparts for many lifesaving and life-enhancing technologies made by U.S. medical device and diagnostics companies because of growing regulatory delays and inefficiencies.

Josh Makower, MD, a consulting professor of medicine at Stanford University and a medical device entrepreneur, is a coauthor of the study.[*] He said that the unpredictability and inefficiencies in the U.S. regulatory process are making it difficult for companies to get life-changing medical products into the hands of clinicians and patients.

But Makower pointed to a recurring problem identified by the surveyed companies: changing reviewers leads to changing requirements and more delays. "As you look at where the issues are coming from," said Makower, "they stem from several inefficiencies to the process and tremendous turnover at the FDA. This creates a lot of uncertainty." Companies that have an agreed-upon protocol, he explained, execute the clinical trial and then return to find that the reviewing group at the FDA is no longer the same. "That group may no longer agree with the group that was there when the study was agreed to," he said. "[The companies] find themselves in the very difficult position of being asked to do another study, even though they thought they were doing the one FDA wanted." This scenario happens in about 44% of reviews, he said.

The survey data showed that the average total cost for participants to bring a low- to moderate-risk 510(k) product from concept to clearance was approximately $31 million, with $24 million spent on FDA-dependent or related activities. For a higher-risk premarket approval (PMA) product, the average total cost from concept to approval was approximately $94 million, with $75 million spent on stages linked to the FDA.

"The current regulatory environment is putting our nation's fragile medical innovation infrastructure at risk," Makower said.

> FDA and innovators share the common goal of improving patient care. To achieve this objective, FDA and industry must work together towards a reasonable and balanced regulatory process for new innovations. This will ensure that patients and clinicians have timely access to safe and effective products. Only then will the most cost-effective advances in medical care be delivered; and only then will the public health and our economy be best served.

In February 2011, the U.S. House of Representatives Energy and Commerce Health Subcommittee held a hearing on the "Impact of Medical Device Regulation on Jobs and Patients." At that hearing, Jeffrey Shuren, director of the Center for Devices and Radiological Health, told the committee, "We recognize that we need to provide greater clarity [to device manufacturers] on what we need from them."[†] However, Shuren also fixed some of the blame on industry, saying that delays are often caused by "poor quality submissions and studies" and he said that device companies ignore

---

[*] "Study paints a grim picture of the future of medical device innovation in America: Is FDA to blame?," Sherrie Conroy, December 6, 2010, http://medicaldesign.com/engineering-prototyping/research-development/study-paints-grim-picture-20101206/index.html.

[†] "Hearing addresses FDA funding, industry accountability, and much more," Joe Jancsurak, February 22, 2011, http://blog.medicaldesign.com/perspectives/2011/02/22/hearing-addresses-fda-funding-industry-accountability-and-much-more/.

CDRH recommendations. "If we are going to fix this," he said, "FDA needs to make changes, but we need industry to be held responsible, too."

SMALL COMPANIES SUFFER

Tom Novelli, vice president of government relations for the Medical Device Manufacturers Association (MDMA), said that MDMA started to hear about problems a couple of years ago, with increasing numbers of its member companies saying that the FDA was being "completely unreasonable."* Novelli said MDMA consistently heard the same comments: "They're not clear in what they want. They're moving the goalpost. We're meeting benchmarks and then FDA comes back and requests more studies." The result, he said, is a significant chilling effect on industry, mostly on the innovation ecosystem and novel breakthrough technologies.

All fingers pointed at the 510(k) process. "Initially, CDRH director Jeff Shuren came out and said the 510(k) process is broken," said Novelli. Shuren has since backed off from that stance, acknowledging that it is a sound process that simply needs to refocus on its original intent. Novelli cited one example from an MDMA member to illustrate the problem identified in the Makower study. The company had submitted a 510(k) for an endoscope, which has been cleared and approved dozens of times by the FDA for similar procedures. The procedure for this company's endoscope would be 1–2 degrees warmer than an endoscope approved by the FDA previously. This change of degree, said Novelli, is within the acceptable range of the international standard for the temperature of endoscopes. On the last day before the device could be approved, the FDA requested a 150-patient clinical study to look at this 1-degree difference. Novelli said,

> This is a small company that was venture backed. A new 150-patient study was going to cost them $50 million. The VC said it could not fund the study. The company died on the vine. That's just one. This happens over and over and over.

SOUND SYSTEM

According to AdvaMed president Steve Ubl, "We believe a strong, properly restored, and well-managed FDA benefits everyone," but he pointed to the reports that began to show a disturbing trend."† Ubl was referring to the reports by PwC, the Boston Consulting Group, and Makower that all were released within weeks of each other at the close of 2010 and the start of 2011. All had similar findings that pointed to an inconsistent and lengthy regulatory review process as the primary factor in our slipping grip on innovation.

"Because of FDA's declining performance, American companies and American patients are increasingly left out and left behind. The report from PwC shows that

---

* Tom Novelli, in his keynote address, "The Evolving Legislation and Regulatory Environment for Medical Device Manufacturers," at the *Medical Design*'s Medical Silicone Conference (MSC) in Minneapolis, March 23, 2011.
† "All signs point to FDA," Sherrie Conroy, March 17, 2011, http://medicaldesign.com/engineering-prototyping/regulatory/all-signs-point-fda-20110317/index.html.

regulatory systems in competing countries were less burdensome and more consistent," said Ubl.

"The data show that the U.S. is at risk of losing its global leadership position in medical technology innovation," said Makower, in reference to the findings from his study. "By overwhelming majorities, the companies surveyed reported that European regulatory authorities were more predictable and more transparent than FDA."

Nexon said the FDA's 510(k) plan moves the FDA in the right direction by recognizing that the 510(k) process is fundamentally sound, benefits American patients, and promotes innovation. "It generally appears that the changes should be targeted, have a corresponding health benefit, and support timely access to new treatments and cures," he said.

But, he emphasized that the plan itself was only the first step in the process. The hard part was the very complicated set of implementation steps, which included development of at least eight guidances.

AdvaMed supports the development of device-specific guidances because existing problems were not typically associated with the overall process in terms of FDA's ability to protect patient safety. "Its record of being able to protect patient safety with this process is extraordinarily good, but certainly there are problems with specific device types, where changes in the regulations or standards might be appropriate," he said. "We think that's the right way to approach it."

According to Nexon, many of the proposals had the potential to ensure that the plan improves the timeliness and the consistency of the review process. AdvaMed wants to work with the FDA to ensure that these particular changes are implemented in a way that is constructive, and that, over time, the FDA addresses the broader concerns about the agency's performance, he said.

The FDA's 510(k) 2011 reform plan focused on proposals that AdvaMed believes will strengthen the already robust 510(k) program. Those proposals included enhancing reviewer training, leveraging the use of external scientific experts, improving the consistency of reviews through the development of device-specific guidance documents, and streamlining the *de novo* process.

According to Trunzo, the FDA made it very clear that there is a need to increase reviewer training on existing guidance documents. The FDA has had a lot of new reviewers over the last several years, and the agency understood the need to reinforce that training with the development of these new guidance documents and the existing guidance documents.

Clearly, there is an important need for reviewer training and a better means of ensuring consistency of review. The FDA is also going to make some recommendations on IDEs, which Nexon said had been a "huge sore spot and a tremendous drag on the United States. It's a matter of how well the training is carried out."

"Much of the agency's plan supports our long-standing position that the 510(k) process is fundamentally sound and benefits American patients," said James Mazzo, president of Abbott Medical Optics and former chairman of AdvaMed.* "The plan also generally adheres to our principles that any changes to the 510(k) process

---

* "All signs point to FDA," Sherrie Conroy, March 17, 2011, http://medicaldesign.com/engineering-prototyping/regulatory/all-signs-point-fda-20110317/index.html.

should support timely access to these technologies." Mazzo said he looks at the future with "guarded optimism." He stressed that it is critical that industry is able to work with the FDA to make things better. The underlying expectation was that the FDA also wants a more collaborative system and thus has made great strides to get the plan implemented and get the process reformed.

JUST ONE OF MANY ISSUES

One particular concern is the issue and definition of *split predicate*. "Describing the meaning of *split predicate* has been challenging," said Trunzo. "FDA had a meaning in mind, and those submitting 510(k)s may have thought that they had a split predicate when indeed they didn't. So the bottom line is that the term meant different things to different people." Going forward, instead of focusing on a term such as split predicate, the focus will be on the 510(k) decision process itself using a 510(k) flowchart, Trunzo explained.

> As long as you have the same intended use and you have differing technological characteristics, if you follow the flowchart, you have a more appropriate way to come about a decision on a 510(k) versus using the term *split predicate*.

As part of the 510(k) Paradigm guidance, the FDA clarified the use of multiple predicates. The guidance clarifies that, in certain circumstances, a manufacturer may use multiple predicate devices to help demonstrate substantial equivalence. If the manufacturer intends to use multiple predicates to address decision points 2–4 on the flowchart, for example, each predicate device must have the same intended use as the new device, and any difference in technological characteristics from the predicate devices must not raise different questions of safety and effectiveness. The guidance describes scenarios to illustrate the possible circumstances. A flowchart in Appendix A aids the decision-making process.

STILL MORE TO COME: IOM RECOMMENDATIONS

Many of the tougher questions were referred to the IOM for review. The IOM issued its final recommendations in August 2011. The resulting report shocked industry with its recommendation that the FDA should scrap the 510(k) process altogether and develop an entirely new program.

AdvaMed's Trunzo noted that the plan defers several proposals to the IOM that could negatively affect industry's "ability to innovate and put products on the market." Those proposals included extending the FDA's 510(k) rescission authority and the consolidation of the terms "intended use" and "indications for use."

AdvaMed's Trunzo explained that AdvaMed objected to the recommendation to expand FDA's rescission authority because the agency already has such authority in very defined and narrow circumstances. "We believe expansion of that authority would require statutory change," she said.

The eye opener for the FDA ought to be its own data, which Ubl called troubling. The FDA has failed to meet its own goals for reviews of PMAs, and the number of review cycles for 510(k) submissions has increased, despite an increasing budget and increased staffing since 2007.

Everyone seemed to agree that one major problem with the 510(k) process is a simple one, and one that even Shuren addressed in his comments to the House subcommittee, saying that the FDA staffing is inadequate. He said the agency has about 1250 full-time employees, with 70 percent involved in the device review process.

"We have to ensure that FDA fulfills both its mission to protect the public health and to promote patient access," said Ubl.

> We're on the cusp of a revolution in life sciences. The next breakthroughs are right around the corner—new wireless technologies, new diagnostic tools, new ways of attacking neurological illnesses, nanotechnology to treat patients at the molecular level—but if FDA doesn't address its problems effectively, we will lose a whole generation of new ideas.

IMPLEMENTING ONE REFORM

Under pressure to find ways to foster innovation, the FDA launched the Innovation Pathway, a priority review program for new, breakthrough medical devices. The FDA also announced plans to seek further public comment before the Pathway can be used more broadly. On April 9, 2012, the CDRH launched its second version of the Innovation Pathway, "Innovation Pathway 2.0." The new version "offers new and modified tools and methods to deepen collaboration between the FDA and innovators early in the process, prior to premarket submission, with the goal of making the regulatory process more efficient and timely," according to the agency. Sharon Segal, vice president of technology and regulatory affairs for AdvaMed, said,

> While we support the goals of the Innovation Initiative, we believe that early and consistent interaction and the focus on a cooperative effort to get safe and effective products developed and reviewed quickly should be available to all innovative products, especially those that currently qualify for expedited review. FDA has a number of tools already available to achieve these objectives and they should be used more broadly and effectively.[*]

According to Segal, the FDA already had identified "several steps it intends to take to bring greater speed and consistency to the current review process, including greater reviewer training, development of more guidance documents, and streamlining the de novo process." Segal continued:

> We support these initiatives and believe FDA should continue to focus on these process improvements to help address the unacceptable delays and inconsistencies that have plagued its review process in recent years and have needlessly delayed patient access to life-saving, life-enhancing medical technology.

---

[*] "AdvaMed cool to FDA's new medical device innovation initiative," Sherrie Conroy, March 21, 2011, http://medicaldesign.com/engineering-prototyping/regulatory/advamed-fda-medical-device-innovation-0321/index.html.

The FDA says its Innovation Pathway is a new way of doing business within the existing regulatory framework that "could yield significant benefits to patients in the U.S. by giving them first-in-the-world access to medical devices, including those with breakthrough technology." According to the FDA, the Innovation Pathway is an evolving system that ultimately aims to shorten the overall time and cost it takes for the development, assessment, and review of medical devices, and to improve how FDA staff and innovators work together.

In explaining the program, the FDA says Innovation Pathway 2.0 incorporates new methods for agency reviewers to analyze the potential benefit and risk of a device, including a decision support tool and the application of a Center process for assessing patient perspectives. FDA reviewers use the tool in evaluating first-in-human (FIH) clinical trials. This tool will help the agency provide clarity to the question of whether the device can proceed to early feasibility studies or whether further preclinical testing is needed to ensure safety and effectiveness. In addition, the FDA says, "The tool helps reviewers explicitly consider the balance between allowing the development of the device to proceed, and its potential benefit to the relevant general patient population upon market release, while considering the safety of the test patient population."

NOT ALL STUDIES ARE CREATED EQUAL

One study analyzing the 510(k) process drew the ire of industry groups AdvaMed and the Medical Imaging and Technology Alliance (MITA). Some have said that the data used in this particular study should not even have been compared with one another in the first place. AdvaMed and MITA both say the study contains factual errors, faulty data analysis, and recommendations that would harm patient access to medical technology with no corresponding safety benefit.

The study, "Medical Device Recalls and the FDA Approval Process," was published in February 2011 by Diana Zuckerman et al.* Both groups reamed the study, saying that it contains dangerous recommendations that, if adopted, would add unnecessary and burdensome hurdles to bringing safe and innovative products to market.

In reaction to the study, AdvaMed's Ubl noted, "Simply put, this paper is seriously flawed and inconsistent with three previous analyses of the same data set conducted by respected researchers."

Led by Zuckerman at the National Research Center for Women & Families and published in the *Archives of Internal Medicine*, the study looked at the number of recalls for a subset of devices cleared by the FDA's 510(k) process, the process used to review and clear devices that are similar to those that have already been cleared by the FDA as safe and effective. It was cited by a number of news organizations including the *Wall Street Journal*, the *New York Times*, and the *Los Angeles Times*. Unfortunately, this is how misinformation often gets to the public without being vetted by industry. Ubl said,

---

* "Medical Device Recalls and the FDA Approval Process," Diana M. Zuckerman, et al. *Archives of Internal Medicine*, June 13, 2011, February 14, 2011, Vol 171, No. 11.

Because of an elementary error in data analysis, the conclusions drawn from the study are faulty, and the paper is marked by a large number of factual errors and misleading inferences. Adoption of the paper's recommendations would actually harm American patients by further delaying access to safe and effective treatments.

Ubl also noted that the other three studies have all found that the 510(k) process has a remarkable safety record with extremely low recall rates—one study reported a rate of less than two-tenths of one percent.

Although the findings of the Zuckerman study indicate that a higher number of 510(k) medical devices are recalled than products cleared through the PMA process, MITA said that the authors failed to put these numbers in context, noting that there are more than 3,000 devices and diagnostics cleared through the 510(k) process every year compared with 20–40 products cleared through the PMA process. Based on their limited analysis, the authors recommended that the FDA overhaul this clearance process and send more devices through the FDAs more costly PMA.

According to Dave Fisher, executive director of the MITA,

The Zuckerman study draws inaccurate conclusions based on a simple count of the number of FDA recalls. This irresponsible research method led to potentially harmful claims and recommendations about a clearance process that in fact has an excellent track record for clearing safe and effective products. . . . Interestingly, the study actually appears to add evidence to the argument that products approved through the 510(k) process are just as safe—if not safer—than those devices approved through the lengthy PMA process.[*]

Furthermore, MITA said that the Zuckerman analysis looked at Class I recalls for high-risk devices and used those numbers to question all 510(k) devices, unjustifiably recommending changes to the clearance process for all classes of devices, including devices that are low risk, such as medical imaging technologies. According to Ubl,

While the overall safety record of the 510(k) system is excellent, there is always room for improvement. The 510(k) reform implementation plan recently announced by the FDA provides for improving reviewer and manager training, establishing a Center Science Council to ensure consistency in the review process, issuing more guidance documents to provide greater clarity to manufacturers, and applying additional requirements on a targeted basis. This is the right way to improve a process that has a demonstrated safety record for more than 30 years and is fundamentally sound.

Fisher noted that the 510(k) clearance program has a track record of protecting public health, but as manufacturers innovate diagnostic technologies, the clearance process will have to improve so that it can continue to spur innovation. "MITA remains committed to working with the FDA to identify efficiencies in the 510(k) process so that patients are never denied the latest treatment," he said.

---

[*] "Reforming the 510(k) process: Industry groups slam new study," Sherrie Conroy, March 7, 2011, http://medicaldesign.com/engineering-prototyping/regulatory/reforming-process-industry-groups-20110307/index.html.

CONCLUSION

As concerns about the 510(k) program emerged, the debate elicited recommendations ranging from staff training to establishment of a new class of devices. With its plan of action in 2011, the FDA tackled a majority of its objectives in its plan to reach its larger goal of fostering medical device innovation and enhancing patient safety. For those items deferred to the IOM, industry may still face new processes, depending on what the FDA does going forward. The IOM's recommendation to scrap the program altogether rightly was disregarded as ludicrous. It is important to remember the distinction between rehabilitating the program and overhauling it. Rehabilitating, updating, and fine-tuning the 510(k) process is necessary, but overhauling it outright is not.

ABOUT THE AUTHOR

Sherrie Conroy is currently director of content, *Medical Design*, at Penton Media. For more than 25 years, she has been an editor specializing in B2B technical publications. Before joining Penton, she was editor-in-chief of *MD&DI* and *Medical Electronics Design*, as well as several other medical-related products and publications. Her background includes editing magazines for medical devices, electromagnetic compatibility, spectroscopy, plastics, and pharmaceuticals. She earned a BA in journalism from the University of Oregon.

RESOURCES

Food and Drug Administration. "Plan of Action for Implementation of 510(k) and Science Recommendations." Washington, DC, January 2011.
PricewaterhouseCoopers. February 2011.
Zuckerman, Diana, et al. "Medical Device Recalls and the FDA Approval Process." *Archives of Internal Medicine.* National Research Center for Women & Families, February 2011.

17 Brief Introduction to Preclinical Research

James Swick

CONTENTS

Overview	347
In Vitro Testing	348
Animal Models	348
Project	348
In Vivo Study	349
Data Collection	349
Team	349
Good Laboratory Practices	350
Conclusion	350
About the Author	350

OVERVIEW

Medical devices must be tested in a living system (in vivo testing) for them to be approved by the Food and Drug Administration (FDA) for clinical trials. This can be a daunting task to some. To minimize the fear and trepidation that comes with this aspect of device development, I will lay out a guide that will allow the reader to map out a schedule for success and to minimize chances for failure.

Once your device has undergone all the rigors of bench-top testing, it is wise to see how it performs in vitro. What I mean by this is to procure explanted tissue to identify any modifications that may need to be made before the in vivo phase. There are several sources for obtaining the necessary organ/tissue, which I will discuss later on.

The most important aspect of preclinical work is identifying where to perform the testing. The right lab is critical to your success. A lab with inexperienced personnel who lack the knowledge to help with the intraoperative portion of your procedure can be frustrating and costly. Therefore, it is extremely important to explore all the options open to you before committing to any one facility or group.

If your device is novel and requires submission for independent device exemption, you may want to consider working with a lab or consultant knowledgeable in good laboratory practices (GLP).

IN VITRO TESTING

When you feel your device is ready for prime time, there a few things you must keep in mind. The first consideration is the organ system you will be targeting. A good example is an intravascular stent with delivery system. You may want to test its mechanical characteristics in explanted tissue. There are several places from which you can procure arterial sections, including butcher shops, meat-packing plants, universities, or an independent lab. In the case of coronary stents, you will need an explanted heart.

This holds true for other organ systems as well. The least expensive route (butcher shop and meat-packing plant) is not always the best, however. The tissue may not be in the best condition. If at all possible, you should try and get your samples from an independent lab or university. The latter two sources will give you tissue that has been removed by someone with a surgical skill and kept as fresh as possible.

Once you have the tissue, you may need to set up an artificial environment to mimic blood flow and other environments. As a physiologist, I cannot help you with this, but you engineering folks should be able to figure this out.

If you need an artificial circulatory system, there are companies and independent model makers that can provide a plastic or glass model that works very well. Some of these models can be a bit pricey, but you can use them over and over. They are also very nice to demonstrate your device to potential investors or end users.

ANIMAL MODELS

You must always be mindful that working with live animals is a privilege and should never be taken lightly. The U.S. Department of Agriculture (USDA) regulates the use of animals for research purposes through the Animal Welfare Act (you can find this at http://www.usda.gov).

The right animal model for your in vivo phase of development is truly the most important decision you will make. You need to take into consideration what models others have used in the past, as well as which particular species is the most similar to human anatomy. You can get direction from the medical literature as well as by talking to researchers knowledgeable in your specific area of interest. Some good questions to ask include the following:

- How many animals will I need?
- What organ system is your focus?
- What have others used?
- What species will give the most human-like anatomy?

PROJECT

The next step is to develop the project. You will need to consider how to begin, that is, survival versus terminal. I always recommend that new projects begin with terminal procedures to develop technique (surgical or interventional) as well as to determine what the device will do to the animal physiologically. You may need to incorporate specific medications to ward off complications.

What equipment will be required? If your procedure is interventional, you will need the proper imaging equipment (e.g., fluoroscopy or ultrasound).

What physiological parameters will need to be measured? You will need to collect the appropriate data for your final submission. It is wise to check any guidance the FDA may have regarding your particular area of interest. Also check with clinicians to find out what physiological parameters they want to see measured—for example, hemodynamics, clinical chemistry, and so on. If you do not plan all aspects of your procedure up front, you may find that you have wasted precious time and money. Not having all the data for your submission to the FDA may require that you go back to the lab or, at worst, start over. I cannot stress this point enough. You must plan every detail of your project and evaluate your progress along the way. If things do not go as planned, be prepared to stop and reevaluate before going forward.

IN VIVO STUDY

Once you have developed your plan of attack and have formalized it in a protocol, submit this to the Institutional Animal Care and Use Committee (IACUC) of the test facility you have chosen for the study. Most preclinical labs have their own template for this submission. After it has been reviewed and approved, you will be ready to begin.

You need to take a myriad of variables into consideration here, including the following:

- What specialty equipment will you need (e.g., fluoroscopy, ultrasound, etc.)?
- Will you need surgical or interventional expertise, and who will provide this?
- How much time will be required for the study?
- What kind of support can you expect from the test facility?
- Will this be a survival procedure or terminal?

In most cases, it is recommended to begin with your first animal being terminal. This is recommended so that you can work out any problem areas you may not have accounted for. By doing this, you will be able to develop needed surgical or interventional techniques so that you will know what to expect going forward.

DATA COLLECTION

You will need to establish all the parameters you want to evaluate before starting your study. Items such as histology, clinical pathology, angiography, and so on must be determined so that you can glean pertinent data from the outset. If you do not plan this aspect of the study, you may find yourself wasting precious time and money. If hemodynamic values are of interest, it is usually helpful to develop a data-collection document so that you can have all the relevant information in one place.

TEAM

The personnel who will be responsible for making your project successful are critical to having a good result. Be certain that everyone on your side of the team knows what their responsibilities and duties are before beginning the procedure. The personnel from the test facility must also know ahead of time what is expected of them as well. You, as the study sponsor, are ultimately responsible for ensuring that there is a direct line of ongoing communication between your staff and the staff at the test facility.

GOOD LABORATORY PRACTICES

GLP refers to the FDA's guidelines for submitting data for review by the FDA to receive investigational device exemption (IDE) or premarket approval (PMA) for clinical trials. Inasmuch as this discussion is meant to be an introduction to preclinical research, I will refrain from any dialogue on this particular subject. There have been volumes written on GLP and how to approach this type of data collection. I will say that once you are ready to enter this realm, be prepared to work very closely with the regulatory department of the chosen test facility. The paper trail here can be daunting. Ensure that the facility you choose has a proven track record before beginning your work. This is a very high bar indeed, and it requires extreme attention to detail and can be very costly.

CONCLUSION

In closing, I would like to stress two important points. First, plan, plan, plan and continue planning before beginning any in vivo work. Discuss your project with the test facility staff and get their input, as these are the folks with the most experience. The second vital point is data collection. Do your homework and know precisely which parameters will be necessary for your final assessment.

ABOUT THE AUTHOR

James Swick has been an active participant in the medical device community for more than 20 years and has helped many companies and institutions develop their respective products. He is the founder and visionary behind LyChron, the most successful preclinical laboratory in the western United States. Dr. Swick was on the faculty of Baylor College of Medicine and UCSF in the departments of neurosurgery and ophthalmology, and also held visiting professorships at the University of Arizona and University of Texas Medical Branch. He is a faculty member of the Stanford University School of Medicine lecturing in the Biodesign Innovations Fellowship program where he mentors up-and-coming entrepreneurs. He is a graduate of the University of California at Berkeley and Baylor College of Medicine.

18 Using Medical Illustration in Medical Device R&D

Theodore R. Kucklick

CONTENTS

Value of Medical Illustration to Medical Device R&D 351
Short History of Medical Illustration 353
Types of Medical Illustration 358
    Textbook Illustration 358
    Surgical Approach Planning 359
    Rendering from CAD Programs 359
    Layer Technique in Photoshop 360
    Blue Screen Trick 360
Device Development 361
Intellectual Property Development (Utility and Method) 363
Regulatory 363
Investor Presentations 363
Marketing, Physician Training, and Patient Information 364
Medical-Legal 365
Medical Teaching and Training Models 365
Three-Dimensional Animation 366
Resources 367
    References: The Medical Illustration Bookshelf 367
    References: Other Books 368
    References: Artistic Anatomy 368
    Vendors: Finding and Using Medical Illustration 368
        Licensed Use versus Buyout 368
    Medical Illustrators and Commercial Resources to Find Medical Illustrators . 369
Endnotes 370

VALUE OF MEDICAL ILLUSTRATION TO MEDICAL DEVICE R&D

Most people that even know what medical illustration is think that it is only for marketing and textbooks. Medical illustration, however, can be an important way to conceptualize and communicate medical device design ideas. Medical illustration is a highly developed specialty that has been an important adjunct to the understanding of anatomy and biological systems, as well as a way to conceptualize and visualize the interaction of medical devices with anatomy and pathology. Medical illustration can help engineers and designers to understand the anatomy for which they are designing a device to treat, to plan appropriate surgical approaches, to conceptualize new devices, to document designs and inventions, and to clearly communicate these device ideas to others.

This chapter will give a short history of medical illustration, the key role it has played in the development of medicine, how it is used now, and how to integrate it into the product development process. A number of practical and time-saving tools will be explained that show how to get engineering data and medical illustration to work together efficiently.

When a surgeon is trained, he studies anatomy. From this training, a proficient surgeon develops the ability to picture in his mind what the patient will look like on the inside, before starting the procedure. Medical illustration in textbooks, surgical atlases, and training models, as well as gross and regional anatomy training, are essential tools to develop this skill.

When an engineer or designer is given the task to develop a medical device, she is often trained and skilled in design and engineering, but may lack detailed knowledge of the anatomy or pathology that the device is intended to treat. Studying anatomical atlases is a good way to begin to understand relevant anatomy. Studying a number of good printed reference materials is a good start. There is no substitute, however, for a basic knowledge of gross anatomy, physiology, and detailed understanding of the regional anatomy in the area with which you are working.

Engineers and designers, like the surgeons, can develop the ability to picture in their minds and sketch and represent how a medical device will interact with the anatomy and structures to be treated. The designer will be able to picture and sketch, for example, how a catheter will enter through the femoral artery, thread through the abdominal aorta, and enter the heart via the aortic arch and into one of the coronary arteries in the aortic ostium. The ability to sketch out this type of approach, as well as describe it, can help to produce better medical device design decisions, determine feasible and infeasible surgical approaches, and conceptualize novel ways to perform a surgical intervention. It helps to answer the question, "Can we get there from here?"

A trained medical illustrator can work with design and engineering to help the advising surgeon communicate his therapeutic concepts to the design team and can work with the design team to understand and communicate how the device will work in anatomy. Engineers and designers can also learn and use the skills and techniques developed by medical illustrators in their own concept generation and communication of design ideas. Medical illustration has developed numerous ways to communicate complex anatomical information in a clear and understandable way. This can help to make the product clear and understandable to management, investors, regulators, patent counsel and patent examiners, and patients.

As important as seeing a good picture reference is to understanding anatomy and physiology, there is no substitute for working with and handling actual tissue and observing actual surgeries relevant to the area in which you are working.[1] This will help you to understand how tissues react, how they feel, how tough or fragile they are, and any number of other features that a textbook cannot adequately communicate. In medical illustration, there are a number of pictorial conventions (or common ways to represent information) that may not correspond with real anatomy but that are used to filter and modify visual information and emphasize what is relevant. One of the most obvious is that arteries are often rendered in red and veins in blue. If you have ever seen the inside of a real person, you know that these structures are not so conveniently color coded. If you think of a medical illustration as having a relationship to real anatomy somewhat like a wiring diagram has to actual wiring, then this can help you to understand how these conventions work. The other thing about medical illustration is that the structures are usually shown clean, and not bloody, as they might be in real life.

Another important distinction with illustration, medical photography, and studying anatomy is that an illustration and a photograph will render the visual information quite differently. In studying real anatomy, live tissue, fresh cadaver tissue, and cadaver tissue preserved in formalin all look and behave very differently. Living perfused tissue is different in color, the structures are inflated with blood, the tissue draws heat away from thermal ablation devices, and the tissue has a different texture. Furthermore, it is different in a number of important ways from even fresh cadaver tissue. Fresh cadaver tissue obviously does not bleed, has no muscle tone, and is usually less elastic than living tissue. It also goes immediately into some stage of decomposition. Preserved cadaver tissue in formalin is relatively tough and leathery compared with fresh cadaver tissue. This is because the formalin cross-links the proteins in the tissue. This also changes the color of the tissue. Fixed tissue tends to have less color than fresh cadaver tissue or living tissue.[2]

Illustrations, photographs, and tissue studies are all important tools to conceptualize, design, refine, and communicate in medical device development. In all of this it is important to remember that we are designing products to be used on real living people, patients, not pictures.[3]

SHORT HISTORY OF MEDICAL ILLUSTRATION

Medical illustration has served a vital role in developing and communicating accurate information about the human body and its physiology. The development of medical illustration has grown together with changing beliefs about the nature of the physical body, the role of learning by observation, the development of the sciences and medicine, and the development of printing technology and electronic communication media.

For most of human history, the workings of the human body have been of great interest; however, until recently, comparatively little information was systematically compiled, preserved, and communicated.

Learning in the ancient Western world centered in Alexandria, Egypt. The first textbooks of medicine and anatomy, *The Usefulness of Parts* and *On Anatomical Procedures*, were produced by Galen, between 130 and 200 A.D. For various reasons, dissection of cadavers was considered a violation of a corpse in ancient Greek times. Vivisection of animals was considered inhumane and virtually unknown. Dissections were likely done (along with chance observations from various injuries) and recorded by Homeric and Hippocratic Greek physicians. However, the practice of dissection was frowned upon by the culture of the time.[*] Little in the

---

[*] Ludwig Edelstein, *Ancient Medicine* (Baltimore: Johns Hopkins University Press, 1994): 247–301.

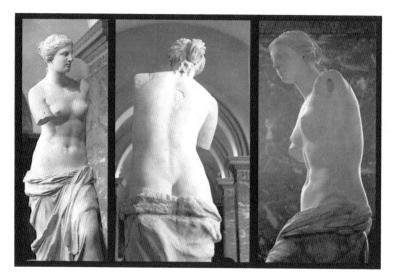

FIGURE 18.1 The Venus de Milo, the Louvre, Paris. A masterful classical handling of surface anatomy. (Courtesy of T. Kucklick.)

way of detailed anatomic knowledge was recorded and transmitted in the ancient world. One reason was the culture, another was the difficulty is distributing visual information, and yet another was the lack of a common nomenclature to describe anatomy. Classical sculptors produced masterful works of the surface anatomy of the exterior of the body, but comparatively little was depicted of the inside (see Figure 18.1).

Recorded learning of the ancients (not destroyed by fires) passed into the hands of the Arabs with the capture of Alexandria in 642 A.D. Texts from Alexandria and works that were preserved in Christian monasteries, such as one in Jundi Shapur, Iraq, which fell into conquered territory, were translated by Averroes, Albumazen, and Al-Kwarizmi, and eventually were transmitted to Europe in the Middle Ages in Latin translations by way of Spain.[*]

The forces of the Renaissance, the Reformation, the Enlightenment, and the development of printing technology revolutionized the understanding of science and medicine, and the dissemination of more accurate knowledge of the human body.

The modern understanding of the structure and function of the human body began with medical illustration. Leonardo da Vinci recorded numerous observations of the dissected human body in his notebooks (see Figure 18.2). These illustrations, however, were not discovered until the end of the 18th century. A near contemporary of Leonardo, Andreas Vesalius (1514–1564), produced the most significant and influential work in the understanding of the human body.

Vesalius, born in Belgium in 1514, studied medicine and settled in Padua, Italy, becoming a respected anatomist. Vesalius produced the landmark *De Humani Corporis Fabrica*, which translates to *On the Structure of the Human Body,* in 1543.

---

[*] James Burke, *Connections* (Boston: Little Brown & Co., 1978): 21–22.

Using Medical Illustration in Medical Device R&D

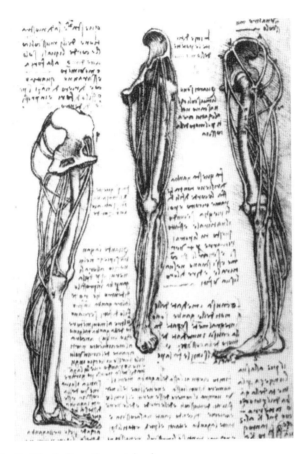

FIGURE 18.2 Da Vinci, dissection notebook page.

One result of Vesalius's work was to overturn the accepted, but erroneous, understanding of anatomy based on the work of Galen* and embedded into the universities through the structure of scholasticism. Vesalius is considered the father not only of modern anatomy, but also of medical illustration.[4]

Not only did Vesalius compile systematic and detailed information on the human body derived from observation, but he also developed ways to realistically present this information by way of engravings and drawings (see Figure 18.3). This information was disseminated by the recently developed technology of printing and made possible an unprecedented understanding of the human body by both scientists and artists.

Work by anatomist artists like Bernard Siegfried Albinus (1697–1770), professor of anatomy at Leiden and an extraordinary illustrator, contributed to the further understanding and visual depiction of the human body.

A link from Vesalius to another landmark discovery in medicine was through the work of William Harvey.† Harvey, the discoverer of the mechanism of blood

---

* Thomas McCracken, ed., *New Atlas of Human Anatomy* (New York: Metro Books, 1999): 15.
† In his work, Harvey dissected both his father and his sister.

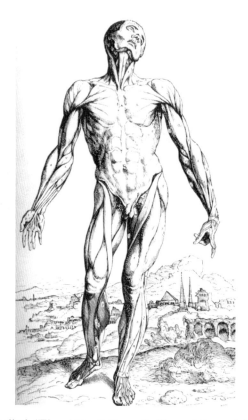

FIGURE 18.3 Vesalius's "Flayed Man." (From *De Humani Corporis Fabrica*, 1543.)

circulation, was trained in Padua by Gabriello Fallopio (1523–1562), for whom the Fallopian tubes are named. Fallopio had been a student of Vesalius and was teacher of Fabricus ab Aquapendente (1537–1619), an influential instructor at Padua, who in turn instructed Harvey.* *Exercitato de Motu Cordis et Sanguinus in Animalbus*, his treatise on the circulation of blood, is one of the most important works in medicine and biology and is illustrated with numerous woodcuts.†

Another medical pioneer was William Hunter (1718–1783), who made extensive and systematic studies of anatomy and is the father of modern obstetrics. Hunter wrote and illustrated *The Anatomy of the Human Gravid Uterus, Exhibited in Figures* (1774), "one of the finest anatomical monographs ever produced."[5]

Despite this impressive record of progress, procurement of cadavers for study in Britain was a thorny problem.‡ A distinct fear through the end of the 19th century

---

* Petrucelli Lyons et al., *Medicine: An Illustrated History* (New York: Abradale Press, 1978): 433.
† A theory proposed by Michael Servetus some 85 years earlier, whose work was cut short by a fatal disagreement with John Calvin over Servetus's Arianism.
‡ For an interesting history on the subject of the procurement of cadavers for anatomical study in Britain, see D. R. Johnson, "Introductory Anatomy," Centre for Human Biology, University of Leeds, http://www.leeds.ac.uk/chb/lectures/anatomy1.html.

was that if one were to die and their corpse were violated, they would thus be denied a proper Christian burial. Parliament passed an act that allowed the dissection of convicted murderers in 1752. Before this, Henry VIII allowed a limited number of hanged criminals to be thus examined. Before the more secular 20th century, cadavers were obtained from the ranks of these criminals or the poor who expired in hospitals at public expense (and thus considered public property). As the profession of surgery developed, and with it the demand for anatomical specimens, the practice of grave robbing and body snatching helped serve the needs of the surgical colleges. There is the nefarious case of Burke and Hare, who procured anatomic specimens for a Dr. Robert Knox in Edinburgh, Scotland, in the 1820s.* Typically, cadavers were procured from persons who had been executed or had expired naturally; however, Burke and Hare accelerated the process with some 16 victims in and around the Hare rooming house.† These were sold to Dr. Knox, who did not inquire very closely where these bodies came from. The resulting scandal and riots in Aberdeen helped lead to the Anatomy Act of 1832. This legislation, promoted by the Utilitarian philosopher Jeremy Bentham, finally provided a regular and legal source of cadavers for scientific study and also established guidelines for their ethical and considerate use. Bentham was also one of the first to willingly donate his body for dissection, a now-common practice.[6]

Another landmark work in the dissemination of understanding of the human body and its systems was the publication of *Anatomy Descriptive and Surgical* by Henry Gray, in 1858, commonly known as *Gray's Anatomy*. *Gray's Anatomy* took the additional step of teaching a form of anatomy useful to medical students and practicing doctors.

Work by 19th-century anatomists and illustrators such as Johannes Sobotta of Germany and Eduard Pernkopf of Austria introduced color illustration and a clean and idealized representation of the dissected body. J. C. B. Grant produced another type of work, *Grant's Anatomy*, which focused on documenting and explaining the relationship of organ systems.

Another medical illustrator worthy of note is Max Broedel, considered the father of modern medical illustration. Broedel was a mostly self-taught medical illustrator. Broedel was driven to understand, not just render his subjects. This led Broedel to make important contributions to medical technology and procedure in his own right.[7] He founded the Johns Hopkins Department of Art as Applied to Medicine in 1911, the oldest medical illustration program in the U.S.‡

One of the best-known modern medical illustrators is Frank Netter, MD. Dr. Netter was both a medical doctor and a trained commercial artist and produced

---

* See http://burkeandhare.com/citytour.htm. The city of Edinburgh's Burke and Hare "Midnight Tour" is a popular contemporary tourist attraction.
† "Up the close and down the stair, In the house with Burke and Hare. Burke's the butcher, Hare's the thief; Knox, the man who buys the beef." Edinburgh Royal Mile, http://www.edinburgh-royalmile.com/famous-scots/burke-and-hare.html (accessed August 12, 2012).
‡ "The curly-headed character also was a bon vivant, a member of the Saturday Night Club, which included some of Baltimore's best conversationalists and beer drinkers, including his close friend, H.L. Mencken." Johns Hopkins University, Johns Hopkins Medicine, http://www.hopkinsmedicine.org/about/history/history7.html.

a prodigious volume of work, especially in his volumes for the Ciba-Geigy Corporation. Netter's work for the Ciba Clinical Symposia illustrated numerous new medical technologies, such as those in the rapidly developing field of cardiology. Dr. Netter was one of the founders of the Association of Medical Illustrators (AMI) in 1945.

One of the important developments in the depiction and understanding of the human body is the advent of digital tools for three-dimensional reconstruction. The Visible Human Project® of the National Library of Medicine has produced a digital data set of anatomy based on the reconstruction of sliced sections of donated cadavers. This has made possible a virtual human that may be dissected any number of ways, and any number of structures or systems studied. One of the more important features of this data set is the ability to rotate the virtual specimen in space to any viewing angle, and the ability to subtract away structures quickly and easily, leaving other structures in the model intact. Previously, this process required laborious and painstaking dissection of structures, especially in delicate organs like the brain. This work was done by a team of computer modelers and programmers, as well as a number of medical illustrators, including Thomas McCracken.

One of the important advances resulting from digital reconstruction of anatomy is the depiction of anatomical variation. Medical illustration, by its nature, usually chooses an ideal, average, or representative depiction of an anatomical structure. In real life, however, there is significant variation in body types, as well as tortuosity of blood vessels and any number of other features. Digital reconstruction from actual anatomy helps to map and document these variations.

Computer-aided radiology and surgery (CARS) is an important tool in surgical planning and detection of variations in anatomy before a procedure. This is especially important in challenging procedures, such as neurosurgery, in which a variation in the location of a blood vessel and hitting it by mistake can be a potentially devastating complication in a craniotomy. Low-cost computing power has made this a more affordable tool in the hands of physicians for procedures, and CARS is beginning to make a difference in the noninvasive screening and detection of disease. The information learned and compiled from CARS is contributing in a revolutionary way to our understanding of anatomy.

Another recent development in the study and popularizing of anatomy is Gunter von Hagens' *Korperwelt* (Bodyworlds). These are donated cadavers that Hagens has taken dissected and has plastinated (preserved in plastic). These cadavers are then placed in life-like poses and publicly displayed.[8]

This work is both fascinating and controversial. For more information on von Hagens and Bodyworlds, see http://www.korperwelten.de or http://www.bodyworlds.com.[9]

TYPES OF MEDICAL ILLUSTRATION

TEXTBOOK ILLUSTRATION

Textbook illustration is the type of illustration with which most people are familiar. These are illustrations that show a surgical procedure. Often these are done in pen

Using Medical Illustration in Medical Device R&D

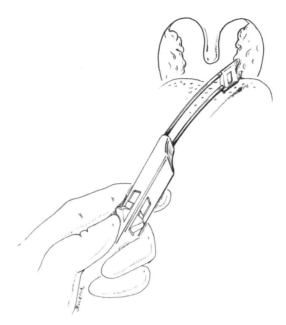

FIGURE 18.4 Example of pen-and-ink procedure training textbook illustration.

and ink for clarity (see Figure 18.4). The illustrator usually works with the surgeon writing a book chapter to produce these drawings. These illustrations help in understanding pathology and treatment of conditions. They are a very useful guide to existing and accepted procedures, and they can help the designer when developing an improved surgical device and method.

SURGICAL APPROACH PLANNING

Medical illustration can be quite useful in developing a new surgical approach. Some medical illustrators specialize in anatomical regions and procedures, such as gynecology or cardiology. A medical illustrator with expertise in the area in which you are working can be an asset in "coming up to speed" on the details of an anatomical region, as well as a source of information for existing clinical practice. The illustrator can produce custom illustrations of the anatomical region and, if the illustrator has the skills, can produce accurate three-dimensional models that can be imported into CAD programs to test ideas (see Figure 18.5).

RENDERING FROM CAD PROGRAMS

Most CAD programs have a built-in or accessory realistic rendering program. This allows the designer to apply realistic materials and finishes to a part, and render the result as an image. Check the documentation of your particular program for information on its renderer.

CAD models, both detailed and rough representative models, can be rendered and then easily trimmed and made into a separate object. Another way to quickly

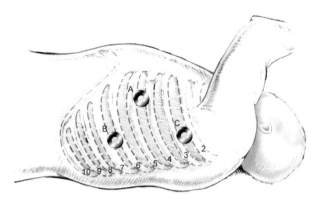

FIGURE 18.5 Thorascopic approach planning illustration. (T. Kucklick for AfX, Fremont, CA.)

grab an image is to use the <Print Screen> key (on a PC). This saves an image on the screen to memory. This can then be pasted in to a bitmap image editing program like Photoshop® by using the <Control + N> "New file" command, and then the <Control + V> "Paste" command. This creates a new file at the size of the screen-rendered image in memory. "Paste" places the image, where it can then be cleaned up.

LAYER TECHNIQUE IN PHOTOSHOP

The layers in Photoshop provide a powerful tool for editing and presenting graphics. An illustration of anatomy can be produced, and each structure can be placed on a different layer, as if on separate sheets of acetate. The layers can then be adjusted for transparency and be made to appear to recede in space. Layers may also be turned on and off. A series of illustrations, showing, for example, a catheter threading up an artery, can be illustrated on different layers and progressively turned off and on, and the resulting image saved to a .JPEG file. These can be used to produce a flip-book animation, which can be made into a digital movie or used as sequential slides in a presentation program such as PowerPoint™.

BLUE SCREEN TRICK

A simple way to trim a rendered object is to render it on a contrasting background, such as magenta or blue. This way the Photoshop "magic wand" tool can be used to select the background, and then the selection can be inversed to select the rendered object. Once the object is selected, use the <Control + X> command to cut the object from the background, use <Contol + N> to open a new file, and then use <Control + V> to paste the object. This places the object in a new file, as a separate object, where it can be easily moved and manipulated in a layered illustration (see Figure 18.6 for an example of this type of illustration).

Using these techniques, CAD data can be easily combined with hand-rendered illustrations, scanned illustrations, or photographs to produce illustrations that show the medical device in an anatomic setting (see Figure 18.7). For a guide to exchanging

Using Medical Illustration in Medical Device R&D

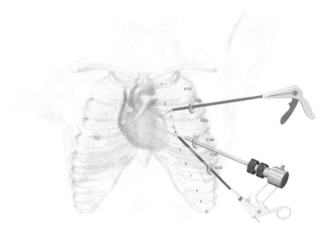

FIGURE 18.6 Surgical approach planning illustration with CAD models and layered illustration. (T. Kucklick for AfX, Fremont, CA.)

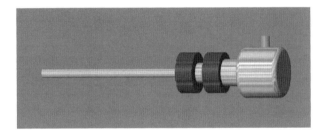

FIGURE 18.7 Rendered CAD model on contrasting background for use in image editing software.

rendered CAD data from three-dimensional programs to two-dimensional image editing and animation programs (see Figure 18.8).

DEVICE DEVELOPMENT

Medical illustration is useful when conceptualizing a device and its usage. It is also a useful part of the design history record (DHR) and design controls, when establishing and documenting user requirements and resulting device designs (see Figure 18.9). In this, Adobe Photoshop or some other good bitmap editing program like Corel Painter™ is quite useful. In the vascular device example, the original drawing was sketched in pencil, and then scanned into a computer and opened in the editing program. The drawing was used as an underlay, and color was added to the illustration in separate layers. Finally, captions and the company logo were added (see Figure 18.10). This method of starting in hand-drawn media and transitioning to digital media can save time when compared with producing the entire work digitally, and it is a method used by many professional medical illustrators.

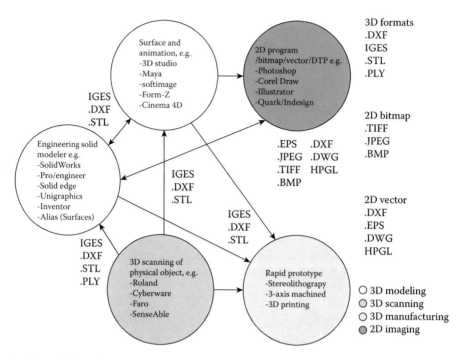

FIGURE 18.8 File exchange map for moving data from CAD to graphics applications.

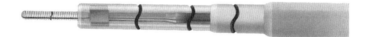

FIGURE 18.9 Catheter illustration. (T. Kucklick for ACS, Sunnyvale, CA.)

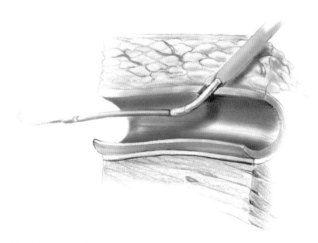

FIGURE 18.10 Vascular closure device concept sketch. (T. Kucklick for Neomend, Irvine, CA.)

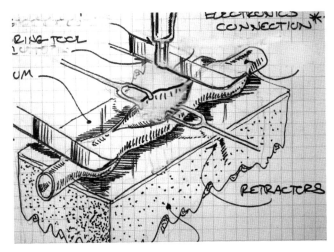

FIGURE 18.11   Lab notebook illustration example. (T. Kucklick)

INTELLECTUAL PROPERTY DEVELOPMENT (UTILITY AND METHOD)

When recording lab notebook information, supporting anatomical illustrations can help clarify and explain complex procedures, and can help document and establish claims for both devices and methods. Good, clear lab notebook illustrations can save time and expense when producing patent drawings. Black-and-white cartooning techniques can work very well to generate clear, direct, and interesting lab book drawings. If the lab drawings are good enough, they might be used as is, or with minimal cleanup in a patent application. This saves the expense of a patent draftsman having to redraw this work. Lab notebook illustrations can capture utility disclosures and claims, and also document novel ways to use a device in concept form or discovered in preclinical and clinical testing (see Figure 18.11).

REGULATORY

Medical illustration can help to clarify device concepts and use for regulatory bodies, such as the Food and Drug Administration (FDA). For example, these illustrations can be included as part of the documentation to claim substantial equivalence in a 510(k) application (see Figure 18.12).

INVESTOR PRESENTATIONS

An old saw in the investment world is "don't invest in what you don't understand." Good technical and medical illustration can help to clearly communicate sometimes-arcane medical information in a compact and compelling way to potential investors. If they can clearly grasp the concept and the value of what you are presenting, and they can see a clear, plausible path to execution, they may be more inclined to invest in your company. In the accompanying example, a CAD solid model of the device and a Foley balloon was composited with a two-dimensional digital illustration of

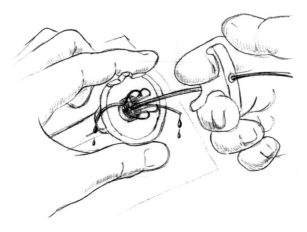

FIGURE 18.12 Drawing for 510(k) regulatory application for a medical device showing function.

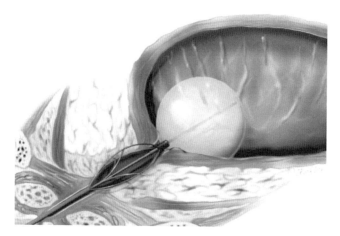

FIGURE 18.13 Illustration combining a CAD model of a medical device and a two-dimensional illustration for an investor presentation.

anatomy for an investor presentation. This helped to communicate the device concept and the company was successfully funded (see Figure 18.13).

MARKETING, PHYSICIAN TRAINING, AND PATIENT INFORMATION

Medical illustration is common in trade show exhibits, medical journal ads, physician training materials, and instructions for use (IFUs). Good medical illustration is not that expensive, especially relative to the cost of space in medical and trade journals or compared with the cost of attending a trade show. Some medical illustration I have seen in some major journals and at major trade shows is of low quality. Your company's image and the reputation are being displayed through the quality of what you put into your graphics. If you are going to take the time and spend the money to put illustration into your marketing and training materials, at least ensure that it is quality work done by a competent professional.

MEDICAL-LEGAL

One established subset of the medical illustration profession is medical-legal. There are medical illustrators who specialize in producing courtroom illustration and are familiar with the procedures and protocol involved with these presentations. This work is usually used by the plaintiff to establish claims of medical malpractice, personal injury, or product liability. This type of illustration may be useful when arguing a defense in a product liability case.

MEDICAL TEACHING AND TRAINING MODELS

The production of medical models is another area of medical illustration. There are numerous varieties of medical models, from the purely visual, to those for training, to those purely for engineering. Rapid prototype models have become a common tool for planning complex surgeries. Examples of these are shown in Chapter 7. Training models mimic some features of a surgical procedure, such as the retraction of tissue for an open procedure, the trackabilty of a catheter, or the insertion force of an introducer (see Figure 18.14). SOMSO Models (Marcus Sommer Somso-Modelle) has been manufacturing medical models in Sonnenburg and Coburg, Germany, since 1876, and the company has been in the Sommer family for five generations. SOMSO makes models of nearly all human anatomy and many zoological and botanical models, which can be purchased in the United States from Holt Anatomical (Miami, FL), the Anatomical Chart Company, and many medical college bookstores. Companies like Pacific Research (http://www.sawbones.com) produce bone models for demonstration and training purposes, as well as carbon fiber bones for realistic engineering testing. Laerdal Corporation (formerly Medical Plastics Laboratory) makes a wide range of medical teaching and training models, specializing in training models for emergency medical services (EMS) and resuscitation. Kilgore

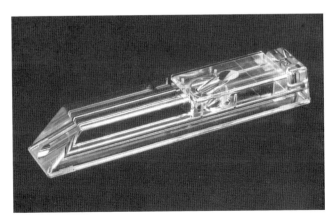

FIGURE 18.14 Femoral artery access training model.

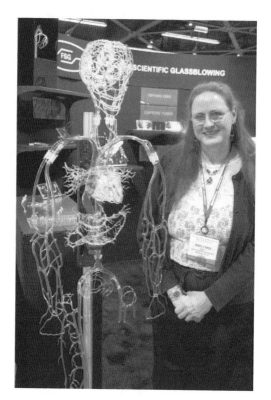

FIGURE 18.15 One of Farlow's glass vascular training models.

International (http://www.kilgoreinternational.com) specializes in dental and skull models. Simulab (http://www.simulab.com) makes models for training surgeons on a variety of procedures. Farlow's Scientific Glassblowing (http://www.farlowsci.com) makes glass vasculature models for testing catheters and other medical devices (see Figure 18.15). Phantoms mimic some characteristic of an organ where radiology is applied,[10] which can include calibration phantoms or imaging phantoms.[11] CIRS, Inc. (http://www.cirs.com) specializes in radiology phantom.

THREE-DIMENSIONAL ANIMATION

Whether threading a catheter, deploying a device, or expanding a stent, three-dimensional animation is a powerful communication tool. One caveat: Three-dimensional animation can be expensive. There is the cost of building the three-dimensional model (especially complex anatomy like the heart) and the cost of rendering the final result to video. Three-dimensional animators typically charge per hour for model building and a per-minute charge for finished video. Importing existing CAD data whenever possible can save some of the expense of three-dimensional model making. Also, some companies sell three-dimensional clip models of body parts, so that some of this work does not need to be done from scratch. Three-dimensional animation is usually reserved for marketing applications for which the return on investment (ROI) from increased sales offsets the expense of the animation. Three-dimensional animation is a specialty all its own requiring expensive specialized equipment to render the animation file to tape, and specialized software like Softimage®, Maya®, or 3DStudio® to produce the animation files. When looking for an illustrator to do this work, find an animator who is skilled in these areas and has a comprehensive understanding of medical illustration and anatomy.

RESOURCES

REFERENCES: THE MEDICAL ILLUSTRATION BOOKSHELF

Medical device designers can benefit from having a complete library of good anatomical reference material. The question is, What is good reference material? A number of years ago, the Association of Medical Illustrators[*] published a suggested reference bookshelf, and some of those recommendations are reflected in this list.

There is no one atlas that covers every structure in the way and in the detail you might require. It is a good idea to go to a school of medicine bookstore and look at each one of these books to see which is most appropriate for your needs. If you buy only one atlas, *Netter's Atlas of Human Anatomy* is probably the best single volume. A recommendation is that you have at least more than one, and over time, acquire several. Comparing the approach and presentation between two or more references will help to build a better understanding of the structures you are studying. Also, there are a number of specialized atlases in areas like cardiology, neurology, urology, and so on (e.g., *Netter's Atlas of Human Neuroscience*), if you need even more detailed information. It is best to start with a good shelf of the general atlases, and purchase an expensive specialized atlas if you have a specific need for one.

Abrahams, P. H., Sandy C. Marks, and Ralph Hutchings. *McMinn's Color Atlas of Human Anatomy*, 5th ed. St. Louis: Mosby International, 2003. This text is another well-done and comprehensive photographic atlas of gross anatomy dissections.

Clemente, Carmine D. *Clemente Anatomy: A Regional Atlas of the Human Body*, 4th ed. Baltimore: Williams & Wilkins, 1997. This text is another excellent and popular anatomical atlas. This atlas was originally published in Germany, and the illustrations are done mostly by a number of German medical illustrators, with a more naturalistic rendering style than Netter's. A companion volume is *Clemente's Anatomy Dissector.*

Drake, Richard, Wayne Vogl, and Adam Mitchell. *Gray's Anatomy for Students*. Philadelphia, PA: Churchill Livingston Publishers, 2004. Richard Drake, PhD., director of anatomy, Cleveland Clinic Lerner College of Medicine, Cleveland, Ohio, worked with a team of authors and illustrators to produce an updated version of *Gray's Anatomy* for medical students. The atlas is different than those by Netter or Clemente, as all of the illustrations were done by one group of artists especially for the book, and thus have more structure and consistency as a group.

Netter, Frank, and John T. Hansen. *Atlas of Human Anatomy*, 3rd ed. Teterboro, NJ: Icon Learning Systems, 2003. This text is the most popular anatomical atlas in print. Icon Learning Systems purchased the Netter collection of work from Novartis in 2000, and publishes and licenses his work at http://www.netterart.com.

---

[*] Association of Medical Illustrators, http://www.ami.org.

Rohen, Johannes, Chihiro Yokochi, and Elke Lutjen-Drecoll. *Color Atlas of Anatomy*, 4th ed. Baltimore: Williams & Wilkins, 1997. This text is a comprehensive photographic atlas of careful and skillful cadaver dissections. This is a good companion to have to the illustrated atlases, as it shows real tissues and not just idealized representations.

REFERENCES: OTHER BOOKS

Gray, Henry, Susan Standring, Harold Ellis, and B. K. B. Berkovitz. *Gray's Anatomy: The Anatomical Basis of Clinical Practice*. Edinburgh: Elsevier Churchill Livingstone, 2005 and Agur, A. M. R., Ming J. Lee, and J. C. Boileau Grant. *Grant's Atlas of Anatomy* Philadelphia: Lippincott Williams & Wilkins, 1999. These classic works are the original modern anatomy books. Grant's has recently had a major revision. *Grant's Dissector* is a companion volume to *Anatomy*. (Tank, Patrick W., and J. C. Boileau Grant. *Grant's Dissector*. Philadelphia: Wolters Kluwer Health/Lippincott, Williams & Wilkins, 2009).

McCracken, Thomas O. *New Atlas of Human Anatomy*. London: Metro, 2000. This atlas is a showcase of computer renderings from the Visible Human Project for a popular audience. It is instructive to compare these renderings to the illustrations and photographs in the academically oriented atlases.

REFERENCES: ARTISTIC ANATOMY

For designers that need to illustrate the external human form, and other structures like heads, hands, and feet, artistic anatomy references can be helpful. Here are some of the better ones:

Barcsay, Jeno. *Anatomy for the Artist*. London: Octopus Books, 1973.
Delavier, Frederic. *Strength Training Anatomy*. Champaign, IL: Human Kinetics, 2010.
Goldfinger, Eliot. *Human Anatomy for Artists: The Elements of Form*. New York: Oxford University Press, 1991. This is considered a classic.
Hale, Robert Beverly, and Terrence Coyle. *Anatomy Lessons from the Great Masters*. New York: Watson-Guptil Publications, 1977. Hale was the dean of figure-drawing instructors.
Robins, Clem. *The Art of Figure Drawing*. Cincinnati, OH: Northlight Books. Robins was a student of Hale and Coyle; a good introduction to life like figure drawing.
Simblett, Sarah, and John Davis. *Anatomy for the Artist*. New York: DK Publishing, 2001. Includes numerous photographs and overlays.

VENDORS: FINDING AND USING MEDICAL ILLUSTRATION

Licensed Use versus Buyout

When hiring a medical illustrator, there are two basic ways to obtain rights to the work. One is a license for a specified use, and the other is a buyout, where the buyer obtains all rights to a work and possession of the original art or file.

The issue of buyouts is a hot topic among illustrators. Traditionally, illustrators are reluctant to sell work outright, unless it was a piece specific to the client. Buyouts are available, but at a higher cost than a license. Illustrators over their career build a library of stock art and license these out. (This is how illustrators are able to even out their income stream and make a decent living.) If you are looking for an illustration of an anatomical structure, there are probably numerous stock examples immediately available from the artist. The artist can also modify the work to meet your specific needs. A professional medical illustrator can be an important partner to an engineering team, if he or she has in-depth knowledge of the anatomy in the area you are working in.

One issue that may need to be clarified with the illustrator is the practice of assigning any intellectual property (IP) and inventions to the company. Some medical illustrators have detailed and valuable experience in medical specialties and can make inventive contributions, but they may not be familiar with customary IP arrangements in engineering groups. To not clarify this issue upfront, and assume the illustrator is "just an artist" and not in a position to make an inventive contribution, may invite potentially acrimonious disagreements over IP ownership.

MEDICAL ILLUSTRATORS AND COMMERCIAL RESOURCES TO FIND MEDICAL ILLUSTRATORS

Anatomical Chart Company, acquired by Lippincott Williams & Wilkins (LWW)
http://www.lww.com/webapp/wcs/stores/servlet/content_h-t-m-l_about_11851_-1_12551
The Anatomical Chart Company (LWW) makes numerous charts describing nearly every important bodily structure and many pathologies, as well as distributing anatomical medical models and books.

Association of Medical Illustrators
201 E. Main Street, Suite 1405
Lexington, KY 40507
U.S.A.
Phone: 1-866-393-4AMI (or 1-866-393-4264)
e-mail: hq@ami.org
www.ami.org
The Association of Medical Illustrators is a professional group of medical illustrators founded in 1945. *The Association of Medical Illustrators Sourcebook* (Serbin Press, Santa Barbara, CA) is an annual publication with ad pages from working medical and natural science illustrators. If you are a qualified buyer of medical illustration, you can call Serbin and ask to be on its distribution list, or purchase a copy when available. Serbin has a limited number of back issues of the *Sourcebook* occasionally available.

Serbin Communications
511 Olive Street
Santa Barbara, CA 93101
Phone: 800-876-6425
Fax: 805-965-0496
admin@serbin.com
http://www.medillsb.com

Indexed Visuals (IV)
http://www.indexedvisuals.com

IV is an online source for medical illustration, with a catalog of thousands of pieces of stock art and ad pages by illustrators. The artists may be contacted directly to negotiate fees for a particular piece of artwork.

ENDNOTES

1. "In collecting the evidence upon any medical subject there are but three sources from which we can hope to obtain it: that is from living subjects, from examination of the dead and from experiments upon living animals." Astley Cooper and Benjamin Travers, *Surgical Essays* (1821), in Ira M. Rutkow, *The History of Surgery in the United States, 1775-1900* (Novato, CA: Jeremy Norman Co., 1988): 394. Quote is attributed to Sir Astley Cooper, 1768–1841.
2. "In dissecting cadavers there may be some fear and discomfort associated with looking at and handling a dead body. First of all, cadaver tissue fixed in formalin is sterile, and not an infection risk, though gloves are strongly recommended. (Fresh cadaver tissue needs to be handled with the same high level of caution as living tissue and blood)." D. R. Johnson, Centre for Human Biology, University of Leeds, "Introductory Anatomy," http://www.leeds.ac.uk/chb/lectures/anatomy1.html (accessed August 12, 2012).
3. When participating in my first dissection of a cadaver arm when designing an orthopedic surgical device, I was doubly uncomfortable that it was cadaver tissue and dismembered at that. I had to work at keeping images from bad B movies out of my mind. The thing that got me over my initial squeamishness was thinking of Ps. 139:14—that the human body is fearfully and wonderfully made—and that I was going to have a privileged opportunity to examine this marvelous work. This helped me get over the initial discomfort, and after the dissection helped build a deep and lasting appreciation for the design and structure of the human body.
4. Much of the controversy between the Roman church and authorities like Aquinas and Albertus Magnus, and investigators like Vesalius and Galileo, had to do with the upsetting of the carefully crafted medieval system of scholasticism, an amalgam of tenets from classical authorities like Galen, Plato, Aristotle, and Ptolemy, and Roman church precepts.
5. "John and William Hunter: Pioneers of Surgery and Medicine," Hoslink: A Resource for Medical and Biomedical Professionals, http://www.hoslink.com/pioneers3.htm, accessed August 12, 2012; "Beginnings," the Hunterian Society, http://www.hunteriansociety.org.uk, accessed August 12, 2012. William Hunter was elder brother to John Hunter (1728–1793), founder of pathological anatomy and known for his fiery temper. He coined many of the terms used today to describe dental anatomy. William is considered the founder of the scientific approach to surgery. Students of William included Edward Jenner, inventor of vaccination, and Sir Astley Cooper, anatomist (Cooper's ligament) and pioneer in vascular surgery. These students, following William's principles, carried out pioneering experimental research and applied their findings to the clinical needs of patients.
6. "The riots, the murders and public opinion meant that something had to be done and the outcome was the 1832 Anatomy Act, which was a key issue in the election of 1832. A key figure behind this was Jeremy Bentham, founder of University College London. His idea was essentially that anyone applying to a hospital for treatment was in effect giving permission for the use of their body, in the event of a poor result, being available for dissection, followed by Christian burial. Although forgoing a Christian burial Bentham was publicly dissected at University College in 1828." D. R. Johnson, "Introductory Anatomy," Centre for Human Biology, University of Leeds, http://www.leeds.ac.uk/chb/lectures/anatomy1.html.

7. "Broedel's determination to understand completely what he was drawing led to his becoming an investigator—and even devising some new surgical approaches. For instance, he recommended that surgeons start fishing for kidney stones from the avascular part of the kidney, in order to limit damage to the organ's filtering mechanisms, which are in the vascular areas. This insight, and a sturdy, triangular stitch still known as Broedel's suture, developed from the artist's in-depth study of a kidney in the autopsy room." Johns Hopkins University, "Art As Applied to Medicine," Johns Hopkins Medicine, http://www.hopkinsmedicine.org /about/history/history7.html.
8. "Anatomical dissection gives the human mind an opportunity to compare the dead with the living, things severed with things intact, things destroyed with things evolving, and opens up the profoundness of nature to us more than any other endeavor or consideration." Goethe, from the body donor solicitation card, Institute for Plastination, Bodyworlds 2 Exhibit, Cleveland, OH.
9. I recently attended the *Bodyworlds2* exhibit in Cleveland, Ohio. The exhibit, which is quite remarkable, includes twenty whole bodies and over 200 anatomical specimens. For anyone who has either seen or done dissections and understands the amount of work that went into the exhibit, the exhibit is impressive. Sectioned cadavers, ones mounted in life-like poses, such as skiers, skaters, and skateboarders, and specimens of pathology such as cancers, stroke, myocardial infarction, and examples of dissections with orthopedic implants are all represented. The exhibit is as close as a person can get to a dissection without performing one and having to smell the formalin.
10. "The International Commission on Radiation Units and Measurements (ICRU) defines a tissue substitute as any material that simulates a body of tissue in its interaction with ionizing radiation, and a phantom as any structure that contains one or more tissue substitutes and is used to simulate radiation interactions in the human body." See http://www.cirsinc.com/technology/publication-references (accessed August 12, 2012).
11. "Calibration Phantoms: are used to establish the response of radiation detectors and for correcting quantitative information derived from digital images. Imaging Phantoms: are used for the assessment of image quality. Within these functional categories phantoms can be further defined: Body Phantoms: have the shape and composition of the human body or part of it. They are also referred to as anthropomorphic phantoms. Phantoms that are used for standardization and inter-comparison of various radiation conditions are often referred to as Standards. Reference Phantoms: include phantoms used to derive radiation dose calculations, mineral density equivalences or other similar type measurements. They can further be defined by their intended modality such as Ultrasound, Mammography, MRI and Computed Tomography (CT)." See Nuclear Medicine Phantoms, http://www.medimaging.gr/cd/pages/phan3.htm (accessed August 12, 2012).

19 Case Study: The BACE™ Mitral Regurgitation Treatment Device

Supplement to Chapter 18, Using Medical Illustration in Medical Device R&D

Theodore R. Kucklick

CONTENT

Acknowledgments... 376

Mardil Medical's (Orono, MN) Basal Annuloplasty of the Cardia Externally (BACE™) device was developed to treat a common heart defect called mitral valve regurgitation, a condition related to many types of coronary heart disease. Mitral regurgitation is a condition in which the weakened mitral valve leaks blood backward into the heart, often leading to congestive heart failure with severe, debilitating symptoms. Current treatments for mitral regurgitation, however, carry a range of serious complications and risks. The BACE is an implanted device that is not invasive to the heart, but it fits around the heart as a custom-fitted sling, providing the extra support the mitral valve needs to close properly and to keep blood from regurgitating back into the heart. The BACE solution is safer than mitral valve repair, or the more extreme solution of heart transplant, because the device is implanted around the heart and has no contact with blood flow like the more invasive surgeries that add to the risks of thrombosis, stroke, and infection.

The BACE device was pioneered by cardiothoracic surgeon Dr. Jai Raman, who has a background in investigating containment systems that address heart failure and an interest in minimally invasive approaches in cardiac surgery. Dr. Raman worked with medical illustrator Beth Croce at the Austin Hospital in Melbourne, Australia, to develop early conceptual drawings illustrating how the device might function. Being very familiar with cardiac anatomy and surgical techniques, Croce worked with Dr. Raman visualizing many of his ideas for devices and techniques, such as radio frequency ablation burn set "maps" and the first versions of the Acorn CorCap™ ventricular support device.

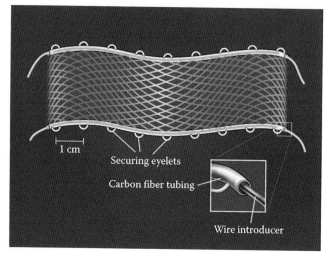

FIGURE 19.1 (**See color insert.**) Conceptual device illustration.

Schematic diagrams of the BACE device depicted a simple mesh band, not unlike the CorCap. While being tested in animal models, Croce was able to illustrate how the band would fit on a human heart—not only its placement but also depicting how underlying structures would be supported using a semitransparent illustration. She also created Flash animations that demonstrated what effect this support might have on mitral regurgitation in a beating heart. These illustrations and animations served not only to convey the current state of development of the device as it evolved but also to make more concrete concepts that might then be explored for further modification before being made into a physical model (see Figure 19.1). In this case,

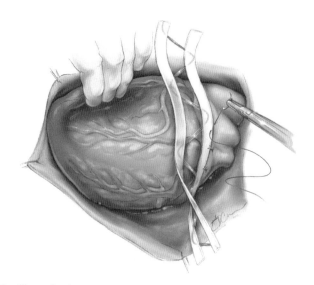

FIGURE 19.2 (**See color insert.**) Surgical planning illustration, step 1.

Case Study: The BACE™ Mitral Regurgitation Treatment Device

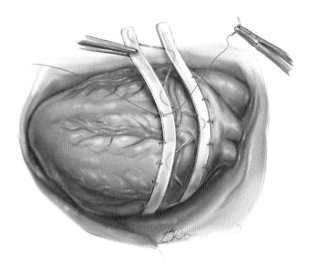

FIGURE 19.3 (See color insert.) Surgical planning illustration, step 2.

the mesh was exchanged for a zigzagging coated wire, and a second option with double crossed wires was depicted as well.

In the version eventually used for worldwide multicenter clinical trials in humans, the double wires replace the polyester mesh and chambers are saline filled on demand to provide adjustable pressure to the ventricle wall and mitral valve.

Dr. Raman, now professor of surgery at the University of Chicago Medical Center, uses the current versions of illustrations and animations in informative talks and presentations on the use of the device and management of heart failure (see Figures 19.2 to 19.4).

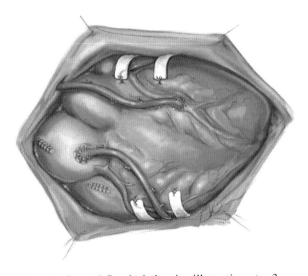

FIGURE 19.4 (See color insert.) Surgical planning illustration, step 3.

ACKNOWLEDGMENTS

The assistance of Beth Croce in the development of this chapter is gratefully acknowledged. Beth Croce is a Johns Hopkins–trained medical artist at the Austin Hospital in Melbourne, Australia, and developed early conceptual drawings showing how the device functioned. At the time, Croce was the in-house illustrator for the Austin Cardiac Surgery Department and had recently completed illustrations for the cardiac surgery atlas, *Ischemic Heart Disease*: *Surgical Management* (Mosby, 1999).

Section IV

Interviews and Insights for the R&D Entrepreneur

20 Interview with Thomas Fogarty, MD

Theodore R. Kucklick

CONTENTS

Resources 386
    References: Other Interviews with Dr. Fogarty: 386

Thomas J. Fogarty, MD, is a legend in the medical device community. He is a retired vascular surgeon, a highly regarded winemaker,[*] a venture capitalist, and a leading medical technology innovator (Figure 20.1). He has founded or cofounded more than 30 companies in the medical device or services field, holds more than 100 patents, and is author of more than 170 scientific and medical articles. Dr. Fogarty invented the Fogarty embolectomy catheter while still a medical student and also developed the stent graft that replaced highly invasive open AAA (abdominal aortic aneurysm) surgery.[†] Dr. Fogarty is one of the most successful medical device innovators of all time. He is a recipient of the Laufman-Greatbatch Prize[‡] for advances in medical instrumentation and received the MIT-Lemelson Prize for Innovation in 2000.[§] He was inducted into the Inventor's Hall of Fame in December 2001.[¶]

MDR&D: You have been a successful practicing physician as well as a pioneering medical device innovator. Could you tell me about some of the innovations and the companies you've founded?

TJF: Yes, I can tell you about a few, but I can't tell you about all. The initial ones were essentially licensing patents. The first was to a company called Edwards, which licensed the first therapeutic balloon catheter. I also licensed a few of the Fogarty clamps, which were the first truly atraumatic vascular clamps. Edwards also had an option to buy a tissue heart valve and had the right to exercise that option in a six-month period. They

---

[*] Thomas Fogarty Wines and Vineyard, http://www.fogartywinery.com.
[†] See "Inventing Modern America: Thomas Fogarty," http://web.mit.edu/invent/www/ima/fogarty_bio.html (accessed August 13, 2012).
[‡] "AAMI Foundation Laufman-Greatbatch Award," Advancing Safety in Medical Technology, http://www.aami.org/awards/greatbatch.html, accessed August 13, 2012.
[§] "Thomas Fogarty 2000 Lemelson-MIT Prize Winner," Lemelson-MIT, http://web.mit.edu/invent/a-winners/a-fogarty.html, accessed August 13, 2012.
[¶] "Inventor Profile," Inventors Hall of Fame, Invent Now, http://www.invent.org/hall_of_fame/162.html, accessed August 13, 2012.

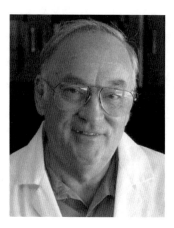

FIGURE 20.1 Thomas J. Fogarty, MD. (Courtesy of Thomas Fogarty.)

chose not to, so I started a company called Hancock Laboratories, where the first successful tissue heart valve reached the marketplace. I became involved with Bentley Laboratories by serving on the board and as a consultant. After that, I got involved in early stage companies.*

MDR&D: You often mention the term "clinical utility" as something that should drive a medical innovation. Could you describe the concept of clinical utility?

TJF: I have people interpret clinical utility as something that helps a physician, but more importantly, it should help the patient. Physicians don't always hear the perspective of a patient, but in order for something to have clinical utility, it has to satisfy both patient and doctor.

MDR&D: You have said that an invention and an innovation are not the same thing—that there's a difference between the two.

TJF: Yes, there is. An invention can be an innovation, and an innovation can be an invention. However, you could innovate a service, but not invent it. In other words, you may come up with a different type of service to benefit the patient, but not invent anything. Or you may come up with a technique and an instrument, which is closer to invention than innovation.

MDR&D: So, if somebody says, "I have a great idea."

TJF: It is an idea and nothing else.

MDR&D: And, it doesn't have a lot of value . . .

TJF: It has zero, unless the idea is implemented.

MDR&D: You have described some of the critical factors to producing medical device innovation, such as having an idea of the market, the people, sales and distribution, and clinical utility.

TJF: Well, that's part of it, but the first thing is recognizing a need. There are certain technologies and inventions to which a physician will say, "Well, I don't need that." One has to accept the fact, which is difficult for physicians

---

* For more information on these companies, see *In Vivo: The Business & Medicine Report* (February 2003), http://www.windhover.com/contents/monthly/ exex/e_2003800031.htm.

MDR&D: to do, that they are lacking because they are intelligent and have been taught to stay out of trouble by doing things the same way to take care of the patient. A lot of doctors have never recognized the need because they are not willing to admit that they are not doing the best job. The same is true of technicians. If you come up with a technology that replaces a technician or replaces a nurse, you're going to have a hard time.

MDR&D: You have also mentioned that it takes different types of people to generate a marketable innovation, such as those who are good at concepts and those who can finish "the last 10%."

TJF: Yes, the finishers are actually the hardest to find, since engineers are all perfectionists. So there comes a time in an engineer's life where somebody has to stop them because they will go on forever. It's a natural tendency of engineers; the enemy of good is better. So there's a fine balance between when to stop and when not to stop. They have to recognize that even when they put it into the marketplace and it gets clinical use, they're going to have additional work. You cannot anticipate everything; you have to acknowledge that. But, if you're going in the wrong direction, you have to make sure you're going in the wrong direction.

MDR&D: What management techniques do you use to keep up a high pace of innovation?

TJF: I think it's a balance of interfering, but not interfering. You have to intercede at the right time with more encouragement than criticism. Innovation surrounding new companies is not a nine-to-five job, period. Commitment is critically important and leaders have to create that environment of commitment.

MDR&D: You have described Fogarty Engineering as a "percolator" rather than an "incubator." What is the difference?

TJF: An incubator implies that there's a certain time frame. For a human, it's nine months. Innovation cannot be scheduled because you cannot create consistently in a time frame. When you say incubate, that means incubate. You cannot do that with innovation. You may work and get there quicker or get there later. With an incubator no matter how you work, it's going to come out in nine months. That's why I call it a "percolator." You can't always tell when the water is going to boil. There are a lot of things that influence the process.

MDR&D: What does "You have to cannibalize yourself to innovate" mean?

TJF: You have to replace it yourself. If the technology is going to replace something, it's better that you do it yourself. It's kind of like you're in a trap, a steel trap. To get out you have to chew your way out. Unless you do it fast, you aren't going to get there. If you have enough vision and have an interest in it, you can. It's hard to cannibalize yourself, but you have to do it. If you don't do it, somebody else will.

MDR&D: One of the characteristics of your innovations is simplicity. Could you speak to the need for simplicity in medical device design?

TJF: That's because that's the way it is. You usually go through a stage of complexity and then return to simplicity. What helps that is when you prototype, you see the issues with making it yourself. And if you start thinking if I make it this way, will it work? And if I make it simple, will it be accepted by more people?

MDR&D: The person doing the design work should be the one doing the prototyping?

TJF: It doesn't have to be, but that has always worked well for me. If I can't do the prototyping myself, the engineers will and then I'll ask, "Let me see you make that." Then I'll say, "Well, maybe I can make it this way." If I change the deployment, the engineer will understand, but he won't understand how a surgeon can use a different technique and achieve the same thing. The first thing that physicians will do, if something doesn't work, is blame the engineer. Then he will immediately want to go back and have the engineer change it. You don't need to always do that; you can change the technique.

MDR&D: Then it's not just the device itself; it's how the physician interacts with the device?

TJF: That's correct.

MDR&D: Are there differences between technology-driven products and clinical needs–driven products?

TJF: There is a difference. If you have a technology that's complicated, then the manufacturing process is going to be too expensive. If you have something that's complicated in terms of physician use, it's going to be difficult. In other words, if he finds it hard to use, he would rather just do what he always did. Then there are clinical needs. Clinical needs should be first from the patient's perspective, not the specialist's perspective. It may help him do something. It may help him make more money. It may help him take one procedure from another specialty.

MDR&D: I understand that when you first came up with catheter interventions, putting balloons on catheters and putting them in blood vessels, you had a tremendous uphill battle.

TJF: Absolutely. The concept was if you manipulated the inside of a vessel with anything, much less scrape it with a balloon, it was totally inappropriate. When I was a medical student at the University of Cincinnati, the professor of surgery said, "Only one so uninformed and inexperienced would dare do such a thing."

MDR&D: You proved the conventional wisdom was not right.

TJF: Right. The golden rule ain't so golden.

MDR&D: What does the statement "First do no harm" really mean?

TJF: It means that's the obligation of a physician. And you do no harm by doing what you were taught to do and always did. That's why physicians aren't so venturesome.

MDR&D: You have said what doctors say they need, and what they want, and what they'll pay for are three different things.

TJF: They are. Absolutely.

MDR&D: Does "First do no harm" mean "do what you've always done?"

TJF: It doesn't mean that. All physicians interpret that as doing what they've always done and not venturing out into what they haven't done or what is not properly documented by someone's criteria. That someone is usually an academic. And what it does for the patient is a fourth different thing. You should look at what's best for the patient.

MDR&D: That's the way to find a real clinical need and find real clinical utility?

TJF: Hopefully the needs match, but sometimes they don't. In other words what's best for the patient and best for the doctor. If they can be therapeutically better and economically better for both the doctor and the patient, that is a good match.

MDR&D: At a medical technology conference, you talked about the different set of priorities between a university teaching hospital and a community-based hospital.

TJF: Most physicians residing in an academic center are focusing close on what they call science and teaching. And, "oh by the way" we do occasionally take care of real patients representing real pathology. There's a difference between science and technology. Science is the explanation of a theory to prove or disprove the validity of the theory explored. Technology is the application of science that is already proven. You may use the scientific method in documenting the technology and you may use the science of epidemiology and the science of statistics to prove the efficacy of a technology.

MDR&D: You have said that the physician–entrepreneur sometimes gets caught in a trap of conflict of interest.

TJF: It's not sometimes, it's always.

MDR&D: Do doctors have difficulty participating in the clinical evaluation of their own technology due to conflict of interest problems?

TJF: Depending upon the institution. At most academic centers it remains an unresolved problem.

MDR&D: How did the Three Arch Partners venture capital fund start?

TJF: I have always been involved in medical technology. When I say always, by that I mean I have had exposure to the hospital environment and physicians since age 12. With this familiarity, I became interested in it. I then became an inventor in the field of medical technology and then finished my training in medical technology. I continued to develop devices over these years. Twelve years ago, I took a year off for the purpose of further developing Fogarty Engineering. In that process some venture groups asked me to be a partner. I looked at the opportunity and felt that most venture firms mostly graded theses. I do not want to spend my life grading theses so I started to explore the possibility of creating what I call an entrepreneurial venture group. This in fact had been done in other areas besides medical technology. I had exposure to two young venture capitalists who were members of the same boards of companies I had founded. I asked if they wanted to start a "different" venture group, which they agreed to. They named the partnership Three Arch Partners.

MDR&D: Are there any particular red flags that would keep you from investing in a company?

TJF: If it's offshore or part of it is. Or if the physician/founder/inventor insists on being a CEO. The fourth thing is obvious unawareness of the regulatory and reimbursement issues. There are probably many, many others.

MDR&D: What's more important when you look at a company to invest in? The people or the technology?

TJF: Both.

MDR&D: How do you overcome reimbursement challenges?

TJF: It depends upon the product. And whether or not it's FDA [Food and Drug Administration] approved, or whether it's in clinical trials. Those sort of challenges aren't consistent. You can actually have a CPT [Current Procedural Terminology] code but have no reimbursement either by a governmental agency, a state, or a national approval or acceptance of payment. Payment and coverage are different. So you could have coverage but no payment.

MDR&D: So there can be a CPT code to cover it but getting the reimbursement from the insurance company is other matter?

TJF: That is correct. FDA approval is not correlated with CMS (Center for Medicare and Medicaid Services). It's quite possible that the whole process will take eight years at a minimum. The rapid pace of technology will exceed the ability of the regulatory agencies that currently exist to keep up.

MDR&D: Do you see the packaging of products and services together as important to the future of medical device technology?

TJF: It's essential. Not important. It's more than important.

MDR&D: How has the medical device field changed over the last 10 years?

TJF: In 10 years, what has really changed back and forth and what has been inconsistent is the regulatory, the reimbursement, social economics, lifestyle, considerations of safety, and who is considering that—the patient, the consumer, the company, the producer of drugs, and the makers of technology by the way of large device companies. And that's only a small sample. They have changed for worse or for better. It is a serious problem. There has been no semblance of consistency.

MDR&D: What advice would you give to someone who is just getting started in this field?

TJF: If you don't have the capacity to listen to others, including the janitor and your secretary, get out.

MDR&D: What are some of the important clinical needs that you see now that don't have good solutions?

TJF: Sleep apnea, obesity, and all areas of preventive medicine are in critical need of being addressed.

MDR&D: You are unique in the sense that you have four successful careers in parallel, a practicing surgeon, medical device entrepreneur, venture capitalist, and winemaker. How do you get them all to work together? (Figures 20.2 and 20.3)

TJF: They're all related. Wine drinking is an extremely valuable preventative medicine. Venture capital is absolutely critical to the progress of technology. Innovation and invention go hand in hand.

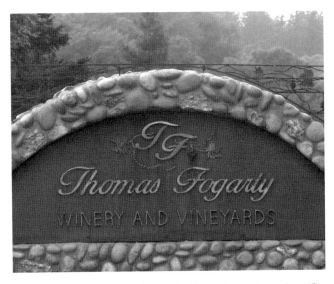

FIGURE 20.2 Fogarty Winery is nestled in the Santa Cruz Mountains. (Courtesy of Ted Kucklick.)

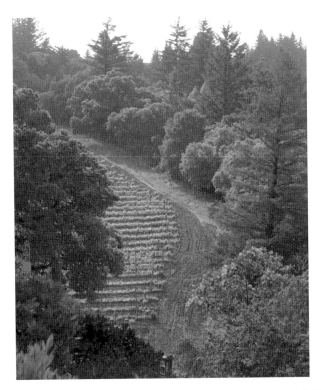

FIGURE 20.3 A spectacular view of the vineyard. (Courtesy of Ted Kucklick.)

RESOURCES

REFERENCES: OTHER INTERVIEWS WITH DR. FOGARTY:

Berlin, Linda. "Stanford Doctor to be Honored for Inventions." *San Francisco Chronicle*, October 5, 2001.
Bestard, Nicole. "Finding a Better Way." *Gentry* (June 2003).
Cassack, David. "The Inventor's Inventor." *In Vivo* (February 2003).
"Doctors of Invention." *Modern Physician* (July 2004).
"Five Questions." *Endovascular Today* (March 2003).
Fogarty, Thomas J. "Physicians as Entrepreneurs." *IEEE Grid* (December 1994).
———. Interview with Inventors Workbench. Stanford Biodesign Program. http://innovatorsworkbench.stanford.edu/store/index.html.
Frost, Bob. "Leading Questions." *San Jose Mercury News*, October 18, 1998.
Hiltzik, Michael. "Medicine's Own Thomas Edison." *Los Angeles Times*, June 5, 2003.
Quinn, Jim. "Failure is the Preamble to Success." *American Heritage of Invention and Technology Magazine* (Winter 2004).
Roggins, Christine. "Transforming Ideas into Products." *Stanford Medicine* (Fall 2000).
Romano, Michael. *Venture Reporter,* October 15, 2003.

21 Interview with Paul Yock, MD

Theodore R. Kucklick

Paul G. Yock, MD (Figure 21.1), is the Martha Meier Weiland professor of medicine and professor of mechanical engineering. Dr. Yock is cochair of Stanford's new Department of Bioengineering and director of the Stanford Program in Biodesign. Dr. Yock is a Stanford cardiologist internationally known for his work in inventing, developing, and testing new devices, including the Rapid Exchange™ balloon angioplasty system, which is the dominant angioplasty system in use worldwide. Yock also invented a Doppler-guided hypodermic needle system, the Smart Needle™, and P-D Access™. Dr. Yock is director of the Center for Research in Cardiovascular Interventions, a Stanford facility that develops and tests new technologies in cardiovascular medicine. The focus of Dr. Yock's research program is the field of intravascular ultrasound. He authored the fundamental patents for intravascular ultrasound imaging and founded Cardiovascular Imaging Systems, now a division of Boston Scientific. In 1998 Dr. Yock developed a new interdepartmental and interschool program at Stanford, the Medical Device Network (MDN). Recently MDN has been expanded under Dr. Yock's leadership into a broader research and educational initiative, the Stanford Program in Biodesign. MDN is now BDN, the Biodesign Network. The primary mission of Biodesign is to promote the invention and implementation of new health technologies through interdisciplinary research and education at the frontiers of engineering and the biomedical sciences.[*]

MDR&D: I understand that you are an inventor on least 36 patents.
PGY: I think that's true. I think there are 40-some now.
MDR&D: Some of the inventions are the rapid exchange catheter and intervascular ultrasound. And you're a practicing cardiologist?
PGY: Yes.
MDR&D: Also, professor of medicine, and cochair of the Stanford Bioengineering Department, as well as cofounder with Dr. Peter Fitzgerald of the Center for Research and Cardiovascular intervention, as well as director of the Stanford Biodesign Program.
PGY: Typical academic list of 47 things.
MDR&D: What first inspired you to go into medicine?
PGY: That's a great question. I hadn't thought about that in a long time. My dad was a dentist. And we grew up appreciating the fact that he got great

---
[*] Stanford Biodesign, http://biodesign.stanford.edu.

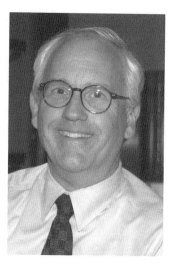

FIGURE 21.1 Paul G. Yock, MD., Stanford, CA, 2004. (T. Kucklick)

satisfaction from taking care of his patients. But he also told us that medicine had a lot more potential, and he kind of nudged us in that direction. I think it was a combination of those influences with the fact that I love the sciences and I loved the biological sciences in high school and college that pointed me in that direction.

MDR&D: Where did you go to school?

PGY: I went to a public high school in Minnesota. Then I went to Amherst College for undergraduate. And then I spent a couple years at Oxford, mainly studying philosophy, actually. And got a master's [degree] there. Then med school at Harvard.

MDR&D: And so from this master's degree in philosophy, what inspired you to combine an interest in medicine and an interest in philosophy with an interest in engineering and invention?

PGY: From reasonably early on, I just liked design itself. If I had the talent, I think I would've been an architect because I loved designing things as a kid. Not building things so much, but just sort of solving problems, design problems. And as I got into medicine, I just kept doing those things. I remember when I was in college I did a summer research project, and it involved an animal technique that was called *ganztierenfrieren*, which basically means you drop a rat in a vat of liquid nitrogen and they get frozen like that. The reason for doing that was to get a snapshot of a metabolic process, knowing when you anesthetize an animal and then sacrifice it, the metabolism changes a lot. So to get a metabolic snapshot, you need to do something quickly.

I designed a device, a little biopsy sucker so that—we were working on kidneys at the time—it froze a section of the kidney rather than freezing the whole animal, and it delivered it in a little vial of liquid nitrogen.

	I always had the inclination to design things like that and just kept doing so through college and medical school, internship, and residency. Most of the ideas were terrible.
MDR&D:	You probably met a lot of people, especially the people you worked with, that you consider to be particularly great innovators and inventors and people who inspired you. Who were some of the most interesting and inspiring people in your opinion in the medical device field?
PGY:	I'd start with the people I had the benefit of working with. I did my fellowship in angioplasty with Dr. John Simpson. That was a marvelous opportunity to have mentoring from one of the great people in the field. John actually helped me to get CVIS, Inc., going, which was the first company I was involved with. It was an intervascular ultrasound company. And I've actually thought a lot about what made him so effective as a mentor, because that's something that we're trying to do now with the Biodesign Program at Stanford. And it turns out that it's not easy to be as good a mentor as he is. And I think the thing that makes him so unique is [that] he has a way of making you feel like it's possible to do big things. Just something about being around him makes you believe that you can do it, too. And I think it's partly that he's a folksy sort of guy and a very friendly guy. Lots of people around him have gone on to start companies. I think he just has this aura that causes people to have the motivation and the gumption to do these things.

Tom Fogarty was another big influence for me. Tom actually also helped start CVIS, invested in it, was a director. And I think Tom is the best needs finder that I've ever met in my life. He understands. He has some kind of sixth sense about identifying important clinical needs and needs that have a market attached to them, too. He does that better, faster, clearer than anybody I've ever met. He's brilliant that way. |
MDR&D:	What are some of the major problems and opportunities you see in medicine?
PGY:	A detection of massive events that are about to occur, like stroke, myocardial infarction, early treatment sensing other metabolic processes. Sensing the early stage of an inflammatory or infectious condition. For example, you've just been seeded with a rhinovirus and can see that you're just starting up that curve, and those technologies will give us some warning about what's happening. That will drive the development of therapies that will hit at the early stage of these diseases. There are huge untapped areas in cardiovascular. We've made minimal progress in congestive heart failure. It is a major epidemiologic problem. Certainly stroke. I mean stroke is appalling the way we treat it now. Atrial fibrillation. Huge problem. We haven't begun to sort it out. Those are some of the areas I would say in cardiology that are worth looking at.
MDR&D:	So you see some of those as maybe some of the grand problems in the field?
PGY:	Yes. Absolutely. And then I think the other big problem, the biggest of all, the granddaddy, epidemiologic problem is the whole obesity, metabolic,

insulin resistance area—it's enormous. And that's upstream a little bit from heart disease and cerebrovascular disease, but it is in some sense the biggest epidemic that we'll deal with in the next 20 years.

MDR&D: How has the medical device development field changed since you first became involved?

PGY: That's a great question, too. I think in my area, cardiovascular, when I first got involved we were at the early stages of catheter interventions, and there were relatively easy solutions to making procedures better, easier, faster. Those mechanical solutions, the gizmo solutions, are a little harder to come by right now. I'm convinced that they're still out there, they're just not as easy to have. One thing I really want to say is that biologic device convergence is really important. But there are still simple device strategies out there that haven't been thought of that are elegant, simple, and important. And there will always be those things. And you see something come along like vascular closure, for example, that just took characterizing the problem, understanding the problem, and solving it. There are several mechanical solutions to that, which are not terribly difficult to come up with. I think those are all still out there ahead of us; it's just again a question of appreciating the need.

MDR&D: How do you identify and develop a new product idea? One thing that you were saying is understanding the problem better.

PGY: You have to start with a need. And the successful, the effective people in medical technology invention start with a clinical need, and they have the ability to find that need and to characterize it and to understand how important it is. That is more than half of the secret to successful inventing.

MDR&D: Another invention that you're known for is the rapid exchange catheter. Could you describe what this is and how it was developed?

PGY: It is a way that a catheter and a guidewire work together that allows a single operator to perform angioplasty and a single operator to change in and out a catheter over a guidewire. I was a fellow with John Simpson when I was learning angioplasty. At that time we were using over-the-wire angioplasty equipment. What that meant was that you had a catheter that was approximately 3 feet long. In order to keep the place in the coronary artery, you had to have a guidewire that was 10 feet long, 5 or 6 feet of which stuck out of the patient, and there had to be two operators. The guy with the skill and experience was upfront moving the catheter up and down, and the flunky, which was me, was at the foot of the bed trying to hold the guidewire in place while the other guy was moving the catheter. You've got a 10-foot-long guidewire, and you're trying to hold it in place where a quarter of an inch matters. You've got a problem with that system, the guy holding the guidewire is always at fault. So I kept being the guy who was screwing up the case. And I couldn't stand that. I said there's got to be a better way to do this that doesn't have this dumb 10-foot-long guidewire. That was my needs statement—I didn't want to be the goat in the procedure anymore. It just occurred to me that there was nothing written that said we had to use an over-the-wire system for the whole length of the catheter. That all we cared about was that it was over the wire inside the artery, and the rest of it didn't have to be over the wire. That was the way that system started. The way I characterize it is that the part of the catheter outside of the guiding catheter in the artery is exactly like an over-the-wire catheter. But back in the guiding catheter, the guidewire exits the catheter so that it functions with a single-operator system with a much shorter guidewire length.

MDR&D: A lot less sterile field problem also.

PGY: Exactly right.

MDR&D: Another intervention you're noted for is intervascular ultrasound. How did this come about and why?

PGY: So that came about because I was around in the early days of atherectomy. And I had just been studying for my cardiology boards, and I happened to know from studying that most plaques in arteries develop on one side of the artery only. The other side is pretty normal. And yet on the angiogram when you get a narrowing it looks like the plaque is all the way around. I got real worried when I saw the directional atherectomy device, the first prototypes, and I said, "Wait a minute. The angiogram is going to teach us to cut around the clock 360 degrees." But for part of that clock we're going to be cutting a normal wall with the atherectomy device. I said, "There's got to be some way of understanding where the plaque is that's better than angiography." I started thinking about techniques that would allow us to look below the surface of the vessel. I had some ultrasound background. It occurred to me that if we could pull it off, ultrasound would be a good way to do that.

MDR&D: I heard that when you went to a certain large company and told them what you wanted, they told you it was impossible.

PGY: It's true that everyone was worried about the fact that we would not be able to make good images, especially when the catheters serve as antennas for noise in the cath lab environment. All the engineers who looked at that problem said there's no way you'll be able to make a clean image with that little tiny transducer at the end of a catheter, the whole catheter serving as an antenna for noise. The cath lab being one of the noisiest electronic environments you can possibly imagine. You've got an unsolvable problem there.

MDR&D: But you did it?

PGY: No, I correct you. The engineers did it. I had the naiveté to think that it should be doable and was lucky enough to partner up with some really good engineers who figured out how to do it.

MDR&D: What advice would you give to somebody starting out in the medical device field? What training should they have? What kind of experience? What kind of education? What would make somebody entering the field successful?

PGY: Well, one important thing is that there is a huge breadth of knowledge in medical technology. It spans medicine and areas of engineering. One trap is to educate yourself real broadly but not have an area of deep expertise.

My one piece of advice would be as you get your education in preparation for going into medical technology, make sure there is one area, and it can be an area of engineering or it can be an area of medicine, where you are really expert—where you can put yourself up against anybody coming out at the same level of training and hold your own. If that's mechanical engineering, you should really understand the fundamentals of mechanical engineering well, and then have the vocabulary of some medical specialties and so on. But don't trade off that deep expertise in one area because, both from a standpoint of companies hiring you and also from the standpoint of your own discipline, and focus, and effectiveness, you need to be an expert. The only way to be a deep expert is to have one area of focus.

MDR&D: What are some of the most common mistakes medical device designers and entrepreneurs make?

PGY: The most common mistake I think by far is to try to develop too complicated a technology. The older I get, the more I appreciate this. At least for procedural technologies, it has to be very simple. It has to be very clean. It has to be easy to learn. Devices that are complicated, demanding, require significant operator training are severely disadvantaged compared to something that's simple. Keep it simple is in my lexicon as rule number one. Another mistake that has nothing to do with technology but is maybe the most common mistake I'm seeing now is not taking into account the regulatory and reimbursement pathways in designing a device. It absolutely doesn't matter anymore if you have the best device in the world if you can't get that paid for. It will not succeed. You need to understand that at the early stages of your design process you need to know what the reimbursement parameters are and what the FDA parameters are. Of those two, reimbursement is actually the more important and the more difficult.

22 Interview with Dane Miller, PhD

Theodore R. Kucklick

CONTENTS

Resources 398
    References: Biomet History 398
    References: Other Interviews with Dane Miller 398

Dane Miller, PhD (Figure 22.1), is president and chief executive officer of Biomet, Inc., a major force in the orthopedics marketplace. From humble beginnings in 1977, Biomet has grown into one of the most respected names in the orthopedics and medical device industries, delivering consistent year-in and year-out double-digit growth. I met with Dr. Miller for this interview at the headquarters of Biomet in Warsaw, IN.

MDR&D: Thank you again, Dane, for this interview. Could you describe how Biomet was founded?

DM: Well, I guess the very starting point was a conversation that Jerry Ferguson and I had in late 1975 when I had made a decision to leave my current employer and Jerry's employer Zimmer, and move to California to join Cutter Biomedical. We talked somewhat facetiously about the prospects of starting a company. By the time we thought about it, I think we realized it was probably impossible. Jerry then called me again in early 1977 and said, "Well, I think it's time." So we began the planning with a group of people. Ultimately Jerry and I were the only surviving partners and we added Niles Noblet and Ray Harroff and incorporated the company in November of 1977, which became our official start date, but began operations in January of 1978. Our original plans were to found a company that could utilize the manufacturing support industry here in Warsaw, IN, and we would simply develop and distribute products to the orthopedic market.

MDR&D: Tell me what Biomet has grown into today from those beginnings in 1975 to 1977.

DM: At the end of fiscal year 2004, we finished with revenues of about $1.6 billion. That's from first-year sales in 1978 of $17,000.

MDR&D: I understand that you did not run in the black that first year.

DM: No, we operated probably our first two or three years in the red, expecting as we got our feet planted, got a product line launched, or a series

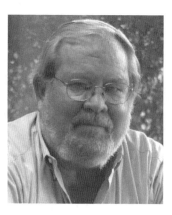

FIGURE 22.1 Dane Miller, PhD, Warsaw, IN, 2004. (T. Kucklick)

of product lines launched, that we wouldn't be making money. It was probably not until fiscal 1981 or 1982 that we had much black ink on the bottom line.

MDR&D: What was the founding team's vision when they started as far as the values that you had and the commitment to innovation and service?

DM: Well, we were strong believers that it all starts with people and the way you treat your people; whether they be customers, distributors, or in-house team members. If you treat people with respect and give them the flexibility to sign on to their own job and make their own decisions, ultimately a company can be successful.

MDR&D: You mentioned in Biomet's corporate history book, *From Warsaw to the World*, that one of the things you learned at big companies is how not to do things. What were some of the things that you didn't want to duplicate at your company?

DM: Most importantly, we didn't want to get in the way of creative people doing their jobs. What often happens with bigger companies, and I should point out that I don't think big is necessarily defined by revenues or the number of square feet a company occupies or number of employees or team members. It's more than that. It's a state of mind. We at Biomet work very hard to create an environment and harbor an environment where people can do their best work. For example, I think with some companies when something goes wrong, the political engines begin to run and people start pointing fingers and trying to find blame. The important thing when something goes wrong is what can be learned from it, not a concerted effort to see to it that it never happens again. We look at what was not predicted at the front end that led to the unfortunate outcome and what can be put in the books as a lesson. Too often when something goes wrong, companies write a new policy that prevents that and lots of other things from happening again, instead of learning from it.

MDR&D: So you don't have a policy manual a foot thick at Biomet?

DM: No, we don't. Certainly there are certain things that have to be documented in the form of policies, such as personnel interactions and so forth. But we try to avoid writing a policy every time something happens.

MDR&D: What are Biomet's principles and approach to medical device research and development?

DM: Because of the technical orientation of Biomet's senior management, I think we take a little more of a technical approach than some companies in health care medical devices. We don't let the market drive technical decisions, I think, because a number of us have backgrounds in science and engineering. We tend to take a somewhat more disciplined scientific approach to issues.

MDR&D: What do you look for in a product development associate at Biomet? Somebody, say, who comes in as an engineer.

DM: Independence and self-motivation. We don't believe in strong day-to-day or hour-to-hour management. We feel that creative people have to be given the flexibility to take possession of their jobs and do them well. And we look for a self-starter, I guess, as much as anything.

MDR&D: Biomet has had a steady march of double-digit growth each year. How has Biomet been able to maintain this growth?

DM: By retaining the founding principles of the company to maintain an entrepreneurial environment, one where you're continuing to make progress with new products and new technologies. And we also happen to be fortunate that we're in a market that's growing nicely, as well.

MDR&D: There have been some growth stages in the history of Biomet from entrepreneurial start-up; then you've had a middle stage at about the $300 million revenue mark. And then today you're over $1 billion in sales and a worldwide market presence and a worldwide manufacturing presence. What did you need to do at each stage to move the company up to the next level?

DM: I'm not sure they are clearly separable stages. I think the important thing is we looked at what worked yesterday and do more of it today. And we look at what didn't work quite so well yesterday, and do less of it. We have a 26- to 27-year history of operating our business in that way.

MDR&D: Describe how Biomet sees opportunity where others see problems.

DM: I think the challenges are not to get consumed by problems. Not to let a negative approach to dealing with problems get in your way. When things aren't going the way you hoped, the key is to redouble your effort and get by it and move on and not get hung up with your problems.

MDR&D: You've had one situation—when you acquired Lorenz Surgical—in which you actually turned what could have been a real problem into a great opportunity. Could you describe how that happened and what you did to turn that into an opportunity and salvage it from a problem?

DM: Well, that was certainly a challenging time. Just a little history of the Lorenz acquisition. We acquired Lorenz, which included a relationship with a German manufacturer, whose products made up the vast majority of the Lorenz revenue stream. Not too long after acquiring them we were informed after working very hard to protect and deal carefully with the relationship that they would no longer supply product to us. We did everything humanly possible to harbor a good relationship with the German manufacturer and did not begin manufacturing our own product in-house, such as to create rift in that relationship, only to find the German manufacturer had chosen not to continue shipping us product. As I recollect, we were informed in early November that at the end of that particular calendar year no more orders would be accepted or shipments made to us. And that probably amounted to 80% of our product line or revenue stream at the time from Lorenz. And only a few days later we found that, in fact, the three senior principals at Lorenz were leaving the company to form a new company to distribute those manufacturers' products. So not only did we lose access to the principal supplier for the company, but also we lost senior management at that point. So, we cranked up our ability to manufacture the product back here in Indiana. They're much smaller products than we produced. It required different tooling and different capital equipment, but we unleashed our engineering and manufacturing teams on making sure that there weren't any blanks in product availability, and I think did a pretty good job of showing the sales force, who had been preconditioned to the thought that if Lorenz lost its supplier, the company was in big trouble. In fact, we proved that was not going to be the case.

MDR&D: And you proved it, actually, in a very convincing way at a sales meeting where you showed them an example of what you could pull off.

DM: Yes, we provided them a couple of competitive catalogs and asked the sales force to pick a product, a particular plate design that we had never manufactured, that Lorenz had never manufactured, and we would unleash our engineering team from late morning to early afternoon and see if they could reverse engineer and produce a product, and do all the design work, all the CNC (Computer Numerical Control) machining, and CNC programming necessary to make it. By the end of that day we handed the Lorenz sales force a prototype of the product.

MDR&D: How has Biomet dealt with the continuing squeeze in reimbursements for innovative medical technologies in the managed care environment?

DM: We have for many years focused on reimbursement and total cost of treatment in our product development activities. After all, if we can provide a total hip or a total knee that costs an additional $500, but help the hospital deliver that treatment for a thousand dollars less, we've all come out ahead. And that's been the focus of I think most medical device product development in the health care field.

MDR&D: So you do start with reimbursement strategy upfront?

DM: Absolutely.

MDR&D: And what about the way that the environment has changed under managed care? Ten to 15 years ago the doctors had a lot more leverage and say so over what they could provide. And now much more is being dictated by insurance companies.

DM: I think doctors are signed on to the concept of saving money in ultimate care and treatment of patients. After all, our big challenge going forward is how we're going to provide this expanding group of baby boomers the increased health care demands that they're going to place on the system for less money. That is, less money on a per unit basis.

MDR&D: So that's an area where you're seeking out new clinical needs, in that aging baby boomer population?

DM: Absolutely. As the wave of baby boomers reach their retirement and orthopedic care age, which is somewhere in the 55 to 65 age category, we're going to need to figure out more economical and efficient means of treating them.

MDR&D: How does Biomet maintain such a rapid pace of new product introduction?

DM: We don't have the largest R&D group in the industry, but I would have to say I think we have the most efficient R&D team anywhere in the industry. Each of our major divisions funds an R&D operation. And I think they're all as efficient as anybody in those markets.

MDR&D: Your company has a motto: "Driven by Engineering." What does this motto mean?

DM: If you look at the rest of the orthopedic industry, much of senior management comes from either finance and accounting or marketing and sales ranks. Here at Biomet most of our senior management comes from science and engineering ranks. And we think its science and engineering that's driving Biomet's decision making, and not marketing.

MDR&D: I've talked to a number of sales reps, and Biomet is known as one of the best companies in orthopedics to sell for. How have you developed and maintained that reputation and that relationship?

DM: First, we have a very talented distribution system. And we just work hard to deliver what they need, what their customers need. And [we] don't treat them like just a sales force. They're part of the team.

MDR&D: You and your fellow founders seem to be driven by strong principles. What are the sources for these principles and ideals?

DM: Oh, I think it's upbringing as much as anything. I think it's unusual today to look at a group of people in their 50s and 60s who are married to their first wives. The company began 27 years ago and we're still married to our first wives.

MDR&D: And maybe a few more toys.

DM: We all have a few more toys and they're a little bigger toys, but we're still the same people we were 27 years ago.

MDR&D: How do you see the development of the combination of biologics and devices? This seems to be an area that Biomet is pioneering in. How do you see the future of biomaterials in orthopedics?

DM: Somewhat oversimplified, I see biomaterials assisting the orthopedic surgeon in doing procedures through needles instead of 6-inch incisions. I think the real advent of minimally invasive surgery, minimally invasive treatment techniques will come through the assistance of biomaterials technology.

MDR&D: And you personally got involved in biomaterials testing early on. Tell me how you personally tested titanium for implants?

DM: I was involved in some preclinical research involving a particular titanium alloy and particular surface treatment. And one afternoon a couple of tornadoes blew through the area, taking out the entire power grid in this county. I couldn't go into my office at work because there wasn't any light. So I called a friend in Fort Wayne and took a small bar of titanium that was designed for animal tests and asked if he would implant it in my arm.

MDR&D: And you kept that in your arm for quite a while?

DM: About 10 years.

MDR&D: So you have firsthand experience with biomaterials testing and trying out titanium. It's like the old story, you didn't just contribute, you got involved.

DM: Yes, as a matter of fact, that piece of titanium came out about 10 years later. We did the histology work, and it looked precisely the way it did when it was implanted 10 years prior. And the tissue response was absolutely minimal. The tissue had grown right up to the implant surface.

MDR&D: If you were a new PhD today or an engineer and you wanted to build the next Biomet, or build a successful innovative medical technology company, how would you go about it, starting today? You just graduated from school.

DM: Well, first make sure you put your formal education behind you and be prepared to start to learn all over again. And second, make sure you never hide behind your education as a shield. Get out there and learn what it takes. Educate yourself beyond what your formal education could ever have provided you. When I started I knew absolutely nothing about stock options or finance, for example. I had to learn all of that.

MDR&D: If you think that your formal education did everything that it needed to do, then that would be a mistake?

DM: Absolutely. Your formal education is only the footing. The rest of it, the rest of the structure, comes through experience.

RESOURCES

REFERENCES: BIOMET HISTORY

Hubbard, Richard, and Jerry Rodengen. *Biomet: From Warsaw to the World.* Ft. Lauderdale, FL: Write Stuff Enterprises, 2002. This is the official corporate history of Biomet and is available from Biomet.

REFERENCES: OTHER INTERVIEWS WITH DANE MILLER

"CEO Says Total Joint Replacement Is the Biggest Growth for Biomet," *The Wall Street Transcript* (January 15, 2004). http://www.twst.com /notes/articles/waj608.html.

Herper, Matthew. "Dane Miller: CEO Value to the Bone," Forbes.com (May 8, 2001).

Miller, Dane. "Executive Interview with Knowledge Enterprises," *OrthoKnow* (July 2004). http://www.orthoworld.com.

23 Interview with Ingemar Lundquist

Theodore R. Kucklick

Ingemar Lundquist (Figure 23.1) is a prolific inventor and was one of the early developers of catheters and manufacturing equipment for Advanced Cardiovascular Systems. He developed the indeflator, the standard device for inflating and deflating an angioplasty balloon, and helped develop over-the-wire angioplasty. One of his first successful designs was an automatic postal meter for Friden (now Friden-Alcatel). He was also a pioneer in the design of steerable catheters for EPT, and a cofounder of Vidamed, Inc. His wife, Linda Lundquist, also participated in this interview.

MDR&D: You came here from Sweden with $200 in your pocket. What year was that?

LL: It was 1948 or 1949.

MDR&D: You worked on postal meters and you worked on taxi meters and different mechanical things. How did you make the jump from that to medical devices?

IL: My father died of a heart attack. He asked me to develop devices for the medical field at that time. But he was thinking mostly of some means of moving a patient from one bed to another and stuff like that because the nurses had such a hard time moving people within the hospital from one bed to the other.

MDR&D: From your background going from postage meters to catheters and medical devices, what are the practical skills you used, the most useful skills that you found translated into developing medical devices?

IL: My skills as a machinist, basically. And my know-how about the machines used to develop things, like lathes, milling machines, and so forth.

MDR&D: Did you ever get something right the first time, or did you have to do it several times?

IL: Well, you develop something, you usually don't get it right the first time. You step one little piece at a time to get it eventually the way you want it. You usually don't get that in one shot. It's more than one try.

MDR&D: So this goes back to your machine shop school that seeing the real thing and holding it in your hands is something that's an essential part of doing product development.

IL: Definitely. I don't think I could've developed products just on paper. I had to develop them by actually making the products. I could not convince myself on a piece of paper that it worked. So I had to develop it and see how it functioned physically.

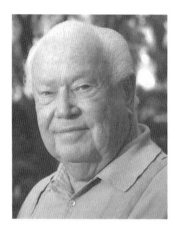

FIGURE 23.1 Ingemar Lundquist Carmel, CA, 2004. (T. Kucklick)

MDR&D: Have you found that using a computer was something that helped you?

IL: It helped a little bit. The thing that really helped me was developing the prototype so I could see with my own hands and eyes if it worked the way I expected it to.

MDR&D: What was a typical workday or a workweek like for you, if there was such a thing?

IL: I don't know if I had a typical workweek. I worked; when I had a project going, I just worked on it all the time usually. I would go to bed and dream about it, so to speak, and wake up the next morning and just continue.

LL: That's true. You stayed down in the basement working and working and working until he got it finished to another step.

MDR&D: Would you work on several projects at one time or would you focus on one thing?

IL: I usually focused on one thing. I didn't spread myself too thin in that respect.

MDR&D: Do you actually consider yourself an inventor, or do you consider yourself more of an engineer or designer or problem solver?

IL: I think I would say for myself as an inventor, and a product development engineer.

LL: Very seldom would he ever mention it to anybody that he had invented.

MDR&D: If you were to, say, define what an invention is, what would you say?

IL: An invention must be something that is different than anybody has developed. An invention is basically a product or a device that is unique and you think you can patent it.

MDR&D: What do you think about the patent process? Is it more difficult to do now than it used to be, or is it easier?

IL: I think it is probably more difficult now because there are more inventions to sort out. It used to be easier. It is quicker now to sort through them because there are more tools available to help you as far as computers and databases.

24 Interview with J. Casey McGlynn

Theodore R. Kucklick

J. Casey McGlynn (Figure 24.1) is one the most experienced attorneys in the medical device industry. Mr. McGlynn is chairman of the Life Sciences Group at Wilson Sonsini Goodrich and Rosati (WSGR) and a nationally recognized leader in the representation of start-up and emerging growth companies in the life sciences field. The Life Sciences Group at WSGR offers focused resources and capabilities to meet the most critical needs of start-up and emerging-growth companies, including private and venture capital financings; public offerings; university licensing; and strategic collaborations and strategic patent counseling. Mr. McGlynn is a frequent speaker and contributor to magazines and newsletters on issues relating to the life sciences industry, and moderates the annual WSGR Medical Device Conference.[*]

MDR&D: How did you decide to go into law originally and what led you to specialize in the life science area?

JCM: Getting into law was just something I was interested in even as a young kid. It was a goal that I set very early on in my life. But with regard to getting into health care law, I knew I was interested in business, and when I interviewed, I interviewed at a number of firms. It turned out that Wilson Sonsini was in this fantastic place called Silicon Valley. As I interviewed here, I realized it was a unique place, so different from the rest of the world. It was only as I began the practice here that I realized how unique it was. One of the first companies that I incorporated was a company in the health care area, and that's really how I began to do things in the life sciences. The first company was called Advanced Cardiovascular Systems. It was incorporated originally as Advanced Catheter Systems, and it became the vascular division of Guidant Corporation. It was first started with angel capital, later funded by venture capitalists, and eventually sold to Eli Lilly to form a piece of their medical device business. Eli Lilly spun off its device business and ACS was spun out as part of Guidant Corporation about 10 years ago.

MDR&D: How is practicing corporate law in the life science area different than other areas, for example high-tech electronics?

JCM: The fundamentals of being a good lawyer are much the same. The issues related to financing and public offerings and mergers and acquisitions are similar. What's different is specific market knowledge about the industry

---

[*] For more information, see Wilson, Sonsini, Goodrich & Rosati, http://www.wsgr.com.

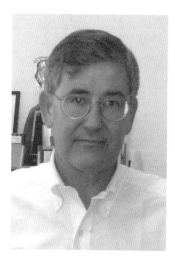

FIGURE 24.1 J. Casey McGlynn, Palo Alto, CA, 2004. (T. Kucklick)

and about what goes on in the industry. Concerns that might be different would be: Who is interested in investing in this sector, or what percentage should officers and directors get of companies, or how have other companies in similar situations dealt with particular issues? When you come to a fork in the road you may have two choices, both of which might actually be logical choices. If you have a long history in the life sciences area, you'll know what roads other people have taken and in many cases which ones worked out and which ones didn't. Industry-specific knowledge is very valuable in the life sciences area. It has allowed me to help clients sort out the business issues they face day to day.

MDR&D: According to a 1997 interview in *Business Week*, Larry Sonsini challenged WSGR to branch out from a concentration in electronics to develop a dominating position in the life science area. According to the article, you took on this challenge and built the WSGR life science practice. Could you tell me about this?

JCM: The firm had a very large practice in life sciences before the life sciences group was formed, but it was a very disparate group. We had several hundred attorneys at that time and everybody had some life science clients. I might have had a bigger practice in the life sciences area at the firm, but there were a number of other attorneys also practicing in the area. One person didn't really know what the others were doing. So the first goal was to figure out what companies WSGR represented. How many of them were there? The next thing was to get people together to begin talking about life sciences. We ran educational programs internally on both the device side and on the biopharmaceutical side. Finally, we began to run an educational program for the industry, aimed at teaching best practices in collaboration, financing, M&A (mergers and acquisitions) regulatory law, and reimbursement.

MDR&D: You took what already existed and organized it?

JCM: That's correct. We did a study. I think we collected 100 key people in the life sciences industry. We hired somebody to go out and interview those people. What came out of that study was that people in the life sciences area really wanted people who were focused on their industry. They didn't want generalists, they wanted specialists that were focused, understood the science, understood some of the quirks in that particular area. That's the feedback we were responding to. We formed an independent group that was just focused on the life sciences.

MDR&D: You were responding to what you saw as a demand and also seeing that the industry had grown large enough to support that sort of an activity?

JCM: We knew it was an important industry, and we had enough clients to form an independent group.

MDR&D: Each year Wilson Sonsini produces the WSGR Medical Device Conference. Could you tell me how this conference came to be and how it has grown over the years?

JCM: We run a lot of different conferences. Probably the largest every year is the WSGR Medical Device Conference. It was actually the first industry-specific conference that WSGR organized. It started off to help entrepreneurs understand the critical issues they would face in starting a new business. It was intended as a workshop to help entrepreneurs understand the nuts and bolts in getting a company organized, funded, public, sold, etc. There were probably 100 people, maybe a little bit less the first time we did the event. I think this last year we probably had about 450 people. We've done it for about 12 years now. It has become an annual event where people get together, when they may not have seen each other for a long time, and have an opportunity to talk about what they're doing and what's new in their lives. We feel that a number of really great companies have had their spark or beginnings at that meeting. So we feel that it's been a very useful thing in terms of entrepreneurs and getting new businesses started.

MDR&D: You mentioned before about how Silicon Valley was an exciting place to be and this is where you wanted to be. What do you think makes Silicon Valley tick? What makes it different?

JCM: What I like about Silicon Valley, what I am amazed at, is that I meet a lot of very technically talented people very early in their careers and they are very driven by their vision of how they want to change the world. They are not focused on creating great wealth for themselves but in changing the world. And in many cases, obviously, they become wealthy. But wealth is not the real driver. And honestly in my early days, when I had a big plate full of electronics companies, I found the people in those industries to be really interesting people with incredible drive. I find there's one additional element in the life sciences area that for me is one of the reasons that I'm still practicing law. It's great to have a great idea, to be passionate about that idea, to create it and to transform the world with it. But the thing about health care that's so fantastic is that in the process you are not just transforming the world. You are actually helping save lives, making the world a much better place than it was before you got there. And to me, that is the one thing about the medical device industry, and the biopharmaceutical industry, that is just fantastic. It just makes me feel really great about a lot of the companies that I've had an opportunity in my career to be a part of and help because I know I've indirectly helped a lot of people live longer and healthier lives.

MDR&D: Do you think that Wilson Sonsini as a firm has helped to shape Silicon Valley corporate culture?

JCM: To say we shaped corporate culture would be too egotistical on our part. But we've been a part of the valley from the very beginning. And our goal has always been to service companies from start up through the large multinational company. Our model is to provide all the services those companies need. Companies need different services at different times. Start-ups need things that are really radically different than a large company like Hewlett Packard might need. The key is to know when to bring those services to bear to help clients move forward and be as successful as they possibly can be. I don't know whether we transformed the valley. That's probably too egotistical, too. But I would say we've definitely been a part of the valley from the very beginning.

MDR&D: How does a life science start-up lay a foundation for growth and success?

JCM: I'd say for me when I look at a new opportunity it's about the people and it's about the idea. And those are the two key pieces. It doesn't mean that you have a complete management team on hand on day one. But it means that there is a special person in that organization. It might be an engineer, it might be a scientist, or it might be a doctor that really, really understands the field that he's moving into and really has a vision of what needs to be changed. It's that one change maker, if you will, that's absolutely critical on the people side. And then again it's this product concept. What I have found interesting on the product concept side is that many of the entrepreneurs that have an idea may not have fully crystallized that idea. It's only through networking with a lot of other very talented people in this industry that they're able to really crystallize the right application. So I guess it's really people first. But it has to be an idea that makes some sense, even though it may not be the final crystallized idea.

MDR&D: How does a company change over time from a small entrepreneurial seed stage company through its growth stages and ultimate exit?

JCM: It changes obviously by hiring people. Each person a start-up hires has such a profound influence on the culture of that company and also on the company's capabilities. And it's a very expensive process. Every employee is a very expensive addition to an enterprise early on in a company's life. So you really have to pick those people very carefully. For me the companies that turn out to be the best are the ones whose founder or CEO has the passion for real excellence and is very, very focused on making sure he gets the best and the brightest into his organization because those are the people that can really transform a good idea into a great idea or can make a company that has potential to really sing. To me the hiring process is really critical in terms of creating a great organization. When I say people, it's not just the people that the companies hire. It is also the investor that they select. Everybody that you bring into your organization, whether it be service providers like lawyers or accountants, whether it be venture capitalists, whether it be your scientific advisory board, all those people tell about who you are and what kind of company you want to become. So I say, focus on the best and the brightest and make sure that you set a very high standard for yourself because people will judge you by the decisions that you make in terms of creating that organization.

MDR&D: What are some of the biggest mistakes start-up companies make?

JCM: It's so interesting because there are so many ways to fail and there's probably only one path to success in a particular given company. In other words, you can make a big mistake by hiring the wrong CEO. You can make a big mistake by raising too much money. You can make a big mistake by getting the wrong venture capitalist associated with your business. You can make a big mistake a lot of other ways. The problem is that every one of these mistakes has a lasting impact on the organization. It's something we can't get rid of for the next four or five years. There are a lot of different mistakes that entrepreneurs can make that can turn out to be very serious. I'd say some of the biggest problems people have run into were when people underestimated the clinical challenges with regard to products. They thought that they could build it and the product would just be fine. And they weren't rigorous enough with regard to clinical development. We had a lot of failures in the late 1980s and early 1990s because of that kind of problem. I don't think today that clinical failure is nearly as likely as it was 10 or 15 years ago. Today I'd say one of the areas where people can continue to under appreciate the seriousness of the problem is in reimbursement. This is not an area I would have been talking about 10 or 15 years ago, but today it's a very serious issue. It's one of those things that the best companies focus on early. In many cases, though, a company will move forward through development, clinical trials, regulatory approval, and release of the product, and it's only after the product gets into the marketplace that management realizes what a huge problem reimbursement is. So again, I think today reimbursement is one of the biggest challenges for the industry as a whole.

MDR&D: You're saying reimbursement issues could kill a company?

JCM: That's right.

MDR&D: Do you see any solutions to the problems with reimbursements any time in the future?

JCM: Companies need to become more sophisticated about reimbursement. It's really a question of understanding what it takes to get reimbursement and putting that process in place. Maybe collecting additional data in early clinicals and getting peer-reviewed articles published. There's a whole litany of things that can be done to make sure that you'll be able to be reimbursed earlier, but you've got to work on it ahead of time. I think that's the process that we're going through right now. The best managers are more sophisticated and are working on reimbursement earlier. I do think we're getting better at it but it's still one of those issues on which we have a lot of work to do.

MDR&D: One of the things that is essential for a start-up is capital, and it's been said that a good venture capitalist (VC) provides more than just money. What else does a good angel or VC provide?

JCM: Today it's almost impossible in my mind to finance a company without venture capital. You have to start with the premise that sooner or later you're going to have venture capitalists in your company. The question is really when do you want to have them? I do think that they bring a lot of experience and a lot of connections. There are a lot of companies out there. When it comes time for people to make decisions, when it comes time for investment bankers to decide which companies they want to take public, or when it comes time for some of the big health care companies to decide who they want to acquire, there are a whole bunch of companies in almost every one of the areas. The question is which one are they going to pick? All I can say is you create signposts with every action you take. One of the signposts is to have a great group of venture capitalists associated with your business. They're going to know the investment bankers and have relationships with them. They're going to know the major health care companies and have relationships with them. They're going to be able to make introductions and help you. Those are signposts for both the investment banker and the health care company. It makes them look a little bit more closely at your company than they would otherwise look. That allows you to create a company that has a better chance of being successful. I do think that their contacts and relationships are very useful for companies and can increase the probability of success. I'd say the best and the brightest venture capitalists can be very useful and can be very helpful in terms of helping you make decisions, thinking about what actions you want to take based on the things that failed for them in the past and the things that were successful for them in the past. As I always tell my CEOs, it's ultimately up to the CEO to make these decisions. You have to call on the venture folk to get their comments and thoughts, but every fact pattern is different. It's up to the CEOs to evaluate what they are hearing from their venture friends and figure out the right course of action. It's never black and white. It's never "It was this way the last time and therefore it has to be this way." I think the VCs have a lot of good advice and a lot of good connections that could be very useful for CEOs.

MDR&D: You said before that choosing the wrong VC partner can be harmful to a company. How can it be harmful to a company to have a mismatch between a company and a VC?

JCM: I've sat on a lot of boards where the management and the VCs did not get along at all. And it wasn't a question of the company not doing the right things or not trying to build the business, or the CEO not being competent. But it was a situation where it was just incredibly adversarial at the board level.

That is a very destructive thing. It's very disheartening for management to try and create value. It's not about being challenged, but it's about being directed or crushed. There are a whole bunch of words we could use. But it can be a very destructive process if the management of an organization and the venture capitalists are really at odds. The venture capitalist can say, "We can change management." as they can, and they can put more money into the company. But these are all sad stories because it takes a long time to fire a CEO and to find a replacement. And it costs a lot of money. And it's just a huge amount of lost time and energy. A lot of the companies that fail, fail because they've got complex personalities inside their organization that are just at loggerheads with each other. So for the CEOs or founders, you have to choose your investors really wisely. And that means you need to really understand who these people are by doing some background checks. If you don't know your investors before the financing, you risk relationships that are destructive.

MDR&D: How does a new company find venture capital? How do you get the partners' attention, and how do you get in front of them to make your pitch?

JCM: Palo Alto and Menlo Park, for example, have a huge number of venture capitalists. So the question really is finding the ones that are interested in your business. If you're a health care company, you don't want to go to a fund that's primarily focused on electronics. If you're interested in medical devices, you don't want to end up at a venture capital firm that's primarily focused on doing biotechnology. You need to find somebody that can help you identify who the key players are in your sector. If you happen to have a CEO that's already done it once before, that CEO is probably going to be very knowledgeable and there is not going to be an issue. But if you are a first-time founder of a company, it's going to be important to find somebody who has a huge network of relationships and really knows who these people are, what kinds of deals they've done in the past, and what focus they have so that you can get an idea about who you should go see. So that's the first thing. Now, getting in to see the right people is simple if you work with somebody who has a relationship with them. The venture capitalists are interested in meeting entrepreneurs and seeing new ideas but they've got so many things crossing their desks. The entrepreneur must find some way to help the VC know this is a project they should spend some time on. The key variable is making sure that somebody who has a relationship with that venture fund is the one that's contacting them for you. You can't send an e-mail or a business plan to them without some prior introduction from some third party that actually knows them. The introduction can come from lawyers, from other CEOs, or from other venture capitalists. The network is pretty broad and it's just a question of identifying some people who can help you make those introductions. The next piece, obviously, is getting in there and having a great story to tell. That story involves your background and who you are and why you're unique and why you're a person that somebody should give millions of dollars to, and why your idea is unique and important and something that's going to transform the world. Assume you've got about 30 to 40 minutes in your first meeting in order to convince them that the founders and the ideas are special, not run of the mill. So you need to spend a lot of time on the presentation thinking about what it is you want to cover in that short meeting. You're not going to get a second chance unless you capture their imagination at the first meeting.

MDR&D: Describe the amount of effort it can take for companies that get that first meeting with a VC to finally get to a term sheet?

JCM: It could be as immediate as your first meeting, if you happen to hit the sweet spot for that venture capitalist, if your project is something that the VCs are already interested in, and if you look like the absolute right person to execute on this particular opportunity. And it could be literally less than a month before you have a term sheet from the venture fund. On the other hand it can take a long time. I think at the last WSGR Medical Device Conference Karen Talmadge, the founder of Kyphon, said it took several years during which time she had over 100 meetings before she found a firm that wanted to invest in her company. So it can take a long time, too. Tenacity is a very important attribute of the great entrepreneurs because not everybody is going to see your vision. In the case of Kyphon, obviously, a lot of people said no. And yet today the company is worth over a billion dollars. Fundamentally the product that they're selling today is exactly the product that the founder of Kyphon was talking about at each one of those initial meetings with venture capitalists. The VCs just didn't see the opportunity because it wasn't quite in their sweet spot.

MDR&D: What are some of the elements of a good term sheet?

JCM: First you'd want to be dealing with a first class venture fund that you feel is going to be a real team player and not an adversary in the company building process. And then you want to get the highest valuation reasonable. And after that you need to look at the stylized terms that financings typically have. One of the provisions that we typically see is dividends. Dividends could be cumulative or noncumulative. We'd like to see them noncumulative, which means that they are only paid if declared, and these dividends will never be declared for start-up companies. So it becomes a benign provision. But if it turns out to be cumulative dividends, then of course that's like having a promissory note with an interest rate. It's going to grow every year. If it has a 9% or 10% dividend rate, you know that in seven or eight years they're going to double the value of their investment. It can be a very expensive provision to give in on and something that we wouldn't want to have in a deal.

The next provision and perhaps the most important provision and the most discussed provision is liquidation preference. I'd say today there's going to be a liquidation preference. You're going to be selling preferred stock. The goal would be to just have a 1X liquidation preference without what is called participating preferred. The goal is to make the investor choose between either getting his money back or getting what the founders and other shareholders, the common shareholders, would be getting for a share of the company. Today the venture capitalists are pushing for participating preferred. It may be a full participating preferred, or it may be a participating preferred that's capped at some maximum number. But participating preferred means that investors get their money back before the other common shareholders get anything, and then they participate along with the common shareholders on a share-for-share basis so that in addition to the liquidation preference they get the same thing that the common shareholders would get. So that at the end of the day if the common shareholders got a dollar back, the preferred investor would have gotten that dollar back on his share plus he would have gotten back his initial investment.

There are a lot of other kinds of provisions. There are voting provisions. There are redemption provisions. And I think with each provision, I could go into a lot of detail, but suffice it to say the way I look at term sheets is I ask myself: "Which things are going to cap the wealth creation opportunity for the entrepreneur?" And: "Which things are really there to help minimize the risk for the investor?" I like to look at those things separately. In my mind the more important issues are those that avoid limiting the upside in the wealth creation process for the entrepreneur as opposed to focusing on some of the fears that the venture capitalist might have. To me if things don't go well, there's probably not going to be anything for anybody. But if things do go well, we're going to be dividing up a pie and we want to make sure that we get as fair a deal as possible for the entrepreneur. Those are some of my thoughts with regard to term sheets.

MDR&D: What percentage of ownership can founders expect to retain after seed rounds and VC rounds?

JCM: It's hard to say. And it's all over the place. I would say there is a lot of dilution in companies. So you have to be real smart about building a financing strategy with regard to your company and also making sure that you use capital really efficiently. It's funny, sometimes people brag about how much money they have raised or how much money they raised in this particular round of financing. But it's not about how much money you raise, it's about how far you get on the least amount of money possible with the lowest amount of dilution possible because that's how we create wealth for entrepreneurs. It really has to be a mind-set from the very beginning that we're going to try to do this as frugally as possible. That being said, the difference in burn rates between companies is radically different. I mean it's absolutely amazing, if you looked at how lean and mean some companies were and what percent of the company they ended up with. There's a company called Cutera that went public. I think that the founders owned over 50% of the company when it went public last year. They did two rounds of financing before the public offering. Just to give you a sense of how capital efficient they were, they never even dipped into the second round of financing. On the other hand, there are companies that have raised over $100 million privately before they got ready for their public offering. In those cases the founders have obviously been decimated by the dilution that they've suffered and own at most 2% of the company. So again I think capital efficiency is probably the most important factor once you've gotten your company financed.

MDR&D: On the subject of legal representation strategy, what should a medical device start-up look for when shopping for good legal representation?

JCM: I'd say a couple of things. One, you would like somebody that's very experienced in terms of representing your industry. So in the life sciences area he or she understands the industry, understands who the players are in the industry, has lots and lots of contacts and relationships so that you can use those relationships and contacts for your benefit. I think next you want a law firm that has the capability of solving your problems now and in the future so you don't feel obligated to move later on. When you are a very young company, you are very capital focused. So you want a firm with lots of experience with private financing, corporate partnering, and licensing, as well as patent prosecution. As you get larger there are other problems that you'll face, so you want a firm with public finance, employment law, tax, M&A, FDA [Food and Drug Administration], and litigation. Finally I think you want a firm that is responsive and that is very motivated to help you succeed.

MDR&D: Going back to your other statement about capital conservation, how does a company conserve capital with respect to its legal costs? How does it get the best representation and the best services while still conserving capital and preserving its capital efficiency?

JCM: I think that's a great question. The way we typically work with our clients is try to build a team. Because lawyers are very expensive, we have a partner, and an associate, and a paralegal on that team so that the most serious strategic issues can be worked on by somebody who has worked on lots of deals, has lots of great experience, and can help get to the right decision. So that's the first level. The second level is implementation of what might be a term sheet, a letter of intent, or whatever. And there I think being able to move it down to a lot less expensive person with adequate supervision will save a huge amount of money for the client. And then finally there are those things that have to get done but are of a mundane nature like preparation of stock certificates or stock option agreements. These can be done by paralegals again at a much lower rate. So the goal is really to find a way to do it as inexpensively as possible. One other way to save money is to work with people who have lots of experience with the work you need done. If you hire experienced people, you're going to get people that don't need to reinvent the wheel when it comes to the next transaction. Those are ways to minimize the cost with regard to lawyers.

MDR&D: How has the financing and business model for the life science company changed since the "class of 1996"?

JCM: In 1996 most of the med-tech companies that went public were development stage without an approved product or sales. They projected when they thought they would get regulatory approval and when they would be able to launch their product, and what the product launch would look like. The analysts carefully wrote down all of those promises and worked it into a model, valued the companies, and then took them public. The problem was that the performance after that public offering in most cases was pretty dismal. When the companies missed their projections, their valuations were slammed. But the companies that we see going public today are companies with real muscle mass. They are companies that have approved products, that have a predictable revenue ramp, and that are approaching profitability. It's a much better place to be if you're going to be public to have products that are in the marketplace, already approved, and where you're able to predict with increased accuracy the growth rate with regard to your company. I think those are important variables that have really changed since the "class of 1996."

MDR&D: How is going public different today with regulations such as Sarbanes-Oxley?

JCM: The actual IPO [initial public offering] process has not changed that much, but the liabilities are much more in people's minds today. It's not that there was not significant exposure in the past for management and the board of directors with regard to misstatements of fact in a registration statement. But recently enacted laws, the focus of the SEC [Securities and Exchange Commission] on management, and the increases in lawsuits from plaintiffs' attorneys make us all a lot more cautious. We see people being much more concerned, and cautious, with regard to the preparation of the registration statement. Because many of the rules in Sarbanes-Oxley focus on reporting after the public offering, we see companies that have gone public need larger accounting staffs, and a lot more work is being done on verification of the financial information that's being reported to the CFO and then finally to the board of directors and the public. The responsibility of management has really increased. The Ken Lay defense of: "I didn't know it was happening" is no longer available. Because of that there is a lot more emphasis on due diligence and making sure of the accuracy of financial statements in order to avoid liability. So it is a period of increased scrutiny, and, therefore, I think increased anxiety for the management of a public company.

MDR&D: Following up on that, describe the relative advantages of a company being acquired versus going public?

JCM: Selling a company allows management to take the money off the table, walk away, and start a new enterprise a short time later. For the CEO and management, it's a great opportunity to cash in and to begin again. In the IPO situation it's not going to be possible for management to cash in and walk away because the world is going to be looking at management to meet the promises it made to the public. And the public is going to be watching all of management's filings so that if you are an active seller into the marketplace, the public is going to wonder why it should be holding your stock. So it is much more difficult for management to find a way to diversify by selling the stock in its company. I will say, however, that some of the biggest and best stories in the medical device industry have been companies that have gone public, have continued as a public entity for two or three years, built real muscle mass, and then sold the company to a large medical device manufacturer. These are some of the largest deals in the industry as opposed to oftentimes smaller deals that get done in a merger and acquisition context prior to a public offering. So it is a complex equation trying to figure out whether or not you want to take your company public, or whether you want to sell it. I would say you need to be opportunistic because you owe your fiduciary duty to your shareholders. And it may be that, for example, you would love to do a merger but that because of the market environment the IPO is really the right thing for you to do for your shareholders.

MDR&D: You have worked with a number of "serial entrepreneurs." What are the qualities of the ones that are really successful, the really great ones?

JCM: I would say they tend to be technically very astute, with vast knowledge about their area of expertise. There's a second category of entrepreneur who is not as technically astute but is a manager as opposed to an engineer, or scientist, or doctor. The manager entrepreneur understands people and markets, and his expertise can supercharge the company.

MDR&D: What advice would you have for someone who is a company founder who has had a great idea, worked hard, executed properly, and has really done well? What do you do after you've "made it"?

JCM: Hopefully, the really successful entrepreneurs will find a way to give back something to the industry. There are a lot of very experienced people interested in helping young entrepreneurs, and I think that's great for our industry and it can be very satisfying for those who do the executive mentoring of the young entrepreneur.

MDR&D: What are some of the exciting med-tech areas that you see on the horizon?

JCM: There is a lot going on in orthopedics and in congestive heart failure. There's always a lot going on in the cardiovascular area, and I am also very excited about women's health. It's an area that 10 years ago the first companies with which I was associated turned out not to be that successful. But we've had some incredible successes since then. I also like the aesthetics field. These products are private-pay and don't have reimbursement issues. The aging population has created a real demand for these products.

25 Keys to Creating Value for Early Stage Medical Device Companies

Richard Ferrari

CONTENTS

Seven Common Characteristics 414
Clinical Impact.. 414
Franchise Value and Strategic Need... 417
Value of Execution 418
Sustainability... 419
When to Exit? 420
Resources 421
About the Author.. 422
Acknowledgments... 422

Companies that exit successfully via mergers and acquisitions tend to share characteristics that enable significant value creation. Start-ups can use these characteristics as a template to gauge their own potential for success.

The 1999 sale of Perclose Inc. to Abbott Laboratories Inc. for $680 million on sales of approximately $50 million established an upper threshold for maximizing value of a medical device company. Perclose, which developed a novel suture technology, ran an especially efficient operation: over its seven-year preacquisition history it raised approximately $23 million in venture capital, another $54.5 million from an initial public offering (IPO) and a follow-on offering and generated a hefty 12-fold multiple of sales on the acquisition by Abbott. Similarly, VidaMed Inc. (acquired by Medtronic Inc.), CardioThoracic Systems Inc. (CTS; bought by Guidant Corp.), Oratec Interventions Inc. (an absorbed division of Smith & Nephew PLC), and PercuSurge Inc. (acquired by Medtronic) all generated exit values, in most cases post-IPO, ranging from $225 million to $350 million on less than $50 million in sales.

The exit values for those five firms make them standouts among the universe of small-cap medical device companies. Importantly, they possess a common set of characteristics that enabled significant value creation and their successful exit through mergers and acquisitions (M&A). Indeed, those characteristics, which include the development of a novel, best-in-breed technology with significant clinical impact; a set of products that delivers a competitive edge; and careful execution of their respective business plans (including managing capital and timelines), can serve as a template for early stage medical device companies and help define the parameters necessary for them to engineer their way toward an outcome that maximizes value. Companies that are able to hit the mark in all or most of those categories can expect the greatest rewards.

That is not to say that every start-up has to hit the ball out of the park, however. Start-ups can still achieve a successful exit for early investors even though their achievements only reflect a few of the key characteristics; the key is to know how far to continue development and how much to expect for their efforts. Indeed, one crucial element of success is to know what window of time is required for a company to validate its work and blossom.

SEVEN COMMON CHARACTERISTICS

The five benchmark companies noted thus far all had significant market caps—above $200 million—and their acquisition prices occurred at high multiples of sales (see Table 25.1). Other companies have maximized return on investment (ROI) for their early investors with exits at lower values in absolute dollars owing to smaller amount of capital invested. In general, these exits occurred earlier, before demonstrating clinical impact, sales revenue, and sustainability (see Table 25.2).

Although no single characteristic is enough to maximize value, experience suggests a combination of certain key characteristics is required to generate an exit value above $200 million. The five successful companies, for example, grade highly in most if not all of the success-enabling activities. Even VidaMed, which for years fell short on execution, stumbled until it brought in a hard-nosed president and chief executive officer (CEO), Randy Lindholm, who had spent more than 15 years at General Electric Co.'s GE Medical Systems. Eventually (after 11 years), it obtained a good exit because of the clinical impact, novelty, and need for its first-in-class product line of minimally invasive radiofrequency devices for benign prostatic hypertrophy (BPH).

These seven parameters are not comprehensive of those things a company must achieve. It's difficult to understand how a franchise can be created and a sustainable business maintained without a strong intellectual property position, for one thing. Other characteristics are similarly implied. Although physician adoption, for example, is not considered a separate characteristic, it is without question a critical underlying element and an intimate part of having successful clinical impact.

CLINICAL IMPACT

Clinical impact is a fundamental characteristic and the most important benchmark for success of a medical device company. Almost all firms that generate premium M&A exits have products that fundamentally alter the preexisting practice of therapy or diagnosis. Take Perclose, whose suture catheter provides a novel method for closing a femoral access wound. Perclose fundamentally changed the clinical thinking and challenged the standard of care in the cardiac cath lab (pressure with sandbags). The improvements in patient care, comfort, and cath lab efficiency were immediate. A new way of thinking emerged, creating an entirely new market.

TABLE 25.1
Benchmark Companies

Company	Clinical Impact	Franchise Value	Strategic Need	Execution	Capital	Sustainability	Years To Acquisition	Exit (Value, acquirer)
Perclose	Substantial	High	High	Excellent	VC-$23 million; IPO-$34.74 million (also $19.7 million follow-on offering)	High	7	IPO, acquired ($680 million, Abbott)
VidaMed	Substantial	High	High	Average	VC-$21 million; IPO-$20.8 million (also $4.3 post-IPO private placement)	High	11	IPO, acquired ($326 million, Medtronic)
Cardio-Thoracic Systems	Medium	High	High	Excellent	VC-$5.6 million; IPO-$74 million	High	4	IPO, acquired ($313 million, Guidant)
Oratec	Medium	High	High	Excellent	VC-$36 million; IPO-$52 million	High	7	IPO, acquired ($310 million, not including a prior $9.2 million investment by acquirer, Smith & Nephew)
Percu-Surge	Substantial	Medium	High	Excellent	VC-$53.75 million	Medium	5	Acquired ($225 million, Medtronic)

Note: These rankings are informal and based solely on De Novo observations.
Source: De Novo Ventures Windhover's *Strategic Intelligence Systems* (Bridgewater, NJ).

TABLE 25.2
Companies with Shorter Exit Routes

Company	Clinical Impact	Franchise Value	Strategic Need	Execution	Capital	Sustainability	Years to Acquisition	Exit (Value, acquirer)
Enteric Medical	Medium	Medium	Medium	Good	VC-$12 million	Medium	3	Acquired ($124 million, Boston Scientific)
Vascular Science	Medium	Medium	High	Excellent	VC-$10.5 million	Medium	3	Acquired ($95 million [including milestone payments], St. Jude)
Embolic Protection	Medium	Medium	High	Excellent	VC-$12 million	Medium	2	Acquired ($75 million, Boston Scientific)
AneuRx	Medium	Medium	High	Excellent	VC-$14 million	Medium	2.5	Acquired ($75 million, Medtronic)
Atrionix	Medium	Medium	Medium	Good	VC-$11 million	Medium	4	Acquired ($62.8 million, J&J/Cordis)

Note: These rankings are informal and based solely on De Novo observations.
Source: De Novo Ventures; Windhover's *Strategic Intelligence Systems* (Bridgewater, NJ).

CTS (CardioThoracic Systems) similarly challenged the standard method of performing bypass surgery and pioneered a new market. It created a technology and procedure that enabled coronary artery bypass surgery to be accomplished while the heart remained beating, with attendant advantages to the patient and overall cost savings to the hospital. (Because the procedure was difficult and time-consuming for surgeons, however, with roughly equivalent results to the standard of care, off-pump bypass surgery only captured about a third of the market.) Oratec, with its heat-generating catheter for treating back pain, was more successful in driving change in clinical practice and expanded the market for its acquirer, Smith & Nephew, as did PercuSurge's embolic protection device for Medtronic.

An acquirer willing to pay a premium multiple of sales more often than not will require best-of-breed, clinically validated products. Each of our benchmark companies had the resources to run clinical trials and establish its clinical impact. But management and directors may rightly decide not to invest the capital or to take the time needed to clinically validate a technology, instead choosing an earlier exit. Atrionix Inc., for example, had only generated equivocal data on its catheter-based system for treating atrial fibrillation at the time of its acquisition by Johnson & Johnson's (J&J) Cordis Corp. Because Cordis badly wanted to expand its franchise, however, Atrionix decided only four years after its founding to accept a buyout at a multiple of just under six. On the other hand, having a best-of-breed technology is not a prerequisite if an early stage company is successful in other aspects. Boston Scientific Corp.'s Enteric Medical Technologies Inc. was able to generate a more than tenfold return primarily based on the novelty of its approach to treating gastroesophageal reflux disease (GERD) and the size of the GERD market.

FRANCHISE VALUE AND STRATEGIC NEED

The industry first began talking about franchise value in the mid-1990s, a time of robust M&A activity in medical devices, as elsewhere. The premiums paid to companies could not be modeled by traditional methodologies because CEOs, bankers, and acquirers needed a means to describe or justify the higher value and multiples being applied.

Franchise value implies that a company's technology and the resulting clinical application are in fact novel and clearly the best of breed. In almost all cases, companies with high franchise value are the first to market in an entirely new category. They establish a dominant presence and create a new clinical franchise. The recent acquisition of Advanced Bionics Corp. by Boston Scientific generated a nine-fold multiple of sales (not including earn out) based largely on franchise value.

A second critical value driver is strategic need. Technologies that may seem strategic from one point of view may not be seen in the same light by an acquirer, and vice versa. More often than not, strategic need is about creating an edge against competition, either by strengthening a patent portfolio or by preventing others from acquiring the intellectual property (IP). Other reasons may fall into the category of broadening a product line or increasing the efficiency of the sales force to maximize the revenue per procedure from each sales call.

Strategic need can create value by way of a competitive threat or offensive move against a competitor. Sometimes the value placed on a technology and company by an acquirer is simply due to the fact that the acquirer is looking forward as a way to protect and preserve its core business. (Recent cases in point: Boston Scientific's acquisition of Advanced Stent Technologies Inc. [AST] for IP and to protect its competitive edge, as well as St. Jude Medical Inc.'s acquisition of Epicor Medical Inc. and Stryker Corp.'s acquisition of SpineCore Inc.)

On the surface, franchise value and strategic need (the extent to which an acquisition furthers the long-term goals of the acquirer) are quite similar. But it is difficult to find high premiums being paid on strategic need alone. Among recent M&A technology plays, J&J's January 2001 acquisition of Heartport Inc. for $81 million was, like Boston Scientific's takeout of AST, driven by a compelling need to lock up competitive IP; the acquisition of Percutaneous Valve Technologies Inc. (PVT) by Edwards Lifesciences Corp. for $125 million netted a good multiple given PVT's equivocal clinical data; however, the purchases by Medtronic Inc. of TransVascular Inc. and Coalescent Surgical Inc., each for approximately $60 million, barely got investors out with a gain.

For the most part, companies that are still emerging and only beginning to establish the other key characteristics command lower exit values. The combination of clinical impact, franchise value, strategic need, and the other characteristics generates significantly more value. Moreover, each of the four technology-based acquisitions noted in this section provided that acquirer with new or better access to a customer base that was a strategic component of its long-term growth plans.

VALUE OF EXECUTION

A company's performance during the early stages of its development is critical to maximizing value. This explains why venture capitalists place so much emphasis on the management team. Not only is execution important, it is controllable; an experienced team knows how to organize itself around key issues, thereby preventing situations such as program misdirection and lack of appropriate development focus from taking hold, while at the same time preserving the ability to change direction on the basis of new information.

Execution, which may also be thought of as organizational focus, is intimately linked to time and money. A poorly run organization wastes precious time and inhibits the company's ability to hit the market at the optimum time. An inaccurate assessment of the time needed to reach a company's key clinical and commercial milestones consumes cash. Windows of opportunity are only open for so long. A mismanaged organization consumes its initial funding without ever hitting the milestones necessary to achieve the next round of financing quickly and at a higher value than the previous round.

Charting the value of execution points to this problem. Well-run organizations move through the inevitable hard-reality low period, reevaluate their business model, and redirect their engineering efforts as needed to keep a program on track for commercialization. These organizations remain focused and answer the product development questions necessary to make a product work and hit their launch date around the three- to four-year time frame. An organization that is wedded to the

Keys to Creating Value for Early Stage Medical Device Companies

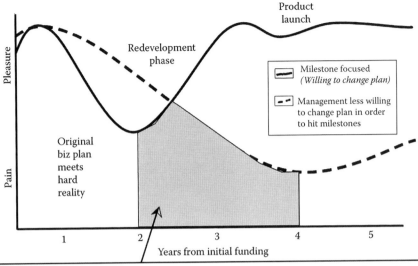

FIGURE 25.1 Value creation curves.

technology and refuses to alter its approach often consumes more cash before it hits hard reality and realizes too late that it must change direction and redesign (see Figure 25.1). Indeed, execution is inexorably linked to management of capital and time, two additional critical factors for a successful exit.

The dynamic has played out countless times in venture-backed companies. Almost all start-ups hit hard-reality points early on; the good ones are capable of changing direction and reengineering quickly to maintain their cash and still achieve their value creation milestones. The companies that refuse to alter direction and reengineer their programs, on the other hand, miss the milestone, run dangerously close to being out of cash, and consequently fall into a state of limbo during which time they lose their edge and miss the window of opportunity. Without question, this scenario produces very poor return for the investors and employees. Too many companies follow a path of being wedded to a technology or market for too long. Consequently they consume much more money than they should before realizing that the company's model, technology, or management are wrong. Companies capable of executing on the value creation milestones within a time frame of two to four years on efficient use of their funds are better positioned to achieve maximum value.

SUSTAINABILITY

In thinking about M&A and the amount of quantitative analysis and models built to justify an acquisition or an IPO, analysts place extensive weight on the sustainable, predictable sales of the acquired technology. Indeed, buyers want to know whether acquiring a company and its technology is going to generate long-lasting profits. A large market, significant clinical impact, and the ability to establish or bolster a franchise for the acquirer is critical to profit sustainability.

Sustainability therefore implies successful management of both capital and time. Maximizing returns is almost impossible without funding that is adequate to give a company the time to demonstrate clinical impact, franchise value, and sustainability. Most companies with successful exits had not only venture dollars but also public money: The five companies in Table 25.1, for example, averaged $66 million in private and public capital. They also had solid cash positions at the time of acquisition, enabling them to run efficient operations and avoid accepting a less-than-optimal deal to ensure survival. The average amount of cash to establish those premium exits appears to be in the $30 to $40 million range and in all cases (except VidaMed) was achieved in a four- to seven-year time frame. The lower exit-value companies in Table 25.2, on the other hand, raised $11 million and their exits were two to four years before any real value was placed on clinical impact and sustainability. In the majority of cases, therefore, companies that achieved higher values had more cash and used it very effectively.

Because it relates to execution and funding, effective time management is also to a large extent controllable. More often than not, poor management creates poor execution and direction—witness the early issues at VidaMed. With the right investors and management team, however, this phenomenon is controllable. Even technologies that require more involved clinical trials and a more complex Food and Drug Administration strategy may appear to be uncontrollable, but if managed well, are.

WHEN TO EXIT?

Benchmarking against the characteristics for success is a way to gauge performance and can be used as a management tool to help determine when, and at what price, to exit. The characteristics for obtaining a successful exit can be plotted against the exit values.

A company with a groundbreaking technology may exit too early. Investors become concerned over the progress against milestones and the timetables without understanding future potential and impact. These situations generally result in exits before hitting the inflection point at which much higher values could be generated (see Figure 25.2). Conversely, a top team that can articulate the requirements in terms of time and money is able to have the company's runway extended to this inflection point. The investors will have to be convinced that extending the company's runway will in fact achieve a much higher exit value. This type of scenario occurs every day. If the management is unable to reinforce and demonstrate that a product will have clinical value; that the market is still underserved, large, and growing; and that over the next few years significant value creation milestones will be achieved, it should take the lower exit value scenario.

In the past four years, market conditions have driven up the amount of money required to bring a company to a maximizing event—a major concern not only to the venture capital community but also to entrepreneurs. As the IPO market dried up

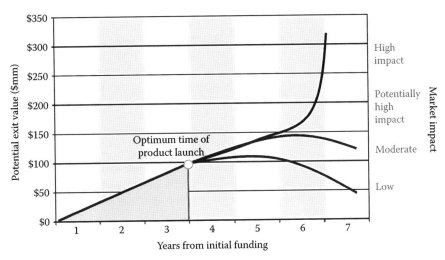

FIGURE 25.2 Market impact and value creation.

and the requirements for going public shifted back to a solid revenue stream, while showing adoption and growth, the timelines required to demonstrate this characteristic have also shifted. The importance of solid execution has always been critical, but over the last few years, it has become even more so.

The IPO market provided Perclose, VidaMed, CTS, Oratec, and PercuSurge access to adequate cash early on, enabling them to prove their models. But today, achieving the exit values that most venture capitalists seek takes much more careful planning because the requirements to tap into the public markets have become much more difficult.

Indeed, market conditions dictate an increasing emphasis on both execution and management of capital. Moreover, there is only a short list of likely acquirers, further reduced by J&J's purchase of Guidant Corp.[*] The good news is that large-cap companies still depend on small medical device companies as a source to expand their offerings without earnings dilution, and therefore, funding will continue to be available for novel, clinically relevant products that serve large and growing markets. The challenge for executives is to manage capital and establish realistic timelines that enable their firms to hit those benchmark characteristics that define a successful creation and exit.

RESOURCES

De Novo Ventures (http://www.denovovc.com) maintains an archive of insightful articles covering numerous subjects critically important to the med-tech entrepreneur and raising venture capital. This article and many more are available at http://www.denovovc.com/articles.html.

Windhover (http://www.elsevierBI.com) publishes *InVivo*, *Start-Up*, *Medtech Insight*, "The Pink Sheet," and "The Grey Sheet" and produces the IN3 Investment in Innovation Conferences.

---

[*] See "Elephant Cha-Cha: The J&J/Guidant Deal," *In Vivo*.

ABOUT THE AUTHOR

Richard Ferrari, a managing director of De Novo Ventures, was formerly CEO of Cardiovascular Imaging Systems Inc., cofounder and CEO of CardioThoracic Systems Inc., and founding CEO of Cryovascular Systems Inc. and Paracor Surgical Inc. He was awarded the Mallinckrodt Award for Excellence in Medicine and twice was a finalist for the Entrepreneur of the Year Award.

ACKNOWLEDGMENTS

The permission of Richard Ferarri, managing director of De Novo Ventures, and David Cassack, vice president of content of Windhover Information Incorporated (an Elsevier Company), to reprint this article is gratefully acknowledged.

26 Female Leadership in the Medical Device Industry

France Helfer

CONTENTS

Female Entrepreneurship in the 21st Century 423
Personal Requirements for a Start-Up 424
Why Start a Company? 425
Key Components for a Medical Device Start-Up 426
    Unmet Need in a Growing Field 426
    Regulatory and Reimbursement Pathway 426
    Funding and Financing 427
Conclusion 427
About the Author 428

Dr. Gabriela Ruiz, head of the Biomedical Engineering Department, School of Biotechnology and Health, ITESM Campus Monterrey, was using the first edition of *The Medical Device R&D Handbook* in her bioengineering curriculum. Of special interest were the interviews with industry leaders, which Dr. Ruiz and her students found inspiring. Dr. Ruiz called me with a special request. She asked if I knew of any prominent female medical device entrepreneurs, and if I could include these in a future edition. I told her that I did, and her inquiry was especially timely, as I was in the process of developing the MDR&D second edition that you are now reading. I asked France Dixon Helfer, serial entrepreneur, to give her perspective as a woman in the medical device industry.

Theodore R. Kucklick

FEMALE ENTREPRENEURSHIP IN THE 21ST CENTURY

The old adage "behind every great man there is a woman" is alive and well in the 21st century in the medical device industry, and this pertains to female entrepreneurship. Only 4% of healthcare companies have female CEOs.[*] The female gender is intelligent, well-educated, driven, and capable; however, in a male-dominated industry—and in the male-dominated world still existing in the 21st century—breaking away from the status quo to take a leadership position and maintain it is difficult at best. It is easy to point fingers, yet each one of us shares much of the blame. Females

---

[*] "Your CEO May Be A Man, But Your Healthcare Customer is a Woman," July 22, 2012, "Venture Valkerie" blog by Lisa Suennen, Psilos Ventures.

generally accept our position as "number two," and if we make it to the top, we spend most of our time politically campaigning to maintain that position, rather than focusing on building that newborn company to its full potential. Funding female-led businesses through the normal venture capital (VC) channels is equally frustrating. According to the Center for Women's Business Research, women-led businesses receive less than 5% of all VC funding[*]; however, women own more than 40% of all privately held companies in the United States, and I would venture to assume that a large number of those women owners have been turned down by the incestuous white male-led venture community. With this sobering statistic, I will provide my beliefs on the basis of my many years of experience, on what it takes to be a successful female entrepreneur in the 21st century.

I did not attend a prestigious university, but I absolutely received a well-rounded education that prepared me for the working environment. I attended a California state university and received an excellent education. My parents encouraged advanced education but did not support it financially. I put myself through college by working a minimum of two jobs—one was always in my industry, the medical sciences, to gain practical skills and understanding when competing for a job in industry. In the 1970s, when I was a university student, I longed to become a physician; however, I did not have the financial means or encouragement to pursue this path, but I took pre-med studies and fulfilled the obligations for a degree in the biological sciences. In 2012, the tides have changed, and since 2003, the number of women applying to medical schools in the United States has exceeded men. Women physicians graduating and practicing in the United States now outnumber men. The pay differential still exists, and it is reported that male physicians out-earn female physicians in the 15% to 20% range. Once working as a full-time employee, I continued my education, technically, and in business management.

An entrepreneur is defined broadly as a risk-taking businessperson who initiates new commercial enterprises. What that definition seems to trivialize is the incredible amount of work it takes to build a new company, but how thoroughly satisfying it is to have developed a start-up from the ground up.

PERSONAL REQUIREMENTS FOR A START-UP

Starting a company includes neither having a defined role nor others to rely on. In a start-up company, as the founder, you do as much groundwork as possible before raising money and bringing in colleagues to round out your team. It is imperative to have worked in management at large and smaller companies before venturing off to become a company founder. The reasons are basic. In a large company—and I had the fortune to work for major medical device companies Johnson & Johnson, and Medtronic—one is taught the discipline that will be required in a start-up company, including the budget process, regulatory and clinical requirements of working with the Food and Drug Administration, product development planning, administrative duties including hiring and firing, employee benefits and employee appraisals.

---

[*] Center for Women's Business Research, 1760 Old Meadow Road, Suite 500, McLean, VA 22102, 703-556-7162; fax 703-506-3266.

The large company environment also teaches interactions with all functional departments, critical in understanding who and what is needed to start a company. In my case, I had worked in research and development (R&D), marketing, operations, and corporate development for large companies, and therefore I had a very broad understanding of what was required to launch a start-up company. I had already been a vice president and a chief operating officer (COO), and I had experience in the boardroom at several companies; therefore, president and chief executive officer (CEO) was my next step. As a vice president of corporate development, I learned about negotiating and licensing. Working in large companies is where you will find your professional network. As a manager, you will know who you need and who you want to work with you at the highest level. Strong leadership is imperative to attract the top talent to your start-up. The right management team and the right product idea are two critical aspects for a new company, of which I cannot say enough. Those top managers will have their own network to fill in. An important mistake to avoid is promising jobs to your friends. The right person is often the one with whom you interact only on a professional level. With that said, if your choice for a key management position is a person you have butted heads with across the table at staff meetings, no matter how talented, the friction will interfere with your ability to get the job done.

WHY START A COMPANY?

Generally, medical device and healthcare start-ups are pursued with either an engineer and doctor getting together to develop an idea created from an "unmet need" or a doctor and a sales and marketing executive doing the same. In this case, the physician and engineer may already have filed the idea for patent protection. The patent process in the United States is an embarrassment; the U.S. patent system is currently undergoing its first significant reform in 60 years. The changes are numerous and beyond the scope of this chapter. However, do not let the lack of an issued patent discourage you if the idea and device are solid. Large companies are other sources for start-ups, which are generated by the ideas developed in the R&D department that the company has opted not to pursue for a number of reasons.

Generally if the market potential is too small, the product is not identified in the company's strategic plan, or the product idea is outside the company's area of core competency, the large company will shelve the idea. With either start, the founder must identify the product and check to see whether there is intellectual property (IP) filed for the idea by the physician, engineer, or other entity (like a large company) and then take the necessary legal steps to license the technology's IP. This is a long and arduous process, and using a good licensing attorney or law firm is critical. I have worked successfully with Wilson Sonsini Goodrich & Rosati (WSGR, Palo Alto, CA) for many years. The Life Sciences practice of the WSGR group is staffed with top notch attorneys and paralegals all who understand the requirements for a start-up organization and work closely with your company to ensure efficiency and speed. I have been impressed with WSGR's ability to provide start-up groups with the same professionalism, attention, and support as provided to large organizations.

KEY COMPONENTS FOR A MEDICAL DEVICE START-UP

Once you have decided that your identified or invented technology is worthy of developing into a product, other key components must be in addressed.

UNMET NEED IN A GROWING FIELD

Determining the market you are in, and staying focused is key for any new company. Take a look at your space in the medical device industry. Is it the spine market that has been overplayed and is now consolidating? Is it a vascular stent with more patents pending and issued than perhaps any other medical product in history? These are generalizations, but they are key considerations, which will be roadblocks in development and in your fundraising efforts. Conversely, some technologies will get the attention of those with the money to fund your company and with end users (customers), such as miniaturization, less-invasive or noninvasive, and remote or wireless technologies. Once you have determined that your device is in a growing field that currently is generating interest, and has a large market potential for growth and revenue, take a look at where that field is expected to be in three to five years— the realistic time frame for your device to get through the development, design, and regulatory hurdles. Know your competitors, respect them, and do what you can to understand their strategies, their limitations, and where you will fit into the field.

REGULATORY AND REIMBURSEMENT PATHWAY

The regulatory and reimbursement pathway is a tough one, for which there is no crystal ball. The Food and Drug Administration (FDA) requirements are undergoing changes, and working with them early on is important. Working with top-notch regulatory experts in the field is critical, and this is not an area for you to make compromises. If you are assuming a Class II 510(k) clearance route, you must do the legwork to determine recent predicates that have not "crept" in and are clean. You must review the predicate files and products for "substantial equivalence," so that the device is clearly similar for FDA reviewers. This is the same for filing with the European regulatory agencies through a Notified Body to get the mandatory CE marking (the *Conformité Européenne*). Once you have determined the equivalent devices, do not scrimp or pass over the testing requirements for the agencies. Work with legitimate test labs, have your regulatory professional audit those labs, and before engaging them, ask for a large number of references to ensure that these outsourced services will conduct pristine studies. It is a significant expense that you do not want to have to repeat because of poor quality controls. Reimbursement is another sometimes overlooked area. *No matter how brilliant your device is, if there is no reimbursement pathway in place from either third-party insurers or Center for Medicare and Medicaid Services (CMS), very few will adopt it.* Many start-ups have failed for just this issue. It is not enough to be covered under an umbrella reimbursement code; it is highly recommended to conduct reimbursement studies with true endpoints that show your device has advantages over current practice, such as saving lives, saving time during the procedure, reducing repeat operations, reducing morbidity, and so on. Once you have conducted well-run reimbursement studies, with clearly successful endpoints, you can apply for a reimbursement code to obtain coverage and a payment level, which will be used by the end user to get reimbursed for your device. This is not an easy process, but it is one that should be understood very early in the life of the company and product.

FUNDING AND FINANCING

There are several ways to fund a new company. These include angel funding (including "friends and family" investors) and large angel organizations, venture capitalists, and corporate investors. Since October 2008, when the stock market dropped to levels not seen in about 10 years, the world of VC funding has changed. When a VC group invests in a company at any stage, they plan to invest for the "life of the company," which generally is when an exit event occurs. For example, if a VC fund has invested $10 million into a "B" round, they will anticipate how much additional money the company needs to get to profitability, and they will set aside that money for investing in later rounds of financing. When the stock market adjusted down, the VC funds took huge hits because the limited partners who were invested in the funds were personally affected and did not want to invest in new funds. Consolidation and closure of many VC firms ensued. It is now harder than ever to secure VC funding; however, as of 2011, the market began to see recovery. As a result of the poor U.S. economy, companies must have the ability to achieve more milestones with less capital investments. Virtual companies and teams are now commonplace and teams of industry professionals are starting more virtual companies without being in a central office location. In a now very wired world, it is easy to function without being together daily in a face-to-face mode. This has resulted in companies getting much further on their goals and significant milestones with less money invested. Additionally, uncommon five years earlier, large corporations are now looking at start-up companies at earlier stages for codevelopment projects or simply for investments. Know who your investors are: During the negotiations, lead investors will want to serve on your board of directors, and this is a long and close relationship. The best board make-up include highly seasoned industry experts, a financially astute individual, an objective product end user, and at least one or two of the company senior executives.

CONCLUSION

Nothing is more rewarding than building something from the ground up. This applies to everything in life—from home projects, to raising children, and relevant to this chapter, to starting a medical device or healthcare company.

The key challenge is to manage your resources intelligently, including both human and capital resources. As a female serial entrepreneur, there are many hurdles that must be cleared, but I imagine that male entrepreneurs face similar ones; however, they are not as steep. Once you have a successful track record, the experience, the lessons, and the successes and failures all culminate in a broad knowledge base.

Starting a company is not something to take lightly. Entrepreneurship is an arduous path but not for everyone. The risks and stakes are inherent and great. The security of a pension and retirement plan that can be earned at a large company are not available in a start-up. "Hitting it big" is not the norm in a start-up; it is the exception. This must be considered at all stages of the company's development. And, finally, look introspectively. Understand your leadership and management skill set and whether you have been successful in building teams and products, and launching them. If your answer is that you are not ready yet, or you do not have the confidence it takes, do not think you can learn on the job. Stay in the industry, absorb as much as you can, and when the time is right, you will know.

ABOUT THE AUTHOR

France Helfer is a 30-year veteran of the medical device industry, with 20 years in executive management roles. She has worked for industry leaders Medtronic, Johnson & Johnson, Sorin, Pfizer-Shiley, and for a number of smaller companies in management roles, including founder, CEO and president, COO, international sales and marketing, business and corporate development, mergers and acquisitions, R&D, and engineering. As a serial entrepreneur, she has raised more than $50 million in angel and VC financing, and she has served on various boards as a member and an observer. She is a frequent presenter at management conferences in the life sciences. In mid-2011, she was recruited as president, CEO, and board chairperson to turn around a southern California-based company in the field of women's health, Halo Healthcare. Halo's current product is a screening and stratification test for detecting breast cancer risk. The company is developing a 3 molecule biomarker lab assay from university developed technology licensed for actual early prediction of breast cancer.

27 Medical Device Sales 101

Devin Hughes

CONTENTS

About the Author 431

> I asked Devin Hughes to contribute this brief article on medical device sales, as the sales representative is one of the most important people in the chain of getting your medical device innovation to the surgeon and the patient, and the one most often overlooked in the innovation process. A good medical device sales rep is far more than a mere "order taker." If they are really doing their job, they will know your product, often better than the surgeon, and be personally dedicated to its success. If the sales rep does not believe in your product, it will not come out of the bag, it will not be presented, and it will not sell, and your innovation will not be adopted. Too often designers that do not spend time in the operating room (OR) design products that are thrown "over the wall" to the sales rep (who spend nearly all their time in the OR) and are asked to risk their "political capital" of surgeon relationships presenting a clunky product. This is a recipe for frustration and failure. This article gives you an idea what to look for in a good sales rep, some of the issues and pressures they face, and how you can think through your innovation to be successful in the sales reps' hands.
>
> **Theodore R. Kucklick**

Selling anything can be difficult enough, but selling medical devices used in the operating room (OR) can be brutal. The easy part is often learning the anatomy and the procedural data. It gets tricky trying to find your place in this vast ecosystem without a GPS and actually applying what you have learned in training. At the same time, you must figure out quickly how to add value to surgeons and staff while helping to improve patient outcomes. The following is a collection of proven tactics that have helped numerous sales reps stand out in the crowd, and this will help the medical device innovator know what will help their product stand out in this environment.

It may surprise a few people, but clinicians and OR personnel lean on their sales reps to get acclimated and trained on medical device products. New products are presented in the office, but more often than not they are presented in the hospital OR. Unless the manufacturer has a huge marketing budget, the surgeon's only reference point to the device is via the sales rep. It is also fairly common for sales reps to introduce a new device just a few minutes before the actual case. Once the surgeon agrees to try it, the sales rep is then asked to stay for the case and get the OR staff up to speed. At this point, the sales rep is under a lot of pressure. They have to perform and show value, and so does the product. The worst nightmare for a sales rep is to have a surgeon struggle to use the new device.

Some context is important: The surgeon typically has a solid relationship with that particular sales rep, trusts his judgment, and has probably worked with them on prior cases. He will listen to the rep coach him through application. Many people might be surprised how much emphasis a surgeon will place on their sales rep. These relationships often last years and include hundreds of cases, so in many ways, the sales rep is viewed as an extension of the surgical team, and his or her judgment is trusted. It takes years for reps to build this level of trust and respect, and they are reluctant to risk this trust on a product that does not perform to expectations.

The tricky part comes down to the actual application of the device itself. If the device is cumbersome, labor intensive, or not that intuitive to use, there is a strong likelihood that the surgeon and staff will refrain from using it, and it will make the rep look bad. Once this happens, the chances of your product coming out of the bag to be presented to another surgeon plummet.

It helps to understand the psychology of surgeons. They develop habits and when something new is introduced, it had better not slow them down or complicate the case. A well-designed product that is easy to use and apply is always well received. Also, the sales rep cannot be there every single time the surgeon operates, so it is critical that the learning curve is not steep.

Following are some key perspectives on what makes a medical device sales rep successful, what to look for in a good rep, and how to design an innovation that will succeed in their hands, because, ultimately, if it does not succeed for them, it will not succeed for you.

1. **Be prepared for some "push back"** about your company, product(s), the last sales rep, your manager, and any other random objection that you might hear from surgeon or staff. Wear your emotional bulletproof vest to work.
2. **Make application easy.** Surgeons will not use the device if they do not know how to use it or if it is perceived as too difficult. More important, it is critical that you know the case and are able to articulate both the how and the why for product usage and placement.
    - Have the residents help—they can teach the surgeons and remind them how to use the device.
    - Teach the scrub technicians and, in turn, they will remind and guide the surgeons.
    - Discuss application tips before the case in the OR lounge or at the scrub sink.
3. **Get your product on surgeon preference cards** (i.e., the product is in the room on every case). Ask the surgeon for permission to inform the circulating nurse to add your product(s).
4. **Be prepared to have difficult conversations.** With many devices, you are not always in the room when they use it, so you often have no idea as to whether they are using your product when you are not around. Prospects will tell you all kinds of stories about how much they use your device and how often.
5. **Work the night shift occasionally (especially in the beginning).**
    - Work at night one or two times per week.

- Establish credibility with staff and surgeons.
- Differentiate yourself from other reps.
6. **Be in surgery (should be obvious).**
    - Work 15 cases per week, at a minimum.
    - Overachieve on effort from the start.
7. **Show a genuine interest in people.** Average reps make a memorable first impression. Great reps usually do that, but they always wear well over time. Why? Their concern for customers is real, and it goes deeper than one case. Surgeons come to value the sales person as much and sometimes more than the device itself.
8. **Understand that context is king.** You must find your advocates as soon as possible. Who is using your product? Why? On what cases? How long have they been a user? Which hospitals do they operate and on which days? Which hospitals have it stocked? Do I have access? *Access* is a major issue right now for most reps, so the quicker you can find out where you have challenges the quicker you can ramp your business.
    - Ask your advocates for assistance (critical for success).
    - Will they introduce you to others in their group, at the hospital, and in your territory?
9. **Take things personally.** Average reps have a job. Great reps are passionate about their positions and it borders on an obsession. They eat, sleep, and drink conversations about their territory, that case, next week, this month, that new doc, this new study, and so on. They never sell enough, never know enough, and never work hard enough. They can always do more and will never be out worked. They do not see rejection and internal resistance as a roadblock but rather as a challenge.
10. **Stay active.** Stay focused on building your brand continuously (what makes you different) and your pipeline. Be in a hospital every day by at least 7:00 A.M. Eat breakfast in the hospital cafeteria. You may run into (OR) staff and "that prospect" who you have been unable to meet.
    - Let everyone know about your solution and why it is different and how it improves patient outcomes.
    - Introduce yourself to surgeons, if you can, between cases, in their offices, in the OR lounge, or anywhere else in the hospital.

ABOUT THE AUTHOR

Devin Hughes is an entrepreneur-in-residence at CONNECT (San Diego, CA). Hughes previously was area director of sales for Genyzme Biosurgery. He attended the UCLA–Anderson School of Management, where he earned an executive certificate in medical marketing in 2009, and the UCSD–Rady School of Management, where he earned a global biotech certificate in 2008. He received his bachelor of arts degree in sociology/anthropology from Colgate University.

28 Invention, Innovation, and Creativity
Or How Thomas Edison Never Changed the World by Creating the Light Bulb

Theodore R. Kucklick

CONTENTS

Science and Discovery 435
Art and Design 437
Finding the Need 439
Endnotes 445

Thomas Edison is perhaps the best-known inventor of all time. Edison also embodies many of the popular myths and misconceptions of invention and the invention process. If you ask the average person, "Did Edison change the world by creating the first light bulb?" he or she would probably say "yes," even though this statement is not correct. Examining this statement provides a convenient framework for discussing some of the misconceptions and challenges in understanding innovation, and how it relates to developing clinically useful medical device technology.

In medical device research and development (R&D), what are we setting out to accomplish? We are seeking practical solutions to clinical problems—solutions with clinical utility. This seeking will involve several unsuccessful attempts before a solution is found. Once that solution is found, it then needs to be turned into a solution that is safe, effective, reliable, repeatable, scalable, and profitable.

From a business point of view it helps if the solution is unique and patentable, so that a company can charge enough for this solution to recoup the cost of finding it, developing it, testing it, and protecting it, and still have enough left to pay a return to the investors who put up the money to make it possible—and maybe a little left over for you, the innovator.

The purpose of this chapter is to give you a practical way to look at invention and innovation, and to try to remove some of the confusion over terms. If terms are defined accurately, it becomes possible to think clearly and logically. If you can define and understand the innovation process better, this will help you to be a better innovator.

One source of misunderstanding comes from the common use of terms that are not quite accurate. Another source of misunderstanding comes from different compartmentalized specialties using similar terms to describe different things or using different terms for the same things.

Vague and insignificant forms of speech, and abuse of language have so long passed for mysteries of science; and hard and misapplied words, with little or no meaning, have, by prescription, such a right to be mistaken for deep learning and height of speculation, that it will not be easy to persuade either those who speak or those who hear them, that they are but the covers of ignorance, and hindrance of true knowledge.

—**John Locke,**
English: An Essay Concerning Human Understanding (1690)

Let us start with a few dictionary definitions (from the *Oxford Universal Dictionary*, 1955 edition):

Invent: From the Latin *invenire*, to come upon, find, or discover. To find out in the way of original contrivance, to devise first a new method or instrument, to find out or produce by mental activity, to find out how to do something.
Innovate: From the Latin *innovare*, to make new. To change into something new, to alter, to renew, to introduce novelties, to make changes in something established, a new shoot at the end of a branch.
Create: From the Latin *creare*. To bring into being, cause to exist. To form out of nothing, to call into existence.

We see from these definitions that the emphasis of invention is discovery. The emphasis of innovation is change.

Here we have a basic conflict between the terms *invent* and *create*. To invent and innovate requires that you start with something to be able to put it into a new form. To create means you start with nothing. As Thomas Edison once said, "To invent, you need good imagination and a pile of junk."

If Edison had not had his pile of junk to start with, he would not have been able to get anything done. Artists talk all the time about creating a work or being creative, yet we know this is not literally true. An artist, inventor, or innovator may be the first human being to put certain preexisting elements into a form that another human being has not done before, make a discovery that another human being has not made, or produce a solution to a problem, but this is very different from calling something into existence from nothing. God creates from nothing. People form and make from that which exists, whether physical objects and forces or from abstract mental processes.

I invent nothing, I rediscover.

—**Auguste Rodin**

An inventor is a person who makes an ingenious arrangement of wheels, levers and springs, and believes it civilization.

—**Ambrose Bierce,**
The Devil's Dictionary

And as James Burke wrote,

The more raw material we have to work with, the better methods we have, and the more focused energy we put into it, the more practical skill, the more times we can try new things, iterate and fail intelligently, the better our opportunity for success at invention.

In the heroic treatment, historical change is shown to have been generated by the genius of individuals, conveniently labeled "inventors." In such a treatment Edison invented the electric light, Bell the telephone, Gutenberg the printing press, Watt the steam engine, and so on. But no individual is responsible for producing an invention "*ex nihilo.*" The elevation of the single inventor to the position of sole creator at best exaggerates his influence over events, and at worst denies the involvement of those humbler members of society without whose work his task might have been impossible.*

The other part of the Edison story most people know is how many thousands of unsuccessful attempts were made before a reliable light bulb was produced. The process of trying many different approaches in a systematic way with a clear goal in mind is an essential ingredient in producing innovation.

Failure is the preamble to success.

—**Thomas J. Fogarty, MD**

Design is a stepwise iterative process. Design starts with a need and then applies technology until the need is solved in the best way possible given the time, resources, talents, and specifications available. This is the way medical device development usually occurs.

An inventor is simply a person who doesn't take his education too seriously. You see, from the time a person is six years old until he graduates from college he has to take three or four examinations a year. If he flunks once, he is out. But an inventor is almost always failing. He tries and fails maybe a thousand times. If he succeeds once then he's in. These two things are diametrically opposite. We often say that the biggest job we have is to teach a newly hired employee how to fail intelligently. We have to train him to experiment over and over and to keep on trying and failing until he learns what will work.

—**Charles F. Kettering**

SCIENCE AND DISCOVERY

Archimedes is known for having the original *Eureka!* moment. He discovered the principles of buoyancy and hydrostaics while contemplating a nondestructive way

---

* James Burke, *The Day the Universe Changed* (Boston: Little, Brown & Co., 1985).

to test the golden crown of King Hiero of Syracuse. Archimedes observed these principles while stepping into his bathtub. Realizing that this was the answer to his problem, the story says he leapt from his tub, *au naturel*, and ran through the streets announcing his discovery to the citizens of Alexandria, shouting "Eureka!" (I have found it!). Whether the Alexandrians were more nonplussed at what he had discovered or that he was uncovered is not known.[*]

Archimedes produced an innovation by matching a physical phenomenon to a problem he needed to solve. He uncovered this phenomenon through his keen powers of observation. Developing these powers of observation and the ability to apply these observations to problems is a key skill of the innovator.

> For what study is there more fitted to the mind of man than the physical sciences? And what is there more capable of giving him an insight into the actions of those laws, a knowledge of which gives interest to the most trifling phenomenon of nature, and makes the student find:
> Tongues in trees, books in the running brooks,
> Sermons in stones, and good in every thing?[†]
>
> —**Michael Faraday**

Scientists, especially those engaged in pure research, are often criticized for the lack of practical use for their discoveries. The United States produces an enormous quantity of publicly funded basic research, which by definition is directed toward the expansion of knowledge, not the production of useful inventions. Universities are becoming more skilled at cataloging these discoveries and offering them for use through their offices' technology licensing.

A fundamental tension in this process is the following: The incentive structure in universities and the sciences rewards basic discovery and publication of results. Commercial application relies on putting a discovery in the form of intellectual property, which requires a degree of secrecy before a discovery is published as a patent. The numerous and complex issues involved in moving basic research from the laboratory bench to the patient's bedside is the subject of intense interest. The National Institutes of Health (NIH) has a Translational Research Initiative (TRI) to help turn basic discoveries into applied therapies.[‡]

> Michael Faraday's interest in knowledge for its own sake often baffled people of a more practical bent. British Prime Minister William Gladstone, observing Faraday performing a particularly unlikely experiment one day, pointedly asked him how useful such a "discovery" could possibly be. "Why," Faraday smartly replied, "you will soon be able to tax it!"[§]

Donald E. Stokes' book *Pasteur's Quadrant* addresses the conflict between basic and applied science. Stokes draws a matrix with curiosity on the x-axis and practicality

---

[*] *Eureka* is also the motto of the state of California. From this anecdote, it may apply to California's reputation for bohemianism, as well as its reputation for discovery.
[†] Michael Faraday, *Harvard Classics*, vol. 30 (New York: P. F. Collier and Son, 1938), 85.
[‡] Science Business, "NIH Adds 5 clinical/Translational Research Centers," http://sciencebusiness.technewslit.com/?p=4734 (accessed August 13, 2012).
[§] Sarah K. Bolton and Barbara L. Cline, *Famous Men of Science* (New York: Crowell, 1960).

Invention, Innovation, and Creativity

on the y-axis. The four quadrants are occupied by Niels Bohr in the upper left, Louis Pasteur in the upper right, Thomas Edison in the lower right, and accident in the lower left. Niels Bohr was entirely theoretical. If a discovery had a practical use, it was of little interest to him. Pasteur was a balance between pure and applied science. Pasteur was driven by an intense concern for the medical needs of people. Edison was by his own admission entirely practical. For Edison there was no "why," but only trial and error until a practical solution with commercial value emerged.[*]

ART AND DESIGN

Another pair of terms that are often used interchangeably are art and design. Again, some definitions:

> **Art:** From *artem*, to fit. Skill as the result of knowledge or practice, human skill, technical or professional skill, perfection of workmanship, application of skill in the areas of taste, poetry, music, architecture, painting. The quality, production or expression according to aesthetic principles (*Oxford English Dictionary* [*OED*], *Webster's*). *Webster's* (1828) makes a distinction between the *polite,* or *liberal,* arts and the *useful,* or *mechanical,* arts or *trades*. One emphasizes mental skill, the other manual skill.

> **Design:** From the Latin *de signo*, to seal or stamp (*Webster's*, 1828). To delineate by outline or sketch, to plan; the preliminary conception of an idea that is to be carried into effect by action (*OED*). Organization or structure of formal elements, composition, plan, blueprint (*Webster's Unabridged*, 1989).

Design helps to make a product logical, usable, and understandable to the end user. Good design is invaluable in making medical technology usable and even safer. It is part of providing complete utility and a satisfying and appealing experience for the user. Design is putting things together in a planned and purposeful way. It can be utilitarian mechanical design, aesthetic design, or a combination of the two. Design can range from the cool rationality of the Bauhaus to exuberant technological Rococo.

In art, the emphasis is on skill applied to aesthetics. Aesthetics is what appeals to the senses or feelings. Aesthetics is primarily subjective and emotional.

In design, the emphasis is on planning and organization. It is primarily a logical and objective activity. It is producing purpose and order.

In his work *The Two Cultures and the Scientific Revolution*, C. P. Snow describes the gulf between the scientific community and the literary intellectual communities. If anything, this gap has widened since Snow wrote his work in 1959.[†] On many levels, the scientific and artistic communities view each other with a mixture of mutual suspicion and disdain. To the scientist, the arts lack rigor and purpose, and to the artist, science lacks feeling.

Why is the artist important to the scientific innovator? Because art communicates and also appeals to the emotions.

---

[*] Donald Stokes, *Pasteur's Quadrant* (Washington, DC: Brookings Institution Press, 1997).
[†] C. P. Snow, *The Two Cultures and the Scientific Revolution* (New York: Cambridge University Press, 1998).

Art is a vital way to communicate scientific information. The medical illustration work of Vesalius, *De Humani Corporis Fabrica*, as well as the work of da Vinci, Albinus, Broedel, and, more recently, Dr. Frank Netter, have been essential to making the human body understandable to generations of clinicians.

Marketers know that buying decisions are primarily emotional. The effective marketer uses the tools of the artist to bring attention and desirability to a product. It turns technical specifications into an appealing emotional story that communicates value. Marketing communicates objective features and subjective benefits. Branding helps people recognize products. Marketing helps to communicate information in a direct and intuitive way. This can help a clinically useful innovation get to the person it is intended to help. People may need what you have invented, but they have to know what you have, want what you have, and like what you have. They have to "buy into" a product before they buy the product. Also, what you have has to ultimately be what people need. All the marketing in the world cannot "push a rope."

It has been said that sales is taking orders for water from thirsty people. Marketing is the art of making them thirsty. Advertising is getting people to crave things they do not yet know exist.

> In art, in taste, in life, in speech, you decide from feeling, and not from reason. . . . If we were obliged to enter into a theoretical deliberation on every occasion before we act, life would be at a stand, and Art would be impracticable.
>
> —William Hazlitt

People operate far more on intuition than logic than they may care to admit. The reason for this is that intuition takes less time. One way marketing persuades us to buy is to communicate the endorsement of a person or institution we trust. We assume that the "expert" has done his homework so that we do not have to.

One difficulty here is that the purists in the academic scientific community as well as the purists in the arts community look on the process of practical commercialization with suspicion or even distaste. In some circles if someone "goes commercial" they have prostituted themselves beyond redemption. Again, the goal is not to be an academic purist, but to develop practical solutions for the real needs of real patients. This will in turn produce value for the workers, owners, and investors of a company and society, and will generate capital for reinvestment and growth. Fields of activity, distilled and isolated, can be as dead as a body part cut off from the bloodstream. Art for art's sake and knowledge for knowledge's sake are no more defensible than profit for profit's sake.

The arts suffer from an internal conflict between pure and applied forms. In his 1891 essay "The Soul of Man under Socialism," Oscar Wilde wrote:

> Indeed, the moment that an artist takes notice of what other people want, and tries to supply the demand, he ceases to be an artist, and becomes a dull or an amusing craftsman, an honest or dishonest tradesman. He has no further claim to be considered as an artist.[*]

---

[*] Oscar Wilde, *The Soul of Man under Socialism*, ed. Linda Lowling (New York: Penguin Books, 2001).

To the aesthete purist, the moment art serves a practical purpose it is no longer fine art. It becomes an inferior applied art. This passage also illuminates the political bent found in some of the fine arts. In the conservative classical view, which prevailed in Western art from Greek and Roman times through the late 19th century, the purpose of art is to evoke noble emotions and teach moral values.* In the modernist view, the ultimate goal of art is to produce social change in the context of class struggle. The classical conservative definition has been virtually eradicated in academic circles. For example, the familiar term *avant-garde* applied to the innovative leading edge of modern art was originally the name for the shock troops of a revolutionary people's army. In this class-warfare model, art that does not annoy or infuriate the conservative middle class is considered a failure, mere illustration, or kitsch. There is a persistent argument over the definition of what is art. The fundamental dispute is actually not over what is art, but a noisy clash between the presentation of fundamentally irreconcilable world views. In the fine art world, Norman Rockwell is recognized for his technical talent but scorned for his idyllic portrayal of bourgeois values. Corporations contribute to and taxpayers are forced to pay for *épater les bourgeois* and *art brut* that is hostile to middle-class values and advocates the overthrow of free-market capitalism. The dissonance this produces in the arts-based industrial design field remains unresolved:

> During the Renaissance, . . . little cleavage was felt between the sciences and the arts. Leonardo passed back and forth between fields . . . that later became categorically distinct. Furthermore, even after that steady exchange had ceased, the term "art" continued to apply as much to technology and the crafts . . . as to painting and sculpture. Only when the latter unequivocally renounced representation . . . did the cleavage we now take for granted assume anything like its present depth.†

FINDING THE NEED

Necessity, who is the mother of invention.

—Plato,
The Republic

Restlessness and discontent are the first necessities of progress.

—**Thomas A. Edison**

Medical innovation usually starts with a need, and then matches an appropriate technology to solve the problem. This is the way the vast majority of medical innovations occur. Some innovations are technology driven. However, according to Beckie Robertson, cofounder of Versant Ventures, a major life science investment fund, these technology-driven products are by far in the minority.

---

* "Christopher L. C. E. Witcombe," Art History Resources, http://witcombe.sbc.edu/modernism/artsake.html (accessed August 13, 2012).
† Thomas Kuhn, *The Structure of Scientific Revolutions* (Chicago: University of Chicago Press, 1996), 161. This influential work popularized the terms *paradigm* and *paradigm shift*.

The ability to find and understand important clinical needs is an essential skill of the medical device entrepreneur. One of the ways to find needs is from thought leaders in a field. This approach has been formalized by Eric von Hippel of MIT into the lead user method. These lead users are leaders and early adopters who anticipate where a technology may be going. Translating this information into a product that one of these early adopters will use is one thing, but making a product that the early and late majorities will adopt is another. Between these early adopters and the majority market is a gap, the so-called valley of death that many technologies fail to cross.

Need finding is not as easy as it sounds. One would think that all you have to do is ask people what they want. Some of the most important needs are latent needs, where people do not know what they want and do not know what they are missing. Market research is especially ill-suited to finding latent needs. How do you predict market share for an innovative product where no comparable product yet exists? Balloon angioplasty and magnetic resonance imaging are two breakthrough technologies initially thought to have no market. Doctors, for many reasons, will seldom admit that they have a need. To admit a need is to say that they are not providing the best standard of care. Gathering and interpreting clinical needs information is another art in itself. For example, Dr. Thomas J. Fogarty, in a talk on this subject, stated that "What a doctor wants, what they say they want, what they need, and what they will pay for are all different things."

Technology-driven products have a seductive appeal. These are products with intriguing technology, with a wide range of potential uses, but with ill-defined clinical utility. The problem with the technology-driven approach is the panacea trap. Medical lasers had this problem. When laser technology became available for medical use, it was applied to a wide range of products. Few of these products were ultimately successful. The most successful medical device products and companies have compelling technology appropriately focused on a specific clinical need, not solutions in search of a problem, and not science projects. Two responses to a new medical technology that you do not want to hear are "that's interesting" or "you have a great solution to a problem I don't have."

Innovation, by definition, is practical, applied, and meets the needs of people. Applied science, invention, applied art, and design work together to produce innovations, solutions to human problems that have commercial value. Peter Drucker wrote the following:

> Above all, innovation is not invention. It is a term of economics rather than technology. Non-technological innovations—social or economic innovations—are at least as important as technological ones. Innovation can be defined as the task of endowing human and material resources with new and greater wealth-producing capacity. Managers must convert society's needs into opportunities for profitable businesses. This too, is a definition of innovation.[*]

Innovation is about finding and solving the real needs of real people, and generating economic wealth in the process. It is taking all of the skills and talents of the

---

[*] Peter F. Drucker, *The Essential Drucker* (New York: Harper Business, 2003), 22–23.

scientist, doctor, engineer, artist, businessperson, and technician to bear on solving the medical needs of patients and building a viable business.

> An idea in and of itself has no value. It's when you implement an idea, by means of an innovation, then you create value for society.*
>
> —Thomas J. Fogarty, MD

To really solve a medical problem, and get it to the people who need it, and you cannot do it all alone. To produce a product of real value, it takes the combined, committed, and organized efforts of people with a range of skills and talents. To get these people to work together and organize their efforts takes skilled management, and this art of management requires very different skills than most innovators have. It takes meticulous science. It takes people with skill at negotiating an ever-changing regulatory landscape. To bring these people together takes capital, and if successful, it produces more capital that can then be put to work solving other problems. Managing capital requires yet another set of specialized and very necessary skills.

Invention is a means to an end, not an end in itself. It does not matter how rapidly you are able to produce iterations of an idea, how cleverly you solve a problem, and how original you are at doing it; what matters in the end is the importance of the human clinical need you are solving and the effectiveness with which you solve it. One needs to get past having a technologically driven solution in search of a problem or trying to market solutions to problems patients and doctors do not have. Medical innovation with real value is the matching of a well-executed solution with an important unmet clinical need.

Edison is known also for his prolific output of patentable ideas. He is credited with 1093 patents during his life. Edison was focused on patenting ideas with commercial value.

> Anything that won't sell, I don't want to invent. Its sale is proof of utility, and utility is success.
>
> —Thomas A. Edison

There is a common misconception that all one needs to have is a patent, and this alone will produce wealth. The truth is that few patents make enough money to cover the cost of filing them. A patent is a fence. You can build a fence around a swamp or a gold mine. A swamp with a fence around it is still a swamp.

The purpose of patents is not to make inventors rich. It is to preserve a record of technology for the benefit of society and for other inventors to build on. The social contract between the inventor and society is a temporary monopoly on the sale of the patented product. This is the compensation given to the inventor in exchange for making the details of his invention public. It is up to the inventor to practice his patent or sell it to someone who generates wealth.

---

* "Celebrating a Lifetime of Innovation" (reception program at Stanford for Thomas J. Fogarty, Lemelson–MIT Award for Invention and Innovation, 2000).

Another more subtle, yet vitally important, issue arises when it comes to patents and intellectual property. This is the concept of freedom to operate. Just because you have a patent on a technology does not mean you can actually practice your invention. A common tactic, especially in crowded fields, is the filing of blocking patents. These are meant to fence off key areas of technology that may not be the product itself, but some of the essential means of practicing the invention. Establishing intellectual property protection as well as verifying freedom to operate are essential to successfully commercializing a medical device innovation.

So, did Edison create the light bulb? According to the literal definition, no. Did Edison invent the light bulb by himself? No. On the contrary, Edison organized a large team of skilled technicians and researchers that made his innovations possible. Employees of Edison Laboratories searched the ends of the earth for a material that would make a reliable light bulb filament. They invented means to insulate and bury reliable electrical cables. They worked on the myriad of challenges to make electric lighting and electrical generation and distribution a reality. In fact, according to James Burke, one of Edison's great innovations was the establishment and structure of Edison Laboratories, which became the prototype of the modern R&D organization. Edison states the structure of his method as follows:

Edison's Six Rules for Invention:

1. Define the need for innovation. If there is no market, don't start.
2. Set yourself a clear goal, and stick to it.
3. Analyze the major stages through which the invention must pass before it is complete.
4. Make available at all times data on the progress of the work.
5. Ensure that each member of the team has a clearly defined area of activity.
6. Record everything for later examination.*

Was Edison even the first to invent the light bulb? Again, the answer is no. The light bulb had been invented some 50 years before. Several inventors, including Sir Joseph Wilson Swan in England, had already developed working light bulbs. Edison even had to share credit with Swan when first marketing electric lighting in England, calling his English subsidiary the Ediswan Company. In fact, the bayonet lock light bulb base used in automobile taillight bulbs today was an invention of Sir Joseph's brother, Alfred Swan.

When discussing Edison, lighting, and electricity, another name that comes up is Nikolai Tesla. Tesla was a mirror image of Edison. Cultured, educated, and a brilliant if eccentric theoretician, he disdained the "empirical dragnet" approach of Edison. Tesla would construct an invention in his mind, and when it was fully formed, build a machine according to his vision, as opposed to the iterative stepwise approach of Edison.

Edison plays to an American saga of the rough, untutored, self-taught, practical natural genius. Tesla was the European-educated, refined, theoretical visionary. Tesla was possibly more technically brilliant; however, commercial success and recognition

---

* James Burke, *Connections* (Boston: Little, Brown & Co., 1978).

eluded him at every turn. Tesla and Edison fought costly and acrimonious battles over the merits of Edison's direct current (DC) versus Tesla's and Westinghouse's alternating current (AC).

In the medical device industry, it is possible to be an innovator with little formal medical education, but it is an uphill battle. Persons entering the field owe it to themselves to get the best relevant education and to get a solid technical foundation as early as possible.

Tesla was further frustrated by Guglielmo Marconi's commercialization of radio. Marconi used inventions and discoveries pioneered and patented by Tesla to make his system work, such as the Tesla oscillator. Tesla thought that his invention of radio was safe because his basic radio patent predated Marconi by three years. The Patent Office, for reasons not entirely clear, invalidated Tesla's 1894 patent, and Marconi became the father of radio and was awarded the Nobel Prize in 1911.

Tesla loved basic research. One of the reasons he was unable to get financial backing for his projects was that he would accept investments (in one example from financier J. P. Morgan) to work on a project and then spend the money on what he felt like working on. This doomed Tesla to penury. Tesla was ridiculed in the press for producing brilliant but eccentric scientific novelties. Society recognizes and rewards those who produce solutions for their problems. Genius, unfortunately, does not speak for itself. Tesla achieved as much success as he did through his association with George Westinghouse, who hired Tesla away from Edison, and recognized the practical potential of Tesla's "polyphase current" and focused his efforts.[*]

Tesla designed intuitively. It took the work of Charles P. Steinmetz to describe the mathematical basis of AC, which eventually allowed AC systems to be understood, designed, and controlled. Among Steinmetz's many accomplishments were the discovery of the law of hysteresis, symbolic calculation methods for predicting the performance of AC circuits, and the invention of three-phase power.[1]

So then, what did Edison do? Edison identified an important unmet market need and focused the resources of Edison Laboratories to solve it. Edison made a practical and reliable light bulb and the methods to produce them inexpensively, in quantity.[2] His R&D team, under his direction, also developed the generating equipment and the wiring infrastructure to deliver electricity to where the light bulbs were. It was not even the ultimate solution. Tesla's AC eventually replaced the DC that originally flowed over Edison's wires. Edison invented the simple and reliable screw-in fixture system that is still used in home lighting today. Edison developed a sales, marketing, and promotion structure. Solutions to problems such as how to generate electricity, how to manufacture the bulbs,[3] and how to insulate wires had to be invented. He formed a research organization that spawned other innovations, such as the phonograph, moving pictures, and a superior way to manufacture Portland cement. Then, perhaps one of the more important parts of the system, and possibly the most overlooked invention in this whole structure, was the electric meter. This, too, was an Edison invention. Not only was a complete, integrated system devised that solved an especially important unmet need, but it also had economic life. Edison devised the linchpin of

---

[*] "Tesla: Master of Lighting," PBS, http://www.pbs.org/tesla/index.html.

the whole system, a way to make money at it, which in turn generated the capital to produce many more breakthrough innovations and gave people lighting that was far superior in cost, performance, and safety to the gas lamps it displaced.*

It was the importance of the need, the effectiveness of the solution, and the sustainability of the system that made Edison a great innovator and earned him a place in history and in the popular imagination.

One significant difference must be noted between the environment in which Edison operated and the one in which the medical device innovator operates. Edison did not operate in a highly regulated environment. In the United States, for example, medical devices have been under the control of the federal Food and Drug Administration (FDA) since 1976 and drugs since 1906.† The purpose of the FDA is to protect the public from unsafe or adulterated medical products. Its charter is to ensure that medical devices and pharmaceuticals are safe and effective before they are cleared for sale. These regulations become increasingly strict as the potential risk to the patient goes up. One person I once worked with referred to the FDA out of frustration as "Forbidding Development in America." Wilson Greatbach, inventor of the cardiac pacemaker, said, "If I did today what I did twenty years ago, I would go to jail. Imagine making pacemakers in a barn, and taking them to a hospital and putting them into patients. We did it, and it worked."‡

Even though the process may be expensive and slow, I recall the statement made to me by a longtime FDA regulator at a medical device materials conference when he was new at the agency. His supervisor told him: "Remember, doctors can only kill patients one at a time. With a bad decision, you can kill them by the thousands."

Another significant difference is that Edison sold his electricity and lights directly to his customer. As medical device innovators, our focus is the patient; however, we rarely, if ever, sell a device to the patient. By law, we sell only to medical professionals. Furthermore, the medical professional to whom we market the device is often not the one paying for it. Discontinuous economic factors, such as insurance reimbursement and managed care, must be understood and dealt with if the medical device innovator is to develop an economically viable product.

The goal of the medical device innovator is to save, lengthen, and improve the quality of life for people, and in doing so, generate economic value and value for society. The focus is the patient and his needs. At a Stanford Innovator's Workbench talk, John Simpson, MD, pioneer in balloon angioplasty, stated the importance of doing right by the patient, and the rewards that can follow, as well as how it will catch up with you if you fail to do so.[4]

We can help people live longer, feel better, and look better. We can help save lives and limbs. We can improve quality of life. We can give a child her grandmother back. It is hard, rewarding work, and it is an important and noble enterprise.

---

* For more information on Edison, see Neil Baldwin, *Edison Inventing the Century* (New York: Hyperion Press, 1995).
† "About FDA: History," U.S. Food and Drug Administration, http://www.fda.gov/oc/history/default.htm.
‡ Kenneth Brown, *Inventors at Work* (Redmond, WA: Tempus Books/Microsoft Press, 1988), 24.

Does a student know how to tackle a problem with no background in the subject? And does he or she know how to get the knowledge needed? Accumulating methodology matters more than accumulating knowledge of subject matter.*

—**Herbert Kroemer,**
Nobel Laureate, on physics and education

It takes a thousand men to invent a telegraph, or a steam engine, or a phonograph, or a photograph, or a telephone, or any other important thing—and the last man gets the credit and we forget the others. He added his little mite—that is all he did.†

—**Mark Twain**

I recognize that many physicists are smarter than I am—most of them theoretical physicists. A lot of smart people have gone into theoretical physics; therefore, the field is extremely competitive. I console myself with the thought that although they may be smarter and may be deeper thinkers than I am, I have broader interests than they have.

—**Linus Pauling**

A good scientist is a person with original ideas. A good engineer is a person who makes a design that works with as few original ideas as possible.‡

—**Freeman Dyson**

ENDNOTES

1. "Institute of Chemistry," The Hebrew University of Jerusalem, http://chem.ch.huji.ac.il/~eugeniik/history/steinmetz.html; John H. Lienhard, "No. 276: Steinmetz," Engines of Our Ingenuity, http://www.uh.edu/engines/epi276.htm. It is interesting to note that Steinmetz was instrumental to the growth and success of one of America's largest corporations, General Electric, a company virtually synonymous with capitalism, although he was a dedicated socialist. Steinmetz kept up a correspondence with V. I. Lenin, and in his office proudly displayed an autographed picture sent to him by the Communist dictator.
2. "In 1876 Maximilian Nitze modified Edison's light bulb invention and created the first optical endoscope with a built-in electrical light bulb as the source of illumination. Like the Lichtleiter from Bozzini, this instrument was only used for urologic procedures." "The History of Laparoscopy," Laparoscopy.com, http://www.laparoscopy.com/shows/lapstry3.htm.

---

* Tekla S. Perry, "Not Just Blue Sky," *IEEE Spectrum* (June 2002).
† Mark Twain, letter to Anne Macy, reprinted in *Anne Sullivan Macy: The Story Behind Helen Keller* (Garden City, NY: Doubleday, Doran, and Co., 1933), 162. Twain was also a friend of both Edison and Tesla.
‡ For more information on Freeman Dyson, see "Freeman J. Dyson," IAS School of Natural Sciences, http://www.sns.ias.edu/~dyson.

3. Matt Hermes, "Silicones," Kennesaw State University Department of Mathematics, ChemCases.com, http://www.chemcases.com /silicon/sil4cone.htm. Edison's bulbs were produced by the Corning Glass Company, pioneers in glass technology, including the glass/phenolic insulation originally used for high-temperature insulation for electric trains. It was the research into high-temperature insulators that led to the synthesis of silicone, a polymer of silicon and carbon, by a young Harvard-trained chemist, Dr. James Franklin Hyde, working for Corning, and the successful development of the methyl silicone polymer by Eugene Rochow in a joint venture between General Electric and Corning. The synthesis of silicates into silicone rubber was a fiendishly difficult chemical engineering problem that eluded the best efforts of chemists for more than 70 years. Silicone found its way into demanding wartime applications, such as high-temperature seals for superchargers in the B-29, and in one of the most famous (or infamous) medical devices of all time, the silicone breast implant, litigation over which eventually forced the bankruptcy of the Dow-Corning Corporation.
4. "The whole concept that you do this for the money is absolutely flawed. If you do it for the patients and it works out really well for the patients, you'll make a ton of money. But if you do it for the money and you figure you've got something and it becomes a scam, then it is really going to be a frighteningly long road. It absolutely does not work." John Simpson, "John Simpson: Reluctant Entrepreneur," interview by David Cassack, *In Vivo* (April 2003). Available at: http://www.denovovc.com/press/denovo-simpson.pdf (accessed August 13, 2012).

29 How to Fail as an Entrepreneur

Theodore R. Kucklick

CONTENTS

Technology-Driven Product 449
Market Too Small 450
"I Just Need a Small Piece of a Big Market" 450
Phantom Markets 451
Sector Inexperience 451
No Reimbursement 451
Regulatory Purgatory 452
Patent Mine Fields 452
Raising Too Little Money 452
Raising Too Much Money 452
Insufficient Margins 453
Lack of Urgency 454
Wrong People Involved 454
Team First, Technology Second 454
Not Shooting the Engineer Soon Enough 455
Innovation as a Panacea 455
Ethical Shortcuts 456
Resources 456
    References: University Biodesign Programs 456
    Vendors: Medical Device Entrepreneurial Services 457

There are any number of "how-to" guides on how to succeed as an entrepreneur. If you are reading this book, and this chapter, you likely are an entrepreneur and would like to be a successful one.

Typically, any successful venture follows a path that in hindsight seemed the only reasonable path to success. This path, however, was likely not known when the journey started. The journey forward was likely similar to a drive down a foggy winding road, at night, with only dim headlights. There were any number of ways to go off the road, but only one way that eventually led to the destination.

The purpose of this chapter is to compile a number of ways a medical device entrepreneurial enterprise can go off the road. A common aphorism states: "walking is falling forward and catching yourself before you fall." There is a well-known maxim known as the "Anna Karenina Principle," that is, there are many ways to fail, few to succeed, and if you eliminate the greatest risks for failure, hopefully, the principles for success remain.*

Happy families are all alike; every unhappy family is unhappy in its own way.

—**Leo Tolstoy,**
Anna Karenina

During World War II, the British would examine battle-damaged bombers that managed to return from raids. They would examine where the bullet holes and flak damage was and then would look for ways to armor the sections of the plane *without* bullet holes. The theory was that if the plane returned *with* a hole, it was assumed that damage was survivable. If it got a hole elsewhere, *that* is what brought down the planes that did not return. This was a clever way to discover and reduce the risks of failing to return from a mission.

This restates the mentioned principle that there are many ways to fail and few to succeed. The goal is to be in the "happy family" of successful entrepreneurs. This principle was also succinctly stated thousands of years before in the Gospel of Matthew:

> Enter ye in at the strait gate: for wide is the gate, and broad is the way, that leadeth to destruction, and many there be which go in thereat: Because strait is the gate, and narrow is the way, which leadeth unto life, and few there be that find it.†

Again, there are many ways to fail, and relatively fewer to succeed.

Some of the principles of success are few and deceptively simple: purpose, focus, persistence, planning, and a bit of providence. Myers and Hurley stated, "The three pillars of bioentrepreneurship are scientific and managerial talent, technology and money."‡ Others have stated this as the various Ps of entrepreneurship: passion, persuasiveness, persistence, priorities, and "pain threshold." This chapter discuses some of the "broad ways" that can lead to entrepreneurial failure. The idea is to identify these potential problems and address them *before* you sink years of your life into the venture and a bunch of money into patents and product development. As found in Proverbs,

> A prudent man foreseeth the evil, and hideth himself: but the simple pass on, and are punished.§

Following is a list of things that I have personally seen lead to entrepreneurial failure in the medical device space. It is hardly exhaustive, but they are distressingly common.

---

* Mentioned in Jared Diamond, *Guns, Germs, and Steel: The Fates of Human Societies* (New York: W. W. Norton & Co., 1999).
† Matthew 7:13–14.
‡ Arlen D. Meyers and Patrick Hurley, "Bioentrepreneurship Education Programmes in the United States," *Journal of Commercial Biotechnology* 14 (2008): 2–12, doi:10.1057/palgrave.jcb.3050078.
§ Proverbs 22:3.

TECHNOLOGY-DRIVEN PRODUCT

In medical device entrepreneurship, one of the most tempting traps to fall into is the "technology-driven product." This is a device that does not address a clear clinical need, or address a clear market, but it has really cool technology. This is the proverbial "solution in search of a problem" or the "science project." These can be the product of grant-based academic research, or the discovery of a company founder. Here the discoverer falls in love with the technology, and all of the time, money and effort are directed to the perfection of the technology. It is believed that the usefulness of the technology will somehow magically become self-evident and that the world will stand in awe of the brilliance of this discovery and beat a path to the door of the company, for this better mousetrap, with dollars in hand. This is the "if you build it, they will come" approach from the movie *Field of Dreams*. Or by having a better mousetrap, you are hoping that the world will beat a path to your door. "Hope" is a prayer, not a plan. There is nothing wrong with hope and prayer, if they are combined with planning, preparation, and crisp execution.

Sometimes the world does beat a path to your door (if you are lucky). More often it is possible to spot the pioneers by the number of arrows in their back.

Symphonix Devices (NASDAQ: SMPX) was a Silicon Valley medical device start-up founded in 1994 to perfect a high-fidelity implantable hearing aid. Virtually all of the funding went to research and development (R&D). Between VCs (including some top-tier firms) and the public market, SMPX raised more than $350 million, and it never produced a marketable product. The technology and IP was eventually sold off in 2003 for $2.5 million. This illustrates the hazard of the technology-driven product.

Pure research projects are perfectly fine if you are doing university or corporate research, and you do not need to immediately build a company that will return a profit. These can even be great licensing deals. If you are taking in investment money that is expected to generate a return on the basis of revenues, these "science projects" are very seductive, but they are best avoided until a clear, compelling marketable need for the technology is identified, and a clear execution path.

Sometimes this can take years. Corning Glass discovered a strong, scratch-resistant glass called "Chemcor" in 1961. For years, this material was intriguing, but it had no market. In 2008, 47 years later, a marketable use for this material was finally identified, and it is now widely used on more than 225 models of mobile phones and liquid crystal displays (LCDs) under the name Gorilla® Glass. Chemcor was a technological breakthrough, only about 40 years ahead of its time. Corning had the good "luck" of patience, remembering what they worked on, and having been in business for 150 years, they knew how to execute when the opportunity came along. It was an example of "success is where preparation meets opportunity."

Josh Makower, MD, has made a science of identifying clinical needs, and is the cochair of the Stanford Biodesign program, and venture partner at New Enterprise Associates. He also suffered from chronic sinusitis. When at an appointment for his sinus problems, he noticed in a magnetic resonance imaging (MRI) image that the convolutions in the sinuses resembled coronary arteries. He began to speculate if sinus blockages could be gently squeezed open with balloons like blood vessels instead of the blockages being resected with rongeurs. The result of this was applying well-know balloon angioplasty techniques and technology in a new indication—ear, nose, and throat (ENT). This focus on clinical need rather than technology has made Acclarent, the company he founded with partner John Chang to make these sinus-clearing balloons, a major medical device success story, acquired by Johnson & Johnson for $785 million.

MARKET TOO SMALL

A basic blunder is attempting to address a market that is too small. Because it often takes as much time and effort to address a large market as a small market, think big and go for the biggest market you can. An entrepreneurial start-up is likely to consume five to eight years of your working life, if not more. Make sure you get into a project with a market size and a payoff that are worth it. Small markets can still be a viable enterprise. You can make this work by having enough niche products to add up to a decent market, and by iterating and commercializing quickly and inexpensively. It typically takes a product with a price tag of more than $300 to get an independent medical device sales rep to focus on it and to get the interest of a corporate acquirer.

Arthrex (Naples, FL) is an example of a company that is in a niche market (arthroscopy and sports medicine) in which many of their products sell for less than $100. Arthrex has a catalog of literally thousands of these products, close relationships with surgeons in the specialty, and an exceptional sales force, tightly focused on the orthopedic sports medicine market. Arthrex booked about $800 million in sales in 2010. You can make a business out of small products; however, this is the kind of effort and marketing execution it takes.

There is nothing wrong with making a meal out of a bucket of chicken wings versus one steak. Just do not try to make a meal out of one chicken wing. It is tempting to go after a small market as it seems there is less competition and fewer barriers to entry, but if you do not scale up after getting your handhold, you may wind up with a business that is too small to generate the revenues to pay its own way, and too small to be of interest to a potential investor or acquirer. Venture capital investors typically will not fund a company in a market less than $1 billion in size. Angel investors usually will not fund an opportunity under $200 million. There has to be enough of a market to scale the opportunity into a real business.

"I JUST NEED A SMALL PIECE OF A BIG MARKET"

This is a tempting fallacy—tempting, oft repeated, but unlikely to succeed. Hospitals are reducing their number of suppliers. They are trying to keep market bit players like you out. Hospital chains like Kaiser Permanente explicitly have put out the "unwelcome mat" for new sales reps and products trying to gain a foothold in their system. You have to have enough critical mass, a compelling enough product, or a distribution partner to get into their purchasing system. This is unlikely to happen when all you want to be is just a "small piece of a big market." Big companies can afford to have small products because they already have the marketing channel in place. You cannot. Also, hospital purchasing organizations are trying to standardize, and keep small vendors out. If you are a potential investor, and this assertion is made in the presentation, you might want to be just a bit skeptical.

PHANTOM MARKETS

It is possible to do "top-down" estimates, twiddle with spreadsheets and clearly identify markets that do not really exist. Back-check your numbers. Make sure that your assumptions of capturing a percentage of a statistically available market does not include selling your product to more doctors than actually exist in that specialty. Do your homework and get current data on the market you plan to enter. Run your numbers top-down (i.e., percentage of a market segment, or overall number of procedures) as well as bottom-up (i.e., how many cases per week a typical surgeon is likely to do in which your product will be used, and how many of these procedures you are likely to capture), and see whether the two agree. Ensure that your total available market (TAM) is also a plausible TAM. Know specifically how you are going to get your product into the hands of these customers, who is going to get them there, how they will be adopted, and how you plan to make these products stick. Know going in what type of a sales force will be needed to accomplish this goal and how much it will cost to develop this marketing channel. Have someone on your team with the sector experience to carry out your plan. Know what a "sales funnel"* is, and have one in place. At some point, you will be selling real products to real customers, not to statistical abstractions.

SECTOR INEXPERIENCE

If you are getting into a medical device market with which you are not familiar, find someone with real sector expertise to give you guidance. This would be someone who knows the chief competitors, their technology, the available distribution channels, the sales cycle, and the available distribution partners. Do you know whether most devices in your market are purchased by hospital buyers under contract? Are devices sold by manufacturer's representatives or agents that are hired directly, are they stocking distributors, or are they independent agents carrying other lines? What are the typical commission levels paid to distributors and agents? How long is the typical sales cycle? Is your product typically bundled and sold with other products that you do not offer? If you do not know the answers to these questions, find them out before you spend money developing your product, or you could be in for an expensive education.

NO REIMBURSEMENT

Some medical device products can be sold without reimbursement. These tend to be consumables and Class I and II exempt products. It is possible to make a business in these product categories, if you understand the economics that tend to be at high volumes and lower margins, or if you can sell into a specific niche in which you can offer exceptional value and have deep expertise. For a therapeutic 510(k) device and especially a premarket approval (PMA) product at higher price point, reimbursement becomes critical. A premium-priced therapeutic device without reimbursement is very unlikely to sell, with the possible exception of patient-pay aesthetic procedures.

---

* Information on the sales funnel is readily available online. For one tutorial, see "The Sales Funnel: Keeping Control of Your Sales Pipeline," Mind Tools, http://www.mindtools.com/pages/article/newLDR_94.htm (accessed August 13, 2012).

It is an unfortunate fact that "what people want, they pay for, and what they need, they expect others to pay for." Study the reimbursement landscape and know what a reimbursement path will require *before* you sink a lot of money into product development.

REGULATORY PURGATORY

Some devices are relatively easy to get approval and clearance for. Others are not. The newer the technology or the more expansive the therapeutic claims, the more difficult and expensive getting Food and Drug Administration (FDA) approval will be. Know what you are getting yourself into before you start.

PATENT MINE FIELDS

Now that you have found a large, attractive market, and have an idea for a technology, there is one more important thing to find out: Did someone beat you to it, and did they patent their technology? The typical layperson that knows about patents and invention typically does not know what a patent really is. It is *not* the right for you to make the invention. It is the right to keep others from making and selling what is claimed in the patent, but it is not necessarily the right for *you* to practice the invention yourself. Others may hold blocking patents that prevent you from making your invention. Knowing if you have "freedom to operate" before you start is a prerequisite to obtaining funding from a knowledgeable or credible investor. This is especially important in crowded therapeutic fields (e.g., cardiology). Also, be sure you have enough money in the war chest to see a patent all the way through from filing in your home country (e.g., the United States) to Patent Cooperation Treaty (PCT) though "National Stage." This subject is handled in detail in Chapter 14, "Intellectual Property Strategy for Med-Tech Start-Ups."

RAISING TOO LITTLE MONEY

One of my favorite quotes is from David Lloyd George, the British prime minister, during World War I: "Take a big step when one is indicated: You can't cross a chasm in two small jumps."[*]

Some things cost as much money as they do, and all of the bootstrapping in the world is not going to close the gap. A variation on this is the "man-year myth" that states: One woman can have a baby in nine months. But you can't get nine women to have a baby in one month. Some things just take as long as they take, and the timeline can only be compressed so far. Tom Fogarty likens this to being a "percolator" rather than an "incubator." The idea of an incubator is that a predictable result happens in a predictable time from known inputs. Innovation rarely happens this way.

RAISING TOO MUCH MONEY

It is rarely possible in med-tech to raise too much money (but you can sell too much of your company and cede too much control). Having too much money (or the illusion of too much money), however, allows you to do the wrong things too easily, for too long. Jim Collins has described this in his book *Good to Great*. Whether you have

---

[*] http://www.brainyquote.com/quotes/authors/d/david_lloyd_george.html (accessed 8/13/2012).

a lot or a little, there is never enough to waste. When dealing with capital, spend money only when it will make more money, or achieve a meaningful milestone, or do not spend it. An anecdote told to me by Joel Pratt, former president of Arthrotek (now Biomet Sports Medicine) illustrates this principle. Dane Miller, chief executive officer (CEO) of Biomet in the early years of the company, was asked by his employees to pave their unsightly gravel parking lot at their headquarters in Warsaw, IN. After bids were obtained the job, Dane held a meeting. He agreed with the employees that a paved parking lot would be nice to have. The same amount of money, however, could also buy a piece of production machinery that Biomet needed. He asked the question: "We can take this money, buy asphalt, and pour it on the ground, or buy a new machine to produce more product that makes all of us money" Needless to say, the new machine was purchased and eventually the lot was paved with the business profits.

The "multiple principle" works in reverse, as well as forward. This is the idea that an investment dollar spent to build value today will yield a multiple in a successful exit. A dollar wasted today, however, destroys a multiple of its value in future returns. This destroyed value manifests itself in down-rounds, reverse stock splits, or the outright failure of the business.

Do not do a job inside that can be done cheaper and possibly better outside, even if you have the money. Do not buy a piece of equipment that does not pay its own way, *after* you have factored in the cost of ownership and the cost of an employee to run it. Do not spend money on non-value-add items like new furniture or class A office space when it is not needed. Fixed expenses are the great enemy in the long run. Given enough time, these expenses can sink even a well-funded start-up.

Beware small expenses. A small leak will sink a great ship.

—Benjamin Franklin

INSUFFICIENT MARGINS

Small volumes require high margins. Low margins require high volumes. No margins or no volume equals no viable business. If you have a product that you expect to be acquired by another company, you will need to be making or be able to make at least 70% gross margin. Here is a simple chart based on a $1.00 cost of goods:

Selling Price	$2	$3	$4	$5	$6	$7
Gross (profit) Margin	50%	60%	75%	80%	83%	85%

For a medical device, you need to be operating in the 60–80% gross margin range to have a viable business. Without these margins, the cost of selling (20–45% commissions and discounts, promotion) while still covering your overhead becomes prohibitive. If you have a product with a small price tag, ensure that there is enough volume to support a business, or if there is a smaller number of potential customers, ensure that the product has a high enough price tag to support a business. If you are contemplating going into a business, or are being presented with an opportunity, this is a quick way to screen what you should and should not be considering. Remember, in the long run, technology is a means to an end. The goal is to build a sustainable business.

LACK OF URGENCY

When running a venture-funded start-up, time is literally money. Think about a start-up with a $200,000 per month burn rate. Divide this into 5.5 working days per week. That is $50,000 per calendar week, and $9,090 per working day. A company like this must have people who know how to get things done. Like the old saying: "Lose an hour, lose a day, lose a day, lose a week" and so on. You burn up money 24 hours a day, seven days a week just standing around thinking about it. Venture money is the most expensive money you will ever have, and the surest way to burn through it is with needless delay and sloppy execution. The penalties for this are down-rounds, layoffs, downsizings, reverse splits, or no follow-on funding rounds and hitting the end of the entrepreneurial road. Take action and ensure that everyone in your organization has a bias toward action.

WRONG PEOPLE INVOLVED

You can have a number of the wrong people involved in a company. One is an "incumbent" or someone who has just "always been there." This person may be a member of the founding team. Sometimes these incumbents give off the message that they will make getting rid of them more painful than keeping them. Do not put up with people that threaten tantrums. Ask yourself, if this person was not already involved, would you bring them into the company now? If the answer is no, then you might think twice about keeping them on. Another wrong person to have involved is an investor, especially as a board member, who does not have the sector experience or who has unrealistic expectations. Educate this person on realistic expectations and help them get up to speed on the business. If, however, you cannot get your interests and expectations and the investor's aligned, you may be headed for trouble. In a corporation, the CEO, even if he or she is a founder of the company, is hired by the board and can be fired by the board. Choose your boss carefully.

Every person in a start-up is critically important. As Jim Collins writes in *Good to Great* you have to "get the right people on the bus and the wrong people off the bus."[*] You are not doing a favor to an employee who cannot advance with the company by keeping them in place. Help them find a situation in which they can succeed and be sure you have the right people for the work the company needs done.

> Executives owe it to the organization and to their fellow workers not to tolerate nonperforming individuals in important jobs.
>
> —**Peter F. Drucker**

TEAM FIRST, TECHNOLOGY SECOND

A good team can navigate their way around a technology roadblock. The wrong team can take the best technology and blow the opportunity with bad execution. The best

---

[*] Collins, James C. *Good to Great: Why Some Companies Make the Leap–and Others Don't*. New York, NY: HarperBusiness, 2001, p. 57.

situation is to have both a compelling technology *and* a sharp team. Ensure that you have "A" players in key roles. Two "B" players do not add up to one "A" player. This is especially critical because the technology and clinical indication you start with at the beginning may not be the one you find success with in the end.

NOT SHOOTING THE ENGINEER SOON ENOUGH

Entrepreneurs are often great starters, but sometimes they are not good at finishing what they start. They always like to do new things and like to live in the fun "fuzzy frontend" of innovation. Engineers and designers love to tinker and iterate. There comes a time, however, when you have to take what you have to market, and if it is successful, start scaling it up and squeezing out the costs. This is the part that entrepreneurs, engineers, and designers often do not like. They want to keep on iterating forever. If you let this happen, the product design will never get frozen, and the company will never have a stable product that earns any money. There comes a time when you have to "shoot the engineer" and stop iterating and run with what you have (provided the product is safe and effective). It takes exceptionally good judgment to know when the product is "good enough" and when to stop adding features that do not add additional incremental value.

INNOVATION AS A PANACEA

Everyone loves innovation. Innovation is great and is the lifeblood of business growth. Innovation is not, however, a substitute for a properly run business. It takes both innovation and a well-run business to have a sustainable advantage. Papering over sloppy practices with "innovation" is just another way of saying you are trying to out-earn stupidity.

A variation on this is the "panacea" technology that is good for everything. Pick one thing the technology does exceptionally well, that meets an important need, and that is within your capability to execute on and focus relentlessly on doing that. Think of a start-up as hunting geese with a double-barrel shotgun. You cannot afford to "wing" the goose and have it fly away, leaving you to starve. Pick the biggest goose in the flock that is within range and shoot it twice.

A classic example of this is Arthrocare (ARTC), the subject of a Harvard Business School case study.[*] Hira Thapliyal and Phil Eggers discovered a unique bipolar radiofrequency modality that generated a cutting and coagulating plasma in saline (Coblation®). At first, this was applied to removing arterial plaque, for which it was found to be unsuitable.[†] Many other uses were envisioned, but the investors informed the founders that although these many indications were interesting, there was only enough capital to execute on one. When it was found that Coblation was especially effective in arthroscopic bursectomies, Arthrocare was formed to pursue this specific orthopedic opportunity, and it continues to do so successfully.

---

[*] Michael J. Roberts, "ArthroCare," *Harvard Business Review* (December 1, 1997), http://hbr.org/product/arthrocare/an/898056-PDF-ENG.

[†] To hear Mr. Thapliyal tell this story, see David Cassack, "Stanford Innovator's Workbench interview with David Cassack," Stanford Biodesign, http://biodesign.stanford.edu/bdn /networking/pastinnovators .jsp#season9.

ETHICAL SHORTCUTS

Skimp on the granola bars in the breakroom. Locate in a class B rental. Skimp on hotels. Fly coach on business trips, but ensure that you are always flying first class when it comes to ethics. This is especially important when it comes to relationships with your surgeon advisors. In the old days, some companies would sign up an influential KOL (key opinion leader) and would expect that advisor to steer business to your company in exchange for a lucrative contract and little real work.[*] Those days are long gone. Giving an advisor a sinecure in exchange for their influence will get you in trouble, either in the short run or in the long run when you are acquired and compliance issues surface during due diligence. Bring in KOLs as advisors but ensure that they are doing real work for fair compensation free of conflict of interest.

I once heard John Abele, founder of Boston Scientific, at the 2006 SMIT [Society for Medical Intervention and Technology] conference in Asilomar, CA, describe *The Simpsons'* Rule and the *60 Minutes* Rule. The *60 Minutes* Rule is this: Don't do anything or say anything that you would not be willing to defend to a hostile reporter from the investigative news show *60 Minutes*. *The Simpsons'* Rule is this: If what you are doing begins to look absurd, as if it could be a skit on the cartoon show *The Simpsons*, it is probably a bad idea and something you should not be doing. Personally I use the Mom Rule, which is this: Never work on or develop a device that you would not be willing to see used on your mother, someone you deeply care about, or yourself.

Remember that electronic data once posted on the Internet never dies, and there is no presumption of privacy. Just ask Tiger Woods. Think twice about committing intemperate comments to e-mail or on social media like Twitter, Facebook, LinkedIn, and the like. Assume that whatever you write or post can appear on the front page of a newspaper or will surface at a deposition.

These are just a few ways to fail as an entrepreneur. There are other ways as well, and some of these likely came to mind as you read this chapter. For more information on how the process of starting and growing an entrepreneurial med-tech business, see Chapter 25, "Keys to Creating Value for Early Stage Medical Device Companies," by Rich Ferrari, in this book.

Fortunately, there are many places to go for good advice. Connect with the angel investor groups in your area. Attend industry conferences, watch and observe investment pitches at meetings like IN3 and OneMedForum, and learn all you can. Because the business and legal environment are always changing, the entrepreneur needs to be always learning.

RESOURCES

REFERENCES: UNIVERSITY BIODESIGN PROGRAMS

Arizona State University Biodesign
http://www.biodesign.asu.edu/about

---

[*] Canon Communications, LLC, "Orthopedics Firms under New Scrutiny from Justice Department," *MD+DI Online* (July 2006), http://www.mddionline.com/article/orthopedics-firms-under-new-scrutiny-justice-department.

"The Biodesign Institute at Arizona State University spurs scientific breakthroughs that improve health, protect lives, and sustain our planet. Our research is aimed at:

- Predicting, preventing, and detecting the onset of disease
- Developing renewable energy and reducing environmental damage
- Developing innovations that safeguard our nation and the world."

Stanford Biodesign
http://innovation.stanford.edu/bdn/index.jsp
http://biodesign.stanford.edu/bdn/india
http://biodesign.stanford.edu/bdn/singapore
"Our mission is to train students, fellows and faculty in the Biodesign Process: a systematic approach to needs finding and the invention and implementation of new biomedical technologies."

Yale University Biodesign
http://dailybulletin.yale.edu/article.aspx?id = 8164

Vendors: Medical Device Entrepreneurial Services

Canaccord Genuity Conferences
http://www.canaccordgenuity.com/EN/about/Pages/Events.aspx
Canaccord Genuity is the global capital markets division of Canaccord Financial Inc., offering institutional and corporate clients idea-driven investment banking, research, and sales and trading services from 16 offices worldwide, and offering musculoskeletal and diabetes and obesity analysts conferences organized by William Plovanic.

The Kauffman Foundation
http://www.kauffman.org
http://www.entrepreneurship.org
The Ewing Marion Kauffman Foundation was established in the mid-1960s by the late entrepreneur and philanthropist Ewing Marion Kauffman and carries out its mission through four programmatic areas: entrepreneurship, advancing innovation, education, and research and policy.

Keiretsu Forum Entrepreneur Academy
http://www.keiretsuforum.com
"The Keiretsu Forum Entrepreneur Academy was designed by the members of our Keiretsu Forum community to provide course offerings taught by seasoned industry executives in the critical elements of start-up companies' business plan."

Medtech Insight
http://www.medtechinsight.com/conferences.html
IN3 events bring together med-tech innovators at every stage of project development, with leaders in investment, venture capital, and business development. IN3

is also a forum for presenting start-up medical device opportunities to prospective investors and corporate partners.

National Venture Capital Association
http://www.nvca.org
The National Venture Capital Association (NVCA), composed of more than 400 member firms, is the premier trade association representing the U.S. venture capital industry. The association's mission is to foster greater understanding of the importance of venture capital to the U.S. economy and to support entrepreneurial activity and innovation.

The NCVA website is an invaluable source of model legal documents, including term sheets, stock purchase agreements, and more. These documents represent the accumulated experience from literally thousands of venture-financed deals and can save you substantial amounts of time and money. The site also includes many other useful links and resources.

OneMedForum and OneMedPlace
http://www.onemedplace.com/forum
OneMedPlace is a gathering of the people leading fast-growing and emerging health care and life science companies in Europe and North America.

Palgrave Journals
http://www.palgrave-journals.com/jcb/journal/v14/n1/fig_tab/3050078t1.html
Arlen D. Meyers and Patrick Hurley compile and publish a list of bioentrepreneurship education programs in the United States.[*]

VC Taskforce
http://www.vctaskforce.com
VC Taskforce has built an organization to which the venture community can give input and direction and from which they get immediate results that benefit both investors and their portfolio companies. VC Taskforce sponsors a number of seminars, panels, and roundtables for entrepreneurs. Their website includes links to numerous resources, VCs, and angel investment groups.

Wilson Sonsini Goodrich & Rosati (WSGR) Medical Device Conference
www.wsgr.com/news/medicaldevice
This conference focuses on understanding how the changing economic climate is affecting the early stage and emerging-growth medical device industry and the venture capital funds that sustain it. In a series of topical panels, presented over the course of one day, industry CEOs, venture capitalists, industry strategists, investment bankers, and market analysts all present information. (See Chapter 24 of this book for an interview with J. Casey McGlynn, chair of the WSGR Life Science practice and organizer of the conference.)

---

[*] Arlen D. Meyers and Patrick Hurley, "Bioentrepreneurship Education Programmes in the United States," *Journal of Commercial Biotechnology* 14 (2008): 2–12, doi:10.1057/palgrave.jcb.3050078.

30 Raising Money for Your Medical Device Start-Up

Theodore R. Kucklick

CONTENTS

Bootstrapping and Resourcefulness 459
Revenues, the Next Best Financing 460
What Is the Anticipated Exit? 460
What Are Investors Looking For? 460
Valuation 461
Rules of Thumb for Funding Rounds 461
Financing Terms 461
How Picky Are Investors? 462
Types of Financing 463
    4F Financing 463
    Government Grants 464
    Angel Financing 464
    Venture Capital 464
    Venture Debt 464
    Bank Financing 465
    Private Equity 465
    Strategic Investment 465
Conclusion 465

So, you have a great idea, now what? Ideas by themselves are worthless. Executing on the idea will take capital. How do you go about getting this?

BOOTSTRAPPING AND RESOURCEFULNESS

Tina Seelig, professor of entrepreneurship at Stanford, wrote a book *What I Wish I Knew When I Was 20*. In the book, she describes an exercise she gives to her students. Student teams are given $5.00 and two hours to generate the best returns they can, given the time and resources. Some of the students get the best results not even spending the $5. The point is that ingenuity and creativity can be worth more than money. Bootstrapping and resourcefulness are always the first and best steps in fundraising.

When you are starting out, look for all of the low-cost no-cost resources you can. Ask for help. Call in favors. Help others with their entrepreneurial projects. Get help from local universities and incubators. Bunk in at other companies' extra space. Look for equipment and furniture at sales and auctions. Thomas Edison once said, "The scope of thrift is limitless." Fixed expenses are the enemy. Bootstrapping—working out of a garage or basement and looking for every possible way to get results without spending money—is the first and most important skill an entrepreneur can have, and a skill to keep using even and especially after you get funding.

REVENUES, THE NEXT BEST FINANCING

It is amazing to me how many start-ups never really intend to make money. The idea is to spin up an idea, get to proof of concept or symbolic sales, and sell to a strategic buyer. If this does not happen before you run out of money, however, you are done. I believe revenues have been the world's favorite source of nondilutive financing for more than 6000 years. When you start a business, build into the plan revenues that will at least cover your basic expenses. This will give you time, and as Rich Ferrari, of DeNovo Ventures, veteran medical device venture capital (VC) investor has said, "If you have time, you have everything."

WHAT IS THE ANTICIPATED EXIT?

There are many different types of structures and exit opportunities for an entrepreneurial business. The most common in the 21st century is a sale of the business to a strategic buyer. It is important that the business structure and goals are aligned with the investor's goals and expectations. For example, an opportunity that is looking for liquidity with an income stream from a licensing deal is a very different investment than a potential IPO (initial public stock offering) or sale to a strategic buyer. Similarly, a business that generates nice cash flow but that will not scale up into a large company (a so-called lifestyle business) may attract the rare angel investor if structured as a loan paying with an abovemarket interest rate. This deal, however, will be of no interest to the typical venture investor. Another type of opportunity that likely will generate no interest is a "science project." Investors are looking for a business that will scale up and into which they can put a substantial amount of money to work. They also are looking for returns of three to five times their investment in three to five years or better. An investor occasionally may be willing to consider a lower return, but this will be in exchange for a shorter investment term and less risk. A deal that can return tenfold in a reasonable amount of time is attractive to anyone.

WHAT ARE INVESTORS LOOKING FOR?

What is an investor looking for? Simply put, the best risk-adjusted returns they can get for their money. They want to put money to work. They want the best technology opportunity and the best team to execute on it that they can get at the most attractive valuation. They are looking for a good horse (technology) and a good jockey (team) to ride into the winner's circle, at a valuation that allows them to make good money. It is not just a good technology *or* a good team, it is a good technology *and* a good team. In short, what investors are looking for is a good investment.

VALUATION

Two key questions you need to be able to answer when fundraising are: What is the valuation of your company? and What percentage of it are you willing to sell? Without a clear, defensible answer to these questions, it is impossible to have an intelligent conversation with a potential investor (yet I have seen entrepreneurs try!). Valuation is critical. Too low, you sell too much of your company and give up too much control. Too high, and you set up unrealistic expectations for the next round of financing or exit, or the potential investor just walks away because they cannot see a way to get a sufficient step-up in value at exit to make the deal worth their while, or worse, they simply do not find you credible. The other issue to consider is dilution. The more of the company is sold, the less of a percentage stake the current owners will have. Dilution is unavoidable if you are raising money. You want to ensure that raising the money will take you to a place where your smaller percentage stake is worth more than before.

Steve Kam, of Cogent Valuations, in San Francisco, suggests the following three valuation questions to which every entrepreneur needs to have quick, clear, snappy answers:

1. What is the expected time and method of anticipated liquidity for investors, complete with underlying assumptions that support projected revenues, earnings, and cash flow?
2. What are your examples of comparable transactions, for the multiple of revenue, EBITDA (pretax earnings), or cash flow used to value the company for the current financing round?
3. What will be the use of the proceeds from the current financing and what will be produced in terms of operations, growth, revenues, and cash flow?

RULES OF THUMB FOR FUNDING ROUNDS

Early stage, prerevenue companies are typically valued at less than $5 million. It is very difficult to price them higher than this and still make a case for decent risk-adjusted returns. Because the average medical device company now takes 8 to 10 years to exit, you want to have a model that shows at least a better than a 10% annual compounded return for the investment to be competitive with other investments that offer these returns and do not have the illiquidity and risk imposed by a venture equity investment. Later valuations are usually based on the net present value (NPV) on the basis of a 5-year discounted cash flow analysis (DVFA), typically using a 30% discount rate. Revenues are typically valued at three to five times this amount, but you need to support this with comparables in your specific market sector.

FINANCING TERMS

Money always comes with conditions. Some of these are antidilution terms, liquidation preferences, participating preferred stock, board membership rights, cumulative dividends, option pools, and others. A detailed discussion of these conditions is beyond the scope of this book; however, you can find more information on these at http://

www.venturebeat.com, and the National Venture Capital Association (NVCA; http://www.nvca.org). Even if you get a valuation that you find acceptable, onerous terms can give you serious headaches down the road. If you get to the stage of getting a term sheet from an investor, you must have people on your team who have negotiated a venture financing before to avoid potential pitfalls. (For information on term sheet provisions, see Brad Feld's blog at http://www.feld.com/wp/archives/2008/06/revisiting-the-term-sheet.html.)

Allan May, founder and chairman of Life Science Angels and chairman of the Kauffman Angel Resource Institute points out that it is critically important to get the financing terms and capital structure correct even at the F + F (Friends and Family) and seed stage, because once the structure is set, it may be painful or impossible to change it later, and getting it wrong can damage the viability of the company or the ability to attract follow-on investment.

HOW PICKY ARE INVESTORS?

The process of raising venture funding can seem daunting. Be prepared to do a *lot* of networking and presentations.

Intel Capital, the VC arm of Intel Corporation, looks at hundreds of potential technology deals per year and will meet with about 100 start-ups. These meetings will be the result of a referral, never from a cold call. Out of 100 opportunities they take the time to meet with, perhaps three will get funded, and all of these will have been told "no" at least once.

Dr. Mark Riley and Karen Talmadge, two of the founders of Kyphon, sold their company to Medtronic in 2007 for $3.9 billion, a very successful exit in anybody's book. In the early days, Dr. Riley and Talmadge were turned down by about every VC there was to turn them down. They all thought introducing the new therapeutic modality of Kyphoplasty to the spine was too risky, and no one had ever used balloons to displace bone. It took exceptional patience and persistence to get the original funding for the company.

The moral of the story is that fundraising for a medical device start-up is a lot of hard work, and you likely will encounter a lot of rejection. For some start-up chief executive officers (CEO), fundraising is their main job. You have to be able to connect with the right investors, tell a compelling story, show how the investors will make money, *and* be able to close the deal. Networking is crucial. No investor I can think of will seriously consider a business plan on a cold call. Getting an introduction is essential.

Using "brokers" that promise to raise money for you can be a problem. Unless someone is registered with the Securities and Exchange Commission (SEC) as a securities broker, this can be legally problematic. Also, investors want to hear the pitch from the CEO. Pitches from a "broker" lose credibility.

When presenting, remember this: The purpose of a meeting is to get the "next meeting" and eventually getting to the one at which you get a term sheet and close the deal. If you have 20 slides, and after 10 slides, a potential investor says, "This looks interesting. Can I have my partners look at this?" Stop presenting, close your laptop, and schedule the next meeting. Do not keep presenting. All you can do from that point on is blow your opportunity.

Right now, the life science financing environment is very tough. A *Wall Street Journal* article from October 6, 2011, "VCs Take Their Case for FDA Reform to Capitol Hill" reports the following:

- 36% of life sciences investors plan to increase investments in European start-ups, while 44% expect to steer more money to Asian companies.
- More than 40% said they would decrease investments in pharmaceutical and device companies, while about half said they would increase investments in information technology and health care services.
- 61% of respondents said regulatory challenges were the top reason they were shying away from life sciences.

These challenges in part are due to the difficulties in getting new therapeutic devices approved in the United States, and also the chilling effect of the impending medical device tax and comparative-effectiveness mandates. Getting funding for life science start-ups is not impossible, but it is clearly more difficult than in years past, especially for PMA (FDA Class III premarket approval) and IND (new drug applications).

The small cap IPOs once common in the 1990s are a thing of the past, with the passage of the Sarbanes-Oxley Act. The difficulty of VCs to get exits has materially inhibited their ability to fund new, early stage deals. It is all the more important to have a compelling value story, and a clear and achievable regulatory and reimbursement strategy. Allan May wrote about the challenges of funding a device start-up with a new technology in a September, 2011, *Atlantic* article, "Why Silicon Valley Is Running Scared from Health Care."[*]

TYPES OF FINANCING

4F FINANCING

The very first money most start-ups get is called 4F Financing, which stands for "Friends, Family, Founders, and Fools." This financing usually is provided in the form of loans. At this stage, a loan convertible later to stock may be the best vehicle, as setting a valuation at this early stage may not be possible or advisable. If the valuation is overly optimistic, disappointment is sure to follow if a later investor insists on a lower valuation. Many times, these are informal deals; however, investors at this stage should meet the requirements of "accredited investors," that is, greater than $200,000 in annual income and more than $1 million in net worth excluding primary residence. Be cautious when raising money from actual family and friends. Will they still talk to you if you do not hit your milestones and cannot pay the money back? Accepting investment money from Aunt Tillie's retirement fund is probably a really bad idea.

Again, even at this stage, setting up a correct company structure is essential, and it pays to engage advisors who have successfully done this before.

---

[*] http://www.theatlantic.com/business/archive/2011/09/why-silicon-valley-is-running-scared-from-health-care/245534/(accessed 8/13/2012).

Government Grants

These can be a good alternative source of nondilutive financing. In the past, medical device entrepreneurs took a pass on this source, as the process to get these funds can be lengthy. With venture financings taking so much longer, or being less available, grants are looking more attractive. For these, it might help to have an academic researcher or consultant on your team who is adept at grant writing. Some of these are SBIR (Small Business Innovation and Research) grants, and if your technology has an important military application, you may be eligible for Defense Advanced Research Project Agency (DARPA) grants. With the dearth of early stage VC money for medical device start-ups, grant funding is generating a great deal of interest, especially if you have some basic science to prove.

Angel Financing

Angels are now taking up the slack in the smaller financings that the VCs do not seem to fund anymore. Angels typically top out at $500,000, although some angel groups are doing deals up to $1.5 million and are starting to syndicate like VCs. Angels are "accredited investors" (high–net worth individuals) who typically individually invest $25,000 to $50,000 in a deal. It can require some management to "herd the cats" to get an angel deal done involving 10 or 20 investors. It may make sense to have them invest as a group under an LLC. Some angel groups like Life Science Angels invest this way, and having small investors on the cap table in a single entity is more attractive to later investors. Angels are less sensitive to market size than the ability of the investment to generate a decent return. Sometimes angels can be surgeons who are enthusiastic about the technology; however, it is important to steer clear of conflict-of-interest regulations. With an angel financing, the entrepreneur is usually expected to construct and provide the deal term sheet.

Venture Capital

There are "tiers" of VC firms, based on the size of their funds. Smaller "boutique" funds can provide smaller fundings starting around $1 to $3 million. Larger funds look to put $10 to $20 million to work in a round. VCs typically will not consider an opportunity with an available market less than $500 million to $1 billion or more. Typically, a VC-funded company will have a "syndicate" or group of VCs invested, so that there is enough capital available to see the company through to an exit. Also, it is important to approach a VC that actually invests in your sector. It is probably a waste of time to take a medical device deal to a VC that makes their investments in things like real estate or social networking. With a VC financing, the VC will construct and offer the term sheet.

Venture Debt

Venture debt is a short-term loan to a start-up that a bank usually will not make. The reason for taking on venture debt is to bridge a short-term need for cash to get to an important value-creation milestone, and selling equity is not available, or desirable. The

BANK FINANCING

For a more mature company with assets and revenues, bank financing can help with smoothing out cash flow. Some companies will finance things like equipment with bank financing. It is a good thing to have a strong allergy to debt. It can leverage and accelerate things on the way up, but it also can sink you if things head down, especially if you fall out of compliance with your loan covenants, or if interest rates jump. You want to have a business that focuses on servicing your customers, not your debt.

PRIVATE EQUITY

Another source of investment can be private equity (PE). PE funds typically will not invest in start-ups or in companies without meaningful earnings. This is because the PE fund is usually interested in an undervalued company that can be purchased, sometimes with a leveraged buy-out (LBO) using the free cash flow of the company, for a later resale of the company at a higher price after restructuring.

STRATEGIC INVESTMENT

Some companies will invest in a technology that they want to have in their portfolio and do not want to develop in-house. The major company investors are starting to take up some of the slack due to lack of VC money. Success in raising this money comes from having something the company really wants to have in their portfolio and from good relationships. Some companies have venture arms, and it can be valuable to reach out to them.

CONCLUSION

The most important thing to remember in fundraising is to have an opportunity that is a fundamentally good investment that can generate value, and generate a good risk-adjusted return for the investors in a reasonable amount of time. This means having the right technology, the right team to execute on its development, and the ability to create customers and revenues, scale the company, and grow value. It is important to know the valuation for your company and the percentage equity you are willing to sell.

Different types of investors have different strategies for generating their returns, different areas in which they invest, and different dollar levels at which they invest. Networking and getting an introduction is critical. It is very important that your opportunity and business model are in alignment with your prospective investor and essential to set up a correct company structure that will not inhibit the prospects of the company in the future.

Grants for development work, such as SBIR grants, are becoming an increasingly popular source of seed money for start-ups and are worth pursuing.

Index

A

Abbott Laboratories, Inc., 413
Abrams' needle, 57
Absorption/distribution/metabolism/excretion (ADME) studies, 86
ABS plastic, 147
Academy of Orthopaedic Surgeons (AAOS), 212
Accredited Persons Program, 304
Acetal, 14
Acorn tip catheter, 118
Acrylic, 11–12, 19
Acrylonitrile–butadiene–styrene (ABS), 11, 18, 137, 219, 223
Acuity, 57
Acute systemic toxicity tests, 77
Adhesive bonds, mechanical testing of, 39–40
Adhesive joint design, 39
Adhesives, 232; *see also* Medical device adhesives
Adobe Photoshop, 361
AdvaMed, 340–343
Advanced Bionics Corp., 417
Advanced Cardiovascular Systems, Inc. (ACS), 100, 120, 121, 401
Advanced Polymers Corporation, 25, 99, 114
Advanced Stent Technologies, Inc. (AST), 418
Advanced Surgical Planning Interactive Research Environment (ASPIRE) system, 204
Agar cutting needle, 57
Agar diffusion assay, 79
Airflow control, 97
Airflow gauge, 97
Air hole punching, for balloon inflation, 112–113
Alias™, 148
Align Technology, 175
America Invents Act, section 102, 292
American College of Surgeons (ACS), 248–249
Ames test, 83
Amplatz catheter, 118
Anatomical Chart Company, 365
Anatomy Act of 1832, 357, 370
Aneurysm needle, 57
Angel financing, 463
Angiography catheter, 118
Angle of rotation, 57
Animal models, 348
Anna Karenina Principle, 447–448
Annealing, 57
Anticipated exit, 460
Anticoring heel blast, 57

Arcam AB, 142, 170, 177
Archimedes principle, 435–436
Arkema Group, 21
Arm probe noncontact scanners, 202–203
Arm probe scanners, 202
Arthrex, 450
"A" side, 237–238
Aspirating needle, 57
Association for Assessment and Accreditation of Laboratory Animal Care International (AAALAC), 69
Association for periOperative Registered Nurses (AORN), 248, 249
Atala, Anthony, 180
Atherectomy catheter, 118
Atrionix, Inc., 417
AutoCAD, 148, 199
Automated adhesive dispenser, 33
Automated fabrication, 129–130
Automated tough probe scanning, 201

B

Back bevels, 57
Bacterial endotoxin test, 82
Balloon blowing, 99
Balloon catheter, 118
Balloon dip molds, 104–105
Balloon inflation, air hole punching for, 112–113
Balloon to catheter assembly, attaching, 114–115
Bank financing, 464
Bard, Charles Russell, 125
Barium, 224
Basal Annuloplasty of the Cardia Externally (BACE™) device, 373–375
BASF, 14
Bass, Lynne, 245–246
Bayer Plastics, 18, 19
BBM-5100, 100, 101
Beahm Designs, 99
Bevel, 57
 length, 57
Bias, 57
Bierce, Ambrose, 435
Bioburden, 234–235
Biocompatibility, 5
 device, 67–68
 matrix, 10, 71–72
 testing, 65–89
  analytical testing, 87–88
  conducting, 67

467

data, need of, 69–70
data evaluation, 67
FDA requirements for, 68
GLP treatment, 73–74
ISO requirements for, 68
materials characterization, 87–88
materials for, 70, 73
methods of, 77–87
planning, 66–67, 74–79
    extraction media, choosing, 74–75
    sample preparation, 76–79
purpose of, 66
selection of, 70
Biocompatible material, choosing, 235–236
Biomaterials
  analytical testing of, 87–88
  availability of, 5–6
Biomaterials Access Assurance Act of 1998, 5–6
Biomet, Inc., 137–138, 175, 175, 393–398
Bisphenol A (BPA), 224
Blue point needles, 52
Blue screen trick, 360–361
Blunt dilators, 55
Blunt end, 57
BMM-2600, 100
Boedeker Plastics, 9, 11
Bohr, Niels, 437
Bonding (heat), 118
Bootstrapping, 459–460
Bosses, 220–221
Boston Scientific Corp., 418
  Enteric Medical Technologies Inc., 417
Bougie tip, 118
Bozeman–Fritsch catheter, 119
BP Amoco, 16
Braasch catheter, 119
Braid, 119
BrainLab System, 171–172, 175, 202
Branson Ultrasonics, 232
Brevet, 113
Bricoleur, 186
Brockenbrough needle, 57
Brush catheter, 119
"B" side, 237–238
Bulk material characterization, 89
Burr, 57

C

California Labor Code, section 2870 of, 258, 261
Cannuflow Extravastat® technology, 245
Cannula, 57
Carcinogenesis bioassays, 78, 84
CardioThoracic Systems (CTS) Inc., 413, 417
Carmon, Park, 155
Casting patterns, of rapid prototyping, 151–152
Cataract needle, 57

Catheter assembly, 107–122
  balloon to catheter assembly, attaching, 114–115
  building, 108–110
  distal tip assembly
    forming, 110–112
    and proximal shaft, joining, 112, 113
  proximal Luer fitting, attaching, 113–114
  proximal steering hub, assembling, 116–117
Catheter drill, punch, 119
Catheter-forming equipment and operations, 93–105
  balloon dip molds, 104–105
  compressors, types of, 96
  features and user controls
    airflow control, 97
    airflow gauge, 97
    cooling air nozzle, 98
    temperature gauge, 97
    thermal nozzle, 97–98
  forming operations
    balloon blowing, 99
    mandrels, 98
    glass molds, 98, 99
      developmental history of, 100–101
    hole punching, 101–102
      automated, 102
  hot-air station, 95
    setup, 95–96
  moisture filters, 96
  particle filters, 96
  safety, 96
  slug ejection, 102
Catheters
  building, 108–110
  defined, 119
Cease distribution and notification strategy, 317
Celanese, 14
Center for Biologics Evaluation and Research (CBER), 298
Center for Bits and Atoms (CBA), 162
Center for Devices and Radiological Health (CDRH), 298, 334–337
  Science Council, 335–336
Center for Drug Evaluation and Research (CDER), 298
Center for Food Safety and Applied Nutrition (CFSAN), 298
Center for Veterinary Medicine (CVR), 298
Central venous catheter, 119
CEREC® system, 155–157, 175
CerLAM™, 139
Certificate for foreign government (CFG), 305
Certification mark, 282
CGI Corporation, 204
Channel sutures, 53
Charriere, Joseph-Frederic-Benoit, 125

Index

Chemcor, 449
Chevalier, 146
Chiba needle, 57
Chilling data, 337–339
Chromosomal aberration assays, 83
CimCore, 202
CIRS, Inc., 366
Clean room molding, 238
ClearVu™, 195, 196
Clinical observation, 241–249
    help in gaining access, 245
    labs and courses, 247–248
    operating room
        access training credentials, 248–249
        as observer, 243–244
        operating room etiquette primer, 245–247
    putting to work, 243
    safety, 248
    value in medical device innovation, 242–243
Clinical utility, 380
Closed eye sutures, 53
Closed patch test, 81
Coagulation assays, 84
Coalescent Surgical, Inc., 418
Code of Federal Regulations (CFR), 311–331
    device listing for manufacturer, 314–316
    establishment registration, 314–316
    exemptions from federal preemption of state and local medical device requirements, 316
    general requirements, 311–312
    individual importers of devices, 314–316
    investigational device exemptions, 318–324
    in vitro diagnostic products, for human use, 316–317
    labeling, 312–313
    medical device classification procedures, 329–330
    medical device recall authority, 317–318
    medical device reporting, 313–314
    medical device tracking requirements, 326–327
    performance standards development, procedures for, 330
    postmarket surveillance, 327–328
    quality system regulations, 324–326
Collective marks, 282
Colony formation cytotoxicity test, 81
Colorants, 236
Commodity plastics, 18–19
    acrylic, 19
    acrylonitrile–butadiene–styrene, 18
    PC/ABS, 18–19
    polycarbonate, 19
    polyethelene, 19
    polyolefin, 19
    styrene, 19

Company, reasons for starting, 425
Complement activation testing, 84
Compliance, 119
Compressors, 96
Computer-aided design (CAD), 76, 128, 129, 187, 192, 218, 230–231
    programs, rendering illustration from, 359–360
Computer-Aided Radiology and Surgery (CARS), 167, 170, 358
Computer numerical control (CNC), 143–146
    full size VMC CNC machines, 146
ConforMIS, 175
Consignee, defined, 317
Continuation-in-part (CIP) application, 277
Continuity, 200
    arm probe noncontact scanners, 202–203
    arm probe scanners, 202
    automated tough probe scanning, 201
    light beam scanners, 201
    three-dimensional image reconstruction, 203
    types of, 200
Conventional cutting needles, 52
Cooling air nozzle, 98
Cope's needle, 57
Corel Painter™, 361
Coring out thick sections, 221
Correction, defined, 317
Coude, 119
Creation, defined, 434
Cross-linked thermoplastics, 7–8; *see also* Thermoplastics
CSA International, 185
Current Good Manufacturing Practice (cGMP), 69, 74
    good clinical practice, 310
    good laboratory practices, 67, 311
    preclinical studies, 311
    Quality System Inspection Technique, 310
    quality system regulations, 309–310
Custom device, 318
CVIS, Inc., 389
Cyanoacrylate adhesives, 35–36, 119
    accelerators, 36
    process considerations, 36
    specialty formulations, 36
    surface primers, 36
Cyberware, 201, 202
Cybyon, 171
Cyro Corporation, 19
Cytotoxicity tests, 77, 79–81

D

Daewoo, 146
Damages, 259
Danforth Biomedical, 100

Decision tool, 214–215
Delrin® acetal, 147
De novo classification, 308, 335
DePezzer, 119
Depth-seeking needles, *see* Reverse cutting needles
Deschamps' needle, 58
Destructive reverse engineering, 204
Detroit Mold Engineering (DME), 229
Device classification, 300–301
Device development, 361–362
Device functional classification, 301
Device listing, 299–300
    for manufacturer, 314–316
Device user facility, 317
Digital capture, 168–170
Digital Imaging and Communications in Medicine (DICOM), 199
Digital light processing (DLP), 141–142
Digital Millennium Copyright Act (DMCA), 187
Digital scanning, 180–182
Digitizing, 189–191
Dimethyl sulfoxide (DMSO), 75
Direct contact cytotoxicity test, 79
Direct Dimensions, 181
Direct metal, 142
Discission needle, 58
Distal tip assembly
    forming, 110–112
    and proximal shaft, joining, 112, 113
Division of Small Manufacturers, International and Consumer Assistance (DSMICA), 299
Dotter, Charles, 94, 119
Dow Chemical, 18, 19
Draft, designing, 222
Drainage catheter, 119
Drew–Smythe catheter, 119
Drill sutures, 53
DTM Corporation, 136
Dukane, 232
DuPont, 14, 25
DXF (drawing interchange file), 149, 199
DymaX, Inc., 30, 114
Dyson, Freeman, 445

E

Early stage medical device companies, creating value for, 413–421
    characteristics, 414
    clinical impact, 414, 417
    franchise value and strategic need, 417–418
    sustainability, 419–420
    value of execution, 418–419
    when to exit, 420–421
EBM (Electron Beam Melting) machine, 142

Echotip, 58
Economic Espionage Act of 1996, 283
Edge gate, 230
Edison, Thomas, 433–445
Edwards Lifesciences Corp., 418
Elastic fabric, 25
Elastomers
    elastometic plastics, 20
    ethylene vinyl acetate (EVA), 21
    Kraton®, 20
    K-Resin®, 20
    Monoprene®, 21
    Pebax®, 21
    polyurethane (PU), 20
    polyvinylchloride, 21
Elastomeric plastics, 20
Electophysiology (EP) catheter, 119
Electroplating, 150–151
eMachineShop®, 147
Emulsifying needle, 58
Enteric Medical Technologies, Inc., 417
Entrepreneur, failure as, 447–458
    ethical shortcuts, 456
    innovation as panacea, 455
    insufficient margins, 453
    lack of urgency, 454
    no reimbursement, 451–452
    patent mine fields, 452
    phantom markets, 451
    raising too little money, 452
    raising too much money, 452–453
    regulatory purgatory, 452
    sector inexperience, 451
    technology-driven product, 449–450
    too small market, 450
    wrong people involved, 454
EntreVu® portal cannula, 245
Envisiontec® Perfactory™, 141–142
Envisiontec GmbH, 158–160
EOS GmbH, 142, 177
Epicor Medical Inc., 418
Epoxy adhesives, 34–35
    chemistry systems, 34
    electrically conductive, 35
    mixed, 34
    one-part, 34
    prepackaged, 34–35
    thermally conductive, 35
    two-part, 34
Equilase 30™, 142
Establishment registration, 299, 314–316
Ethicon Endosurgery, 245
Ethylene vinyl acetate (EVA), 21
Existing device
    building on, for higher performance, 194–196
    cannibalizing, 193–194
Ex-One Corporation, ProMetal™ process, 142

Index

Expanded Polystyrene Styrofoam (EPS) molding, 237
Expanded PTFE (EPTFE), 24
Exporting devices, 305
Export Reform and Enhancement Act of 1996, 298
External communicating device, 80
Extractable material, tests procedures for, 88
Extraction media, choosing, 74–75
Extruded polytetrafluoroethylene, 23
Extrusion, 119

F

Fab Lab program, 162
Fadal, 146
Faraday, Michael, 436
Farlow's Scientific Glassblowing, Inc. (FSG), 99, 100, 366
FARO Arm, 169, 182, 202
Fastening, 232–233, 238
Federal Food, Drug and Cosmetics Act (FD&C) of 1938, 298, 305
Female entrepreneurship, in 21st century, 423–424
Female leadership, 423–428
Fenestrations, 120
File formats, 149–150
File preparation, 148–149
Financing
   angel financing, 463
   bank financing, 464
   4F Financing, 463
   government grants, 463
   for medical device start-up, 427
   private equity, 464
   strategic investment, 464
   terms, 461–462
   venture capital, 463
   venture debt, 463–464
Finding need, of medical innovation, 439–445
Finish and draft angle, 229
Finite element analysis (FEA), 229–230
First-inventor-to-file system, 292, 293
510(k) premarket notification, xiii, 73, 247, 301–304
   abbreviated, 307–308
   "Special 510(k): Device Modification," 306–307
   strengthening, 339–341
Flared end, 58
Flaring, 120
Flatbed scanner, for three-dimensional construction, 192–193
Fluorinated ethylene propylene (FEP), 15, 112, 120
Foam molding, 237

Foam parts, UV cure sealing of, 151
Foam sheet material, 25
Fogarty, Thomas J., 379–384, 435, 441
Fogarty Balloon Embolectomy Catheter, 120, 124
Foley catheter, 120
Food and Drug Administration (FDA), 87, 444
   Blue Book Memorandum G95-1, 68
   CDRH 2012 Strategic Priorities, 334
   centers, 298
   Class III devices, 211
   de novo classification, 308
   device classification, 300–301
   device functional classification, 301
   device listing, 299–300
   Division of Small Manufacturers, International and Consumer Assistance (DSMICA), 299
   establishment registration, 299
   on exporting devices, 305
   Export Reform and Enhancement Act of 1996, 298
   Federal Food, Drug and Cosmetics Act (FD&C) of 1938, 298, 305
   510(k) premarket notification, xiii, 73, 247, 301–304, 333–345
   GMP requirements
      Class I devices, 306
      Class II devices, 306
   humanitarian device exemption, 309
   humanitarian use device, 309
   importing into United States, 304
   Innovation Pathway, 342–343
   investigational device exemption, 303–304
   Medical Device Amendments of 1976, 298
   Medical Device User Fee Modernization Act of 2002 (MDUFMA), 299
   Modernization Act of 1997, 298, 306
   Notice to Industry Letters, 336
   offices, 298
   online assistance, 299
   Plan of Action for Implementation of 510(k) and Science Recommendations," 333–337
   premarket approval, 224, 302–303
   product development protocol, 308–309
   reorganization of, 298
   requirements, for biocompatibility testing, 68
   Safe Medical Devices Act of 1990, 298
   Special 510(k): Device Modification, 306–307
   substantial equivalence, 302
   thirty-party submission review, by accredited parties, 304
   Tripartite Guidance, 68
Food and Drug Branch (FDB) mission, 305

Foreign filing, 278
Forssmann, Werner, 120
4F Financing, 463
Freedom of Creation (FOC), 162
Free length, 58
Freeman Manufacturing and Supply, 147, 212
French (catheter scale), 120
French (Fr) sizing, 63
French catheter size, 55
French eye sutures, 53
Friendliest-to-mold and least expensive material, specifying, 223–224
Full size VMC computer numerical control machines, 146
Funding, for medical device start-up, 427
Fused deposition modeling (FDM), 136–137

G

Ganz, William, 122
Gate(ing), 229–230, 238
  edge, 230
  post, 230
  subgate, 230
  tab, 230
  to part, locating, 230–231
  tunnel, 230
Gauge, 58
GE, 18, 19
Genotoxicity tests, 77
Gershenfeld, Neil, 162
GG-N-196, 58
Gibbs CAM, 146
Glass, 224
Glass catheter molds, 98, 99
  developmental history of, 100–101
Glendo Accu-Finish® grinder, 50
Glendo Corporation, 47
GLS Corporation, 20
Gluing, 232–233
Good clinical practice (GCP), 310
Good laboratory practices (GLP), 67, 311, 350
  regulations, 311
  treatment, for biocompatibility testing, 73–74
Good manufacturing practice (GMP), 58
  current, 69, 74
  requirements
    Class I devices, 306
    Class II devices, 306
Gouley's catheter, 120
Government grants, 463
Grit blast, 58
Grossman, Bathsheba, 142
Gruentzig, Andreas, 120, 125
Guidewire, 120–121
Guiding catheter, 121
Guinea pig maximization test, 81

H

Haas Automation, 146
Hagedorn's needles, 58
Hasson cannula, 58
Hasson trocar, 58
Hazlitt, William, 438
Health Insurance Portability and Accountability Act (HIPAA), 246
Health professionals, 317
Heartport, Inc., 418
Heat stacking, 232
Hemocompatibility, 78, 84
Hemolysis assay, 84
Hemostasis valve, 121
HGPRT assay, 83
High-performance engineering plastics
  for machining, 15–18
    injection-molded and extruded plastics, 17–18
    PEEK™, 15–16
    polyphenylsulfone, 16–17
    polysulfone, 16–17
    polytetrafluoroethylene, 16
    Ultem® polyetherimide, 15
  for molding, 23
Histopathology services, 87
Hole punching, 101–102
  automated, 102
Holt Anatomical, 365
Hook burr, 58
Hot-air station, 95
  setup, 95–96
Hot tip method, 230
HP, 204
Hub, 58, 121
Humanitarian device exemption (HDE), 309, 322
Humanitarian use device (HUD), 309
Huntsman Advanced Materials, 146
Hydrophilic, 121
Hydrophobic, 121
Hypodermic tubing, 54, 55–57
  features of, 48
  materials of, 57

I

Identical molded shells, fitting, 226
IDEO, 186
IGES (Initial Graphics Exchange Specification), 149, 199
Immersion, 202
Implant, defined, 319
Implantation tests, 78, 83–86
Implant device, 80
Impra, 24
Incubator, 381

Index

Individual importers of devices, 314–316
Indwelling catheter, 121
Initial importers, 304–305
Injection-extruded plastics, 17
    considerations, 17–18
Injection-molded plastics, 17
    considerations, 17–18
Injection molding, defined, 238
Injection molding style elements, for medical device R&D, 217–239
    adhesives, 232
    bioburden, 234–235
    draft, designing, 222
    fastening, 232–233
    gate to part, locating, 230–231
    gluing, 232–233
    heat stacking, 232
    identical molded shells, fitting, 226
    inserts, 232
    inspection and acceptance criteria, 237
    interference press fit bosses, 232
    joining, 232–233
    methods of, 223
    molded flow
        edge gate, 230
        gating, 229–230
        hot tip, 230
        post gate, 230
        subgate, 230
        tab gate, 230
        tunnel gate, 230
    molded-in hinges, 228
    part ejection, 231–232
    product design principle, 226
    radius corners, 222–223
    side hole without side pull, 226–227
    snap fits, 232
    straight parting lines, 224, 226
    sterilization, 234–235
        effects on plastics, 235–237
    surface finishes, 228–229
        finish and draft angle, 229
        notes on, 229
        preengineered molds, 229
        in thermoplastic elastomers, 229
    ultrasonic welding, 232
    wall thickness, 219–221
        bosses, 220–221
        coring out, 221
        ribs, 220–221
Inkjet proteins, 161–162
Inner diameter (ID), 55, 58
Innovation
    defined, 434, 440
    vs. imitation, 184–185
    as panacea, 455
    reporting on, 279–281
Innovation Pathway, 342–343
Inserts, 232
    threaded, 151, 232
Institute of Medicine (IOM), 334, 335, 337
    recommendations to 510(k) process, 341
Institution, defined, 319
Institutional review board (IRB), 247, 303, 319
Intel, 204
Intellectual property development, 363
Intellectual property rights, 263–291
    identifying, 286–288
    licensing, 291
    patents, 266–269
        enforcing, 289–291
        options, 275–276
        program, starting, 270–271
        trigger, pulling, 276–277
    research and development, protecting
        foreign filing, 278
        internal IP controls, 278–281
        patenting, 275–277
        planning for inventing, 269–275
    start planning for, 264–266
    trademarks, 281–282
    trade secrets, 282–283
    watch out for others' property
        designing around patents, 285–286
        noninfringement study, 284–285
        state-of-the-art study, 284
        validity study, 285
Interference press fit bosses, 232
Internal business concerns, 271–275
Internal IP controls, 278–281
International Anti-Counterfeiting Coalition, 185
International Commission on Radiation Units and Measurements (ICRU), 371
International Organization of Standardization (ISO)
    ISO 8573, 96
    ISO 9626, 58
    ISO 10993, 26, 32, 50, 66, 68–70, 83, 84, 87
    requirements, for biocompatibility testing, 68
International Polymer Engineering, 24
Interpore Cross International, 139, 153
Intracutaneous test, 82
Invention, 266
    defined, 434
    planning for, 269–275
        internal business concerns, 271–275
        patent program, starting, 270–271
        working with others, 275
    rewards, 279
Invention Disclosure Form, 277
Investigational device exemptions (IDE), 73, 247, 303–304, 318–324, 336, 350
Investigator, defined, 319
Investment cast orthopedic implants, 153–155

Investor presentations, of medical illustration, 363–364
Investors, expectations of, 460
InVision™ multijet modeling (MJM), 133
In vitro diagnostic products, for human use, 316–317
In vitro testing, 348
  animal models, 348
  project, 348–349
In vivo study, 349
  data collection, 349
  good laboratory practices, 350
  team, 349–350
Irritation tests, 77

J

Javelin 3D, 139, 170, 203
Jigs, 174–175
Johnson, Lanny, 241
Johnson & Johnson (J&J), 185, 424
  Cordis Corp., 417
Joining, 232–233, 238
Judkins, Melvin P., 119, 121
Judkins catheter, 121

K

Kettering, Charles F., 435
Kilgore International, 365–366
Knife needle, 58
Knit line, 239
Konica Minolta, 201
Kraton®, 20
Kreon, 203
K-Resin®, 20
Kroemer, Herbert, 445

L

Labeling, 312–313
Labs and courses, for clinical observation, 247–248
Lancets, 58
Lanham Act, section 43(a), 282
Laser Design, 203
Laserform®, 147
Latex, 22–23
Layer technique, in Photoshop, 360
Licensed use versus buyout, 368–369
Licensing, 291
Ligature needle, 58
Light beam scanners, 201
Light-cure adhesives, 37
Loctite, Inc., 30, 114
LOM™, 139
Luer, Otto, 121

Luer fitting, 58–59, 121
Lumen, 59
Lundquist, Ingemar, 399–400

M

Machinable prototype materials, 146–147
Machining, 151
Magnetic permeability, 59
Maintaining records, 260–261
MAKO Surgical, 175
Malleable, 59
Mandatory recall strategy, 317
Mandrels, 98
Manifold, 121
Massachusetts Institute of Technology (MIT), 140
Mastercam, 146
Master file, 321
Master Unit Die (MUD) Base tooling, 214, 229, 238
Material characterization, 87–89
  bulk, 89
  traditional extractable, 88
Materialise NV, 148, 170, 177, 199
Material-mediated pyrogen test, 82
Materials performance, 6
Mazak, 146
McGlynn, J. Casey, 401–412
McNeil PPC, 281
MDX 15, 145
MDX 20, 145, 189
MDX 500, 145
MDX 650, 145
Medical Applications of Rapid Prototyping (MARP), 168
Medical device adhesives, 29–40
  adhesive bonds, mechanical testing of, 39–40
  adhesive joint design, 39
  cyanoacrylate adhesives, 35–36
    accelerators, 36
    process considerations, 36
    specialty formulations, 36
    surface primers, 36
  epoxy adhesives, 34–35
    chemistry systems, 34
    electrically conductive, 35
    mixed, 34
    one-part, 34
    prepackaged, 34–35
    thermally conductive, 35
    two-part, 34
  light-cure adhesives, 37
  silicone adhesives, 38
  silicone dermal adhesives, 38
  solvent adhesives, 33–34

Index

urethane adhesives, 38–38
UV adhesives, 36–37
   chemistry system, 37
   cure lights, 37
   process considerations, 37
Medical Device Amendments of 1976, 298
Medical Device and Manufacturing Show (MD+M Show), 215
Medical device classification procedures, 329–330
Medical Device Manufacturers Association (MDMA), 339
Medical device recall authority, 317–318
Medical device reporting (MDR), 313–314
Medical device sales 101, 429–431
Medical device start-up
  components of
   financing, 427
   funding, 427
   regulatory and reimbursement pathway, 426–427
   unmet need in growing field, 426
  personal requirements for, 424–425
  raising money for, 459–465
   anticipated exit, 460
   bootstrapping, 459–460
   financing, *see* Financing
   funding rounds, rules of thumb for, 461
   investors, expectations of, 460
   resourcefulness, 459–460
   revenues, 460
   technology dealing, 462–463
   valuation, 461
Medical device tracking requirements, 326–327
Medical Device User Fee Modernization Act of 2002 (MDUFMA), 297, 299
Medical-grade plastic, 8–9
Medical illustration, 351–367
  blue screen trick, 360–361
  device development, 361–362
  history of, 353–358
  intellectual property development, 363
  investor presentations of, 363–364
  licensed use versus buyout, 368–369
  marketing, 364–365
  medical-legal, 365
  medical teaching and training models, 365–366
  patient information, 364–365
  Photoshop, layer technique in, 360
  physician training, 364–365
  rendering from CAD programs, 359–360
  surgical approach planning, 359
  textbook illustration, 358–359
  three-dimensional animation, 366–367
  used by regulatory bodies, 363
  value of, 351–353

Medical Imaging and Technology Alliance (MITA), 343, 344
Medical-legal, 365
Medical plastics, 3–25
  biocompatibility, 5
  biomaterials, availability of, 5–6
  commodity plastics, 18
   acrylic, 19
   acrylonitrile–butadiene–styrene, 18
   PC/ABS, 18–19
   polycarbonate, 19
   polyethelene, 19
   polyolefin, 19
   styrene, 19
   finding, 9
  high-performance engineering plastics for machining, 15–18
   injection-molded and extruded plastics, 17–18
   PEEK™, 15–16
   polyphenylsulfone, 16–17
   polysulfone, 16–17
   polytetrafluoroethylene, 16
   Ultem® polyetherimide, 15
  high-performance engineering plastics for molding, 23
  materials performance, 6
  medical-grade plastic, 8–9
  plastics for machining, 9, 11
  plastics for processing by machining, 11–15
   acetal, 14
   acrylic, 11–12
   acrylonitrile–butadiene–styrene, 11
   fluorinated ethylene propylene, 15
   nylon (polyamide), 14–15
   polycarbonate, 12–13
   polyethelene, 13–14
   polypropylene, 13
   polyvinylchloride, 12
  polymer, 7
  polyurethane, 20
   ethylene vinyl acetate, 21
   Kraton®, 20
   K-Resin®, 20
   Monoprene®, 21
   Pebax®, 213
   polyvinylchloride, 21
  processability, 6–7
  sheet and film and foam plastics
   elastic fabric, 25
   foam sheet material, 25
   polyester film, 24–25
   polyethelene film, 24
   polyethylene terephthalate, 24
   polyethylene terephthalate glycol, 24
   polyimide, 25
   polyvinylchloride, 24

styrene butadiene rubber foam, 25
Tyvek®, 24
specialty plastic material forms
expanded polytetrafluoroethylene, 24
extruded polytetrafluoroethylene, 23
thermoplastics, 7
cross-linked, 7–8
thermosets, 7
latex, 22–23
pitrile, 22
polyisoprene, 22
Santoprene®, 22
silicone, 22
Medical teaching and training models, 365–366
MedLAM™, 139
Medtronic, Inc., 418, 424
MEM elution assay, 79
Memry Corporation, 47
Menghini needle, 59
Merit, 113
Metal tube drawing methods, 47
Metric units, 55
Metris, 203
Microelectromechanical systems (MEMS), 142
Microlumen Company, 25
Mikhak, Bakhtiar, 162
Miller, Dane, 393–398, 453
Mimics™, 148, 170, 199
Mironov, Vladimir, 180
ModelMaker™ systems, 153
Modernization Act of 1997, 298, 306
Modified Polymers Corporation, 8
Moisture filters, 96
Mold analysis, 238
Molded-in hinges, 228
Moldflow®, 230
Mold release, 238
Molecular modeling, 153
Monitor, defined, 319
Monoprene®, 21
Mori Seiki, 146
Mouse micronucleus assays, 83
MTT cytotoxicity test, 81
Mucous membrane irritation tests, 82
Multicavity tool, 239
Murine local lymph node assay (LLNA), 81

N

National Center for Toxicological Research (NCTR), 298
National Institute of Medicine, xiii
National Sanitation Foundation, 16
Natural absorbable sutures, 54
Natural nonabsorbable sutures, 54
Needles

French catheter size, 55
gauge size, 54–55
grinding
fixtures, 48, 50
R&D, 47
metric units, 55
suture, 49–55
terminology, 56
types and applications of, 49
Nitinol Devices Corporation (NDC), 47
Nominal wall thickness, 238
Noncircumvention, 257–258
Noncontact devices, 79
Nondisclosure, defined, 259
Nondisclosure agreements (NDAs), 251–261
as employee, signing, 258
lab notebook, keeping, 252–253
mutual, 259
noncircumvention, 257–258
one-way, 259
presenting ideas for evaluation, 256
read and heed, 256–257
references and reputation of people, checking, 257
two-way, 259
value of, 253–256
case example, 253–254
when not to sign, 254–255
who should sign, 255–256
who will not sign, 255
Noninvasive, defined, 319
Nonswaged sutures, 53
Nonuse, defined, 259
Norton Performance Plastics, 21
NovaGen MMX, 180
NovaSom QSG™, 144
NuSil, 22
Nutter, Arthur, 204
Nylon, 14–15, 27, 137

O

Obomodulan®, 147
Obo-Werke GmbH, 147
Obturator, 59
Occupational Safety and Health Organization (OSHA) regulations, 96, 247
Office action, 268
Office-based rapid prototype machines, 133
Office of Regulatory Affairs (ORA), 298
Office of the Commissioner (OC), 298
Olive tipped, 121
Operating room
access training credentials, 248–249
etiquette primer, 245–247
as observer, 243–244
safety, 248

Index

Oratec Interventions Inc., 413
Organisation for Economic Co-operation and Development (OECD), ENV/MC/CHEM(98)17, 73
Organovo, 180
Orthopedic Design + Technology shows (ODT), 215
Orthopedic Learning Center (OLC), 247
Orthopedic Manufacturing and Technology Show (OMTEC), 215
OsiriX, 170–171
OtisMed, 175
Outside diameter (OD), 55
Overall length (OAL), 59

P

Pacific Research Laboratories, 189–190, 365
Pacing catheter, 121
Painting, 150
Palmaz, Julio, 122
Parsons, John, 143
Part ejection, 231–232
Partial thromboplastin time (PTT) assay, 84
Particle filters, 96
Parting line, 238
Parylene, 112
Passivate, 59
Patent(s/ing), 266–269
    committees, 278–279
    defined, 266
    designing around, 285–286
    enforcing, 289–291
    mine fields, 452
    options, 275–276
    program, starting, 270–271
    specification, 267–269
    trigger, pulling, 276–277
Patent Act, 293
Patent Cooperation Treaty (PCT) application, 278
"Patents and Startups 101," xv
Patient Protection and Affordable Care Act of 2010 (PPACA), xiii
Pauling, Linus, 445
PC/ABS, 18–19, 223
P-D Access™, 387
Pebax®, 21, 121
PEM® inserts, 232
Pencil point, 59
Penn Engineering Corporation, 151, 232
Perceptron, 203
Perclose, Inc., 413
Percolator, 381
PercuSurge, Inc., 413
Percutaneous Valve Technologies, Inc. (PVT), 418

Performance standards development, procedures for, 330
Perkins, Rodney, 253–254
Phantom markets, 451
Pharmaceuticals, rapid prototyping applications in, 160
Pharmacokinetic (PK), 86
Pitkin bevel, 59
Pitrile, 22
Pixmeo, 171
"Plan of Action for Implementation of 510(k) and Science Recommendations," 333–337
Plastics
    additives, 224
    commodity, 18–19
    finding, 9
    high-performance engineering, 15–18, 23
    injection-molded and extruded, 17–18
    for machining, 9, 11
    medical, *see* Medical plastics
    medical-grade, 8–9
    for processing by machining, 11–15
    properties and moldability of, 225
    sterilization effects on, 235–237
    thermoplastics, 7
        cross-linked, 7–8
Plastics.com, 9
Plastic sharps, for disposables, 55–57
Plato, 439
PLY format, 149, 198
Polhemus, 202
Polyamide, 14–15
Polycarbonate (PC), 12–13, 19, 219
Polyester film, 24–25
Polyethelene (PE), 13–14, 19, 110
    film, 24
Polyetheretherketone (PEEK™), 15–16, 23, 224, 235
Polyethylene glycol (PEG), 75
Polyethylene terephthalate (PET), 24
Polyethylene terephthalate glycol (PETG), 24
Polyimide, 25
    rod, 17
    sheet, 17
Polyisoprene, 22
PolyJet Objet™ printer, 137, 140–141
Polymer, defined, 7
Polymer Plastics Corporation, 9, 11, 147
Polymethyl methacrylate (PMMA), 27
Polyolefin, 19
Polyphenylsulfone, 16–17
Polypropylene (PP), 13, 137
Polysulfone, 16–17, 23, 235
Polytetrafluoroethylene (PTFE), 16, 98, 112
    expanded, 24
    extruded, 23
Polyurethane (PU), 20

Polyvinylchloride (PVC), 12, 21, 24, 139, 224
PolyWorks™, 191
Port Plastics, 9, 147
Post gate, 230
Postmarket surveillance, 327–328
Preclinical research, 347–350
   in vitro testing, 348
      animal models, 348
      project, 348–349
   in vivo study, 349
      data collection, 349
      good laboratory practices, 350
      team, 349–350
Preclinical safety testing, 86–87
Preclinical studies, 311
Preengineered molds, 229
Premarket approval (PMA), 73, 322, 350
   amendment, 322
   submission, 302–303
   supplement, 322
   third party, 322
Presenting ideas for evaluation, 256
PricewaterhouseCoopers (PwC), 337, 339
Primary skin irritation test, 82
Principal investigator, defined, 319
Printed food, 161–162
Private equity, 464
Pro/Engineer™, 148, 199
Processability, 6–7
Prodigy Plus™, 133
Product design
   principle, 226
   rapid prototyping applications in, 142–143
Product development protocol (PDP), 308–309
Production tooling, 214
Programmable rapid prototype molding, 161
Prothrombin time (PT) assay, 84
Protomold, 147, 214
Prototype casting materials, 174
Proximal end, 59
Proximal Luer fitting to catheter assembly, attaching, 113–114
Proximal shaft and distal tip assembly, joining, 112, 113
Proximal steering hub, assembling, 116–117
Purpose, defined, 259
Pushability, 121
Putnam Plastics, 25

Q

Quality System Inspection Technique (QSIT), 310
Quality system regulations (QSR), 309–310, 324–326
QuickCast™, 135
Quincke bevel, 59

Quintron, 154
Quosina, 113

R

Radiation, 248
Radiation stability, 235, 236
Radiofrequency, 248
Radiology, 224
Radius corners, 222–223
Raman, Jai, 373, 375
R&D needle grinding, 47
Rapid prototype (RP) technology
   short-run injection molding, 213–214
   short-run manufacturing options, 213
Rapid prototyping (RP), 127–164, 168, 187
   additive, 129, 130
   analysis of, 160–162
      Center for Bits and Atoms, 162
      Freedom of Creation, 162
      inkjet proteins, 161–162
      printed food, 161–162
      programmable RP molding, 161
   applications of, 131–132
      CEREC® system, 155–157
      pharmaceuticals, 160
      product design, 142–143
      surgical planning, 152–153
      tissue engineering, 157–160
      training models, 153
   casting patterns, 151–152
   computer numerical control, 143–146
      full size VMC computer numerical control machines, 146
   cost-saving tips, 150
   digital light processing, 141–142
   direct metal, 142
   file formats, 149–150
   file preparation, 148–149
   foam parts, UV cure sealing of, 151
   fused deposition modeling (FDM), 136–137
   LOM™, 139
   machinable prototype materials, 146–147
   office-based RP machines, 133
   PolyJet Objet™ printer, 140–141
      produced medical products, 153–155
      resolution, 137–138
      reverse engineering, 153
      secondary process to RP parts
         electroplating, 150–151
         machining, 151
         painting, 150
         threaded inserts, 151
   service bureaus, 132–133
   sintering, 142
   SLS™, 136
   Solid Creation Systems, 133, 135

Index

stereolithography apparatus, 133–134
stereolithography materials, 134–135
subtractive, 129, 130
surface finish, 137–138
technology selection, 148
three-dimensional printing, 139–140
tooling and molding, 147–148
Rapid technologies, 167–182
   biomedical reverse engineering, 170
   digital capture, 168–170
   digital scanning, 180–182
   innovators, 175–177
   jigs, 174–175
   OsiriX, 170–171
   prototype casting materials, 174
   RTAM custom-made veterinary orthopedic implants, 178–179
   surgical GPS, 171–173
   3D geometry reconstruction, 180–182
   and tissue engineering, 180
Rapid Technology and Additive Manufacturing (RTAM), 167
   custom-made veterinary orthopedic implants, 178–179
Reaction injection molding (RIM), 236
Read and heed, 256–257
Reasonable probability, 317
Recall, defined, 317
Regulatory affairs, 295–331
   cost-effectiveness of, 296–297
   judgment, 297
Regulatory pathway, for medical device start-up, 426–427
Regulatory requirements, 296
   for device safety and effectiveness, 297
Reimbursement pathway, for medical device start-up, 426–427
Removal, defined, 317
Ren Shape®, 146
Repliform, 147
Reproductive and developmental toxicity, 78, 84, 86–87
REPtrax, 249
Research and development, protecting
   foreign filing, 278
   internal IP controls, 278–281
   patenting, 275–277
   planning for inventing, 269–275
Resourcefulness, 459–460
Revenues, 460
Reverdin's needle, 60
Reverse cutting needles, 52
Reverse engineering (RE), 129, 153, 167, 183–205
   biomedical, 170
   continuity, 200
      arm probe noncontact scanners, 202–203

      arm probe scanners, 202
      automated tough probe scanning, 201
      light beam scanners, 201
      three-dimensional image reconstruction, 203
      types of, 200
   defined, 184
   destructive, 204
   digitizing, 189–191
   existing device
      building on, for higher performance, 194–196
      cannibalizing, 193–194
   inspection, 203–204
   in patient care, value of, 187–189
   radiology, 224
   surgical planning, 224
   three-dimensional reconstruction, 198–199
      file formats, 198–199
      flatbed scanner for, 192–193
   used medical devices and equipment, finding, 196–198
Reverse modeling, 184
Rhino™, 148, 202
Ribs, 220–221
Roland Corporation, 145, 201
Roland DGA, 130, 169
Romer, 202
Room-temperature vulcanate (RTV) molding, 212
Rotational symmetry, 226

S

SAFE®, 203
Safe Medical Devices Act of 1990, 298
Saint-Gobain, 21
St. Jude Medical, Inc., 418
Santoprene®, 22
Schatz, Richard, 122
Science and discovery, 435–437
Scientific Notebook Company, 252
Scope, defined, 259
Seldinger, Sven-Ivar, 121
Seldinger needle, 60
Seldinger technique, 121
Sensable, 175
Sensitization assays, 77
Sharps, 248
Short-run injection molding, 213–214
Short-run manufacturing options, 213
Side action, 238
Side cutting needles, 52
Side hole without side pull, 226–227
Side port, 60
Side pull, 238
Signature™, 175

Significant risk device, defined, 319
Silicone, 22
    adhesives, 38
    dermal adhesives, 38
    molding, 236
Silverman needle, 60
SimPlant, 199, 203
Simpson, John, 121, 444
Simulab, 366
Single-cavity tool, 239
Sink marks, 238
Sintering, 142
Sirona Dental Systems, 155, 175
Sleep Solutions, Inc., 143
Slit sutures, 53
SLS™, 136, 151
Slug ejection, 102
Small Parts, Inc., 111
Smart Needle™, 387
Snap fits, 232
Society for Manufacturing Engineering (SME) RAPID show, 215
Society of Plastics Industry Mold Polish Finishes, 228
Softimage®, 367
Solid Creation Systems (SCS®), 133, 135
Solidica, 142
Solidscape, Inc., 138–139, 153
SolidWorks™, 148, 199
Solvay Advanced Polymers, 16
Solvent adhesives, 33–34
SOMSO Models, 365
Sones, Mason, 121–122
Sony, 133, 135
"Special 510(k): Device Modification," 306–307
SpineCore, Inc., 418
Split predicate, 341
Sponsor, defined, 319
Sponsor-investigator, defined, 319
Spring sutures, 53
Sprue, 238
Stanford Biodesign Fellowship Program, 245
Status Blue, 249
Steel safe, 238–239
Steerable catheter, 122
Steinmetz, Charles P., 443
Stent, 122, 196
Stent delivery catheter, 122
STEP (Standard for the Exchange of Product Mode Data), 149, 199
Stereolithography apparatus (SLA), 133–134, 151, 152
Stereolithography materials, 134–135
Stereoniks Corporation of Carson, 139
Sterilization, 234–235
    effects on plastics, 235–237
Stokes, Donald E., 436–437

Stopcock, 122
Stop needle, 60
Straight parting lines, 224, 226
Stratasys Corporation, 133, 136–137, 140, 141, 148, 151, 177
Strategic investment, 464
Stryker Corp., 418
Stubs iron wire gauge, 54
Stylet, 60
Styrene, 19
Styrene butadiene rubber foam, 25
Styrofoam molding, 237
Subchronic toxicity tests, 77
Subgate, 230
Substantial equivalence, 302
Subtractive rapid prototyping (SRP™), 129, 130, 133–134
Surface area calculation, 76
Surface characterization, 89
Surface device, 80
Surface finishes, 137–138, 228–229
    finish and draft angle, 229
    notes on, 229
    preengineered molds, 229
    in thermoplastic elastomers, 229
Surfcam, 146
Surgical approach planning, 359
Surgical GPS, 171–173
Surgical planning, 224
    rapid prototyping applications in, 152–153
SurgiGuide®, 203
Sustainability, 419–420
Suture needles, 49–55
    attachment methods of, 52–53
    identification chart, 51
    size of, 53, 54
    types of, 52, 53–55
Swaged needle, 60
Swaging, 60
    sutures to needles, 52
Swan, Alfred, 442
Swan, H. J. C., 122
Swan, Joseph Wilson, 442
Swan–Ganz catheter, 122
Symphonix Devices (SMPX), 449
Synthetic absorbable sutures, 54
Synthetics nonabsorbable sutures, 55

T

Tab gate, 230
Taeus International, 204
Taper cutting needles, 52
Technical Innovations, 101, 112
Technology-driven products, 440, 449–450
    vs. clinical needs–driven products, 382
Temperature gauge, 97

Index

Term, defined, 259–260
Tesla, Nikolai, 442–443
Texas Instruments, 204
Texloc Corporation, 19
Textbook illustration, 358–359
Therics Corporation, 160
Thermal nozzle, 97–98
Thermodilution catheter, 122
Thermoplastic elastomers (TPEs), surface finishes in, 229
Thermoplastics, 7
    cross-linked, 7–8
Thermosets, 7
    latex, 22–23
    pitrile, 22
    polyisoprene, 22
    Santoprene®, 22
    silicone, 22
Third Party Review Pilot Program, 304
Thirty-party submission review, by accredited parties, 304
Thomas Register, 151
Threaded inserts, 151, 232
    installing, 151
Thre Arch Partners, 383
Three-dimensional animation, 366–367
Three-dimensional printing, 139–140
Three-dimensional reconstruction, 198–199, 203
    flatbed scanner for, 192–193
    geometry, 180–182, 198–199, 203
3dMD, 201, 202
3DStudio®, 367
3D Systems, 133–134, 136, 147, 175
Thrombogenicity, 84
Tipping, 122
Tissue engineering
    rapid prototyping and, 157–160
    rapid technologies and, 180
Tissue substitute, 371
Tool(ing)
    hard, 239
    multicavity, 239
    single cavity, 239
    soft, 239
Torqueability, 122
Trade dress, 282
Trademarks, 281–282
    defined, 281
Trade name, 282
Trade secrets, 282–283
Traditional extractable material characterization, 88
Traditional model-making tools, 211–212
Transitional device, defined, 319
Transseptal needle, 60
TransVascular Inc., 418
Trephine, 60
Triple grind, 60
Trocars, 55, 60
    for disposables, 55
    Hasson, 58
    point, 60
Tunnel gate, 230
Tuohy–Borst valve, 122
Tuohy needle, 60
Tyvek®, 24, 27

U

Ultem® polyetherimide, 15, 23, 235
Ultra-high-molecularweight polyethelene (UHMWPE), 13–14
Ultrasonic welding, 232
Unanticipated adverse device effect, 319
Underwriters Laboratories, Inc., 15, 282
Uniform Trade Secrets Act, 283
Units conversion chart, 46
Unscheduled DNA Synthesis (UDS), 83
Urethane adhesives, 38–38
U.S. Department of Agriculture (USDA), 348
Used medical devices and equipment, finding, 196–198
U.S. International Trade Commission (ITC), 290
U.S. Patent and Trademark Office (USPTO), 265, 268, 269, 276, 281, 285, 292
U.S. Pharmacopeia (USP), 26, 53, 68
    Class VI, 5, 8, 9, 16, 50, 135
UV adhesives, 36–37, 114
    chemistry system, 37
    cure adhesive, 122
    cure lights, 37
    process considerations, 37

V

Valley of death, 440
Valuation, 461
Value Plastics, 113
VendorMate, 249
Venture capital, 463
Venture debt, 463–464
Venture Manufacturing, 108
Venue, defined, 261
Veress needle, 60–61
Vertebrated catheter, 122
V-Flash™, 175
VG Studio Max, 149
Vidamed, Inc., 399, 413
Visible Human Project®, 203
VisionTrak, 202
Visonaire™, 175
Vitrea, 149
VRML (virtual reality modeling format), 149, 198–199

W

Wall thickness, 219–221
 bosses, 220–221
 coring out, 221
 nominal, 238
 radius corners for, 222–223
 ribs, 220–221
Watch out for others' property
 designing around patents, 285–286
 noninfringement study, 284–285
 state-of-the-art study, 284
 validity study, 285
Weld line, 239
Westlake Plastics, 9, 14, 19
White, Dawn, 142
WinZip™, 149
W. L. Gore & Associates, 24
Wohlers, Terry, 177
World Health Organization (WHO), *Handbook on Good Laboratory Practices*, 73

Y

Yock, Paul G., 387–392

Z

Z-cast process, 140
Z Corporation, 133, 139–140, 148, 151, 153, 169
Zeus Corporation, 24